Current Practices in Ophthalmology

Series Editor
Parul Ichhpujani, Department of Ophthalmology
Government Medical College and Hospital
Chandigarh, India

This series of highly organized and uniform handbooks aims to cover the latest clinically relevant developments in ophthalmology. In the wake of rapidly evolving innovations in the field of basic research, pharmacology, surgical techniques and imaging devices for the management of ophthalmic disorders, it is extremely important to invest in books that help you stay updated. These handbooks are designed to bridge the gap between journals and standard texts providing reviews on advances that are now part of mainstream clinical practice. Meant for residents, fellows-in-training, generalist ophthalmologists and specialists alike, each volume under this series covers current perspectives on relevant topics and meets the CME requirements as a go-to reference guide. Supervised and reviewed by a subject expert, chapters in each volume provide leading-edge information most relevant and useful for clinical ophthalmologists. This series is also useful for residents and fellows training in various subspecialties of ophthalmology, who can read these books while at work or during emergency duties. Additionally, these handbooks can aid in preparing for clinical case discussions at various forums and examinations.

Hajirah N. Saeed • Rohan Bir Singh
Editors

Corneal Disorders

Springer

Editors
Hajirah N. Saeed
Department of Ophthalmology
and Visual Sciences
Illinois Eye and Ear Infirmary,
University of Illinois Chicago
Chicago, IL, USA

Rohan Bir Singh
Department of Ophthalmology
Massachusetts Eye and Ear,
Harvard Medical School
Boston, MA, USA

ISSN 2523-3807 ISSN 2523-3815 (electronic)
Current Practices in Ophthalmology
ISBN 978-981-96-5293-8 ISBN 978-981-96-5294-5 (eBook)
https://doi.org/10.1007/978-981-96-5294-5

This Springer imprint is published by the registered company Springer Nature Singapore Pte Ltd.
The registered company address is: 152 Beach Road, #21-01/04 Gateway East, Singapore 189721, Singapore

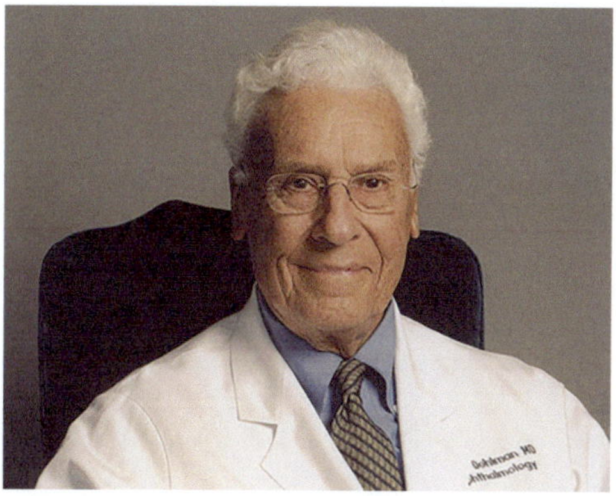

This book is dedicated to Dr. Claes Henrik Dohlman, the pioneer and father of modern cornea. His unwavering commitment to the advancement of ophthalmology has profoundly shaped the lives of so many: our careers on a personal level, the field at large, and the patients whom he so relentlessly served.
The numerous chapters of this book that are authored by those he mentored are a testament to his enduring legacy;
Dr. Dohlman will forever be remembered as an exceptional mentor, a brilliant scientist, and a guiding light in our professional journeys.

There is no phrase that more accurately captures what he would want us to do, and what he exemplified, than his own mantra: "Onward, and Forward!"

– Hajirah N. Saeed, MD, MPH
– Rohan Bir Singh, MD

Foreword

It is a great honor and privilege to introduce the latest addition to the Current Advances in Ophthalmology series, entitled *Corneal Disorders*, authored by Dr. Hajirah Saeed and Dr. Rohan Bir Singh. This comprehensive textbook is a testament to their dedication and expertise in the field of corneal diseases and treatments, providing invaluable insights for both trainees and experienced ophthalmologists.

The field of cornea research and clinical practice has seen remarkable advancements over the years. This textbook meticulously covers a wide array of topics, from the fundamentals to the latest innovations. The chapters span critical areas such as bacterial and fungal keratitis, herpes viral keratitis diagnosis and management, acanthamoeba keratitis, and neurotrophic keratitis. The inclusion of novel interventions in severe dry eye disease highlights the ongoing efforts to enhance patient care through innovative therapeutic approaches.

A standout feature of this book is its detailed discussion on limbal stem cell disease and management, and the comprehensive examination of end-stage corneal disease. These chapters reflect the authors' commitment to addressing complex clinical scenarios with practical solutions.

The text also delves into endothelial disease and management options, covering cutting-edge techniques including Rock inhibitors. This is complemented by sections on endothelial and pediatric keratoplasty, ocular burns, Stevens-Johnson syndrome, and keratoconus. One of the distinctive features of this textbook is its forward-looking approach to technology in ophthalmology. The chapters on artificial intelligence in the diagnosis and management of corneal disease are particularly timely, reflecting the rapid technological advancements transforming our field.

Corneal Disorders by Dr. Saeed and Dr. Singh is a testament to their profound understanding of corneal pathology and their commitment to enhancing patient care through knowledge dissemination. This textbook is set to become a cornerstone reference for ophthalmologists worldwide, bridging the gap between current research and clinical application.

I commend Dr. Saeed and Dr. Singh for their exceptional work and am confident that this book will serve as a vital resource for advancing our understanding and management of corneal diseases.

Kyoto, Japan
June 5, 2024

Shigeru Kinoshita

Contents

About the Editors

Hajirah N. Saeed is currently an Associate Professor of Ophthalmology at the Illinois Eye and Ear Infirmary, University of Illinois Chicago. She is a cornea specialist who has a particular clinical and research interest in complex ocular surface disease, particularly pediatric ocular surface disease and surgery, and Stevens Johnson syndrome and ocular burns. She has over 60 peer-reviewed publications and is an internationally recognized expert in Stevens Johnson syndrome. Her work is funded by the National Eye Institute.

Rohan Bir Singh is a senior fellow at the Laboratory of Ocular Immunology, Transplantation and Regeneration at the Schepens Eye Research Institute of Massachusetts Eye and Ear, Harvard Medical School, Boston, MA, USA. He graduated from the Government Medical College and Hospital, Panjab University, Chandigarh, India. His research interests include the immunopathogenesis of dry eye disease, immunology of corneal graft rejection and ocular graft versus host disease, and epidemiology of ocular disorders in the United States. He is a PhD candidate at the Leiden University Medical Center, The Netherlands, specializing in corneal immunology. Dr. Singh is also an Honorary Associate Professor in the Division of Ophthalmology and Visual Sciences, Adelaide Medical School, University of Adelaide, Australia. He has published more than 100 peer-reviewed publications and chapters in leading ophthalmology and vision science journals.

Bacterial and Fungal Keratitis

1

Sonal S. Tuli, Lauren Jeang, Ankit Shah, and W. Allan Steigleman

Summary

- Infectious keratitis is the major cause of ocular morbidity worldwide though organisms vary geographically.
- Clinical features may help clinicians narrow the differential diagnosis but are not sensitive or specific.
- Cultures and smears are gold standards for diagnosis, although molecular studies and imaging are being increasingly used.
- Topical therapy is the first-line treatment for infectious keratitis. Ancillary procedures should be considered for severe or recalcitrant disease.
- Future directions for the diagnosis and treatment of infectious keratitis are described.

1.1 Introduction

Infectious keratitis or corneal ulceration is a medical emergency with an incidence ranging from approximately 10 per 10,000 individuals in tropical and developing nations to 10 per 100,000 in more temperate climates in developed nations [1]. Corneal infection is normally prevented by the ocular adnexa; rapid tear turnover from blinking and antimicrobial properties in the tear film reduce pathogen exposure to the cornea surface [2]. However, risk factors such as trauma, contact lens wear, ocular surface disease, and corneal surgery can cause breakdown of the corneal epithelial barrier and promote adherence and penetration of an infectious pathogen [3]. Specifically for contact lenses, overnight wear, failing to wash and dry hands prior to handling lenses, and poor storage case

S. S. Tuli (✉) · L. Jeang · A. Shah · W. A. Steigleman
Department of Ophthalmology, University of Florida, Gainesville, FL, USA
e-mail: stuli@ufl.edu; ljeang@ufl.edu; ashah@ufl.edu; asteigleman@ufl.edu

H. N. Saeed, R. B. Singh (eds.), *Corneal Disorders*, Current Practices in Ophthalmology, https://doi.org/10.1007/978-981-96-5294-5_1

hygiene can increase the risk of infection [4]. This results in an inflammatory cascade that produces inflammatory cells and cytokines such as interleukins and matrix metalloproteinases. While these have antimicrobial functions, they also degrade the corneal structural proteins and result in ulceration of the corneal stroma [5]. Progression of this process can cause corneal perforation and intraocular extension of infection that may result in loss of the eye from endophthalmitis. Even with appropriate treatment, there is a high incidence of visual loss due to the development of corneal scarring and irregularity. Thus, rapid diagnosis and aggressive management of infectious keratitis are needed to maintain the integrity of the eye. The estimated yearly incidence of blindness from corneal ulceration is 1.5 million worldwide, and over 840,000 in India alone [6]. In addition, the financial burden and time invested in treatment cannot be ignored. Microbial keratitis costs the US health care system an estimated $175 million in direct health expenditures [7].

Corneal infections can be caused by a myriad of pathogens with incidence based on region. Aside from viral infections, bacterial infections constitute the majority of cases in most areas [8]. The exception is in less developed countries (LCDs), where fungal infections are seen more frequently than bacterial infections [14]. Bacterial and fungal keratitis share some common risk factors and can appear similar, but some distinguishing features can help guide treatment and determine prognosis. However clinical examination alone is not a reliable indicator of the etiology. A study found that cornea specialists can clinically distinguish between bacterial and fungal keratitis only about two thirds of the time [9]. Therefore, diagnostic testing is often needed to assist in disease identification. Herein we summarize the risk factors and clinical features of bacterial and fungal keratitis. Diagnostic and treatment modalities are discussed with a highlight of more recent developments in management.

1.2 Clinical Features

1.2.1 Bacterial Keratitis

Patients with bacterial keratitis typically present with acute onset pain, conjunctival injection, and reduced vision. Clinical examination reveals a corneal infiltrate, epithelial defect, and often corneal thinning at the site of ulceration. Anterior chamber reaction is often present and can be robust with associated hypopyon and posterior synechiae. Patients presenting with anterior chamber reaction of more than 1+ cells, ulceration >2 mm in diameter, and lesions within 3 mm of the visual axis may be more likely to develop vision threatening complications [10]. Although uncommon, severe infectious keratitis may progress to infectious endophthalmitis with profound vision loss and even potentially loss of the globe [11]. Therefore, prompt, efficacious treatment is necessary to preserve vision and prevent potential loss of an eye.

Some clinical parameters upon presentation may suggest a bacterial etiology. Gram-negative infections are associated with a larger baseline infiltrate size and deeper infiltrate that is soupy in appearance due to rapid necrosis of the cornea and associated robust inflammatory response. They are often associated with a rapidly increasing layered hypopyon (Fig. 1.1). *Streptococcus pneumoniae* can be associated with smaller baseline infiltrate and concomitant dacryocystitis, while *Streptococcus* viridans may have a crystalline appearance and usually occurs in patients on chronic topical steroids (Fig. 1.2). *Staphylococcus* species tend to be in mid-peripheral and peripheral locations. *Nocardia* may be associated with shallow infiltrates, longer duration of symptoms before presentation, and better baseline visual acuity [12]. Hypopyon, superficial neo-vascularization, and ulceration area > 20 mm^2 have been reported more frequently in bacterial keratitis vs fungal keratitis. Concomitant ocular disease, coexisting systemic diseases, and previous ocular surgery may be more frequent in cases of bacterial keratitis, while corneal injury is more frequently described in fungal keratitis [13].

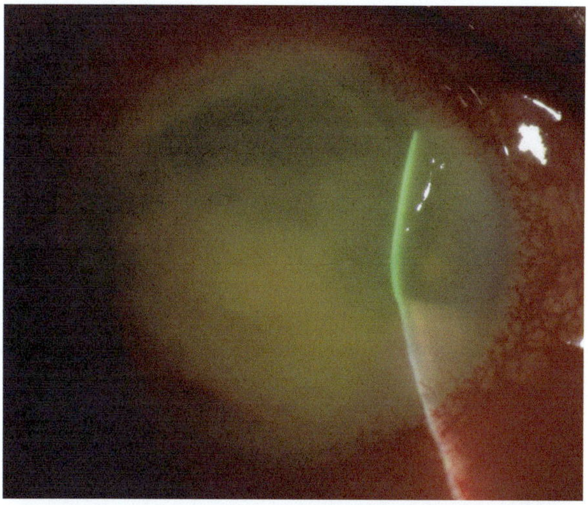

Fig. 1.1 Pseudomonas ulcer showing soupy infiltration of the corneal stroma, purulent discharge, and a layered hypopyon

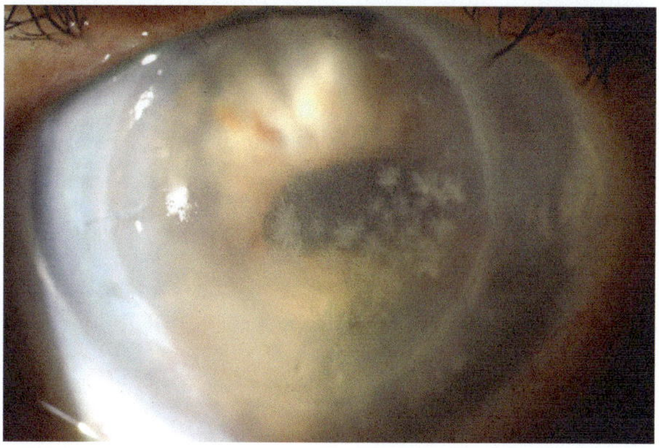

Fig. 1.2 Cystalline keratopathy in a patient on chronic steroids

1.2.2 Fungal Keratitis

Fungal keratitis (FK), also known as keratomycosis, is a disease primarily of the tropics and subtropics, although it is found in all areas of the world. The global annual incidence of fungal keratitis is estimated to be approximately one million, with the highest numbers in Asia and Africa, and the lowest in Europe [14]. In the United States, the percentage of corneal ulcers that are fungal can vary from 1% in the Northeast to 20% in the Southeast, but these are likely underestimates as the isolation rate of keratomycosis is as low as 50% [15]. While trauma has traditionally been considered the major risk factor for this condition, contact lenses are the primary cause in developed nations [16]. The majority of fungal keratitides are filamentary fungi (molds) except in patients with fungal keratitis post-corneal transplantation where the incidence of yeast is slightly higher (52%) than molds [17]. *Fusarium* species followed by *Aspergillus* species were the most common causes of the disease, although over 50 distinct species of fungi have been identified in corneal ulcers. Fungal elements in corneal infections are characterized by branching hyphae that may be septate or nonseptate. Yeasts, on the other hand, are usually seen as budding cells but can form pseudohyphae or even true hyphae on occasion.

The presentation and features of FK differ somewhat from that of bacterial keratitis and can be clues to the diagnosis. The duration of symptoms is often longer and onset not as abrupt as bacterial keratitis. While the pain and redness are similar, FK patients often complain of increased photophobia but less discharge from the eye compared to bacterial keratitis. On examination, fungal ulcers typically appear drier and less necrotic and have been classically described as having feathery borders and satellite lesions. The feathery borders appear pseudopodal and not as fine as those seen in crystalline keratopathy, and the ulcer may appear raised with sloughing. Deep immune rings are seen frequently, and often, the epithelium can heal as the fungus penetrates deeper [15]. One pathophysiological feature that contributes to increased morbidity and decreased response to treatment is that fungus can penetrate intact Descemet membranes and enter the anterior chamber without perforation. Thus, it causes endothelial plaques, and the hypopyon associated with FK often has a form to it as opposed to the reactive hypopyon seen in conjunction with bacterial infection that is layered in the anterior chamber due to gravity (Fig. 1.3). Pigmentation in the ulcer implies infection with dematiaceous fungi such as *Curvularia* and clinches the diagnosis of a fungal infection (Fig. 1.4) [18]. Yeast infections may also have satellite lesions but often present differently. They are most often found in patients on topical steroids or those that are immunocompromised. These ulcers typically appear creamy yellow and may have a crystalline appearance [19]. Keratomycosis can cause significant morbidity from glaucoma, corneal pannus, and penetration of the fungus into the eye.

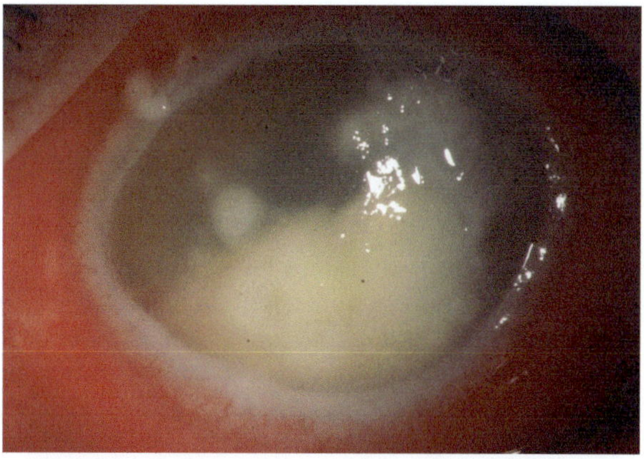

Fig. 1.3 Fungal ulcer demonstrating endothelial plaque and satellite corneal lesions

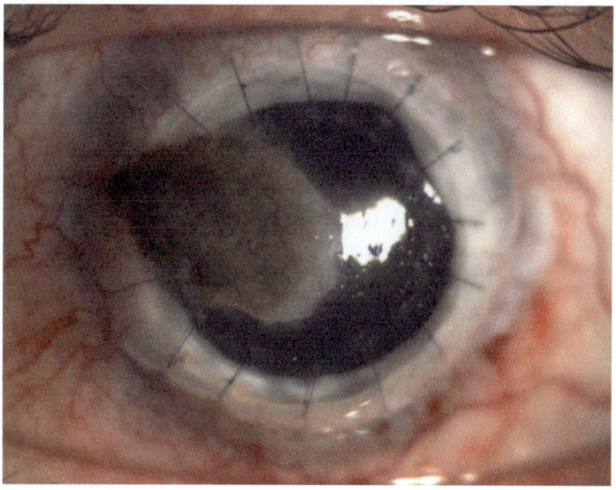

Fig. 1.4 Pigmented fungal lesion on the cornea

1.3 Differential Diagnosis

Herpes simplex virus (HSV) necrotizing keratitis: This presents with an epithelial defect and a rapidly developing suppurative infiltrate that can cause progressive corneal thinning and perforation [20]. Lack of foreign body sensation and discharge associated with a relatively quiet eye would raise the suspicion of this condition, especially in a patient with a history of HSV keratitis. Confirmation with polymerase chain reaction (PCR) is most sensitive, but viral cultures, direct fluorescein antibody, or a Tzanck smear can also be used.

Acanthamoeba: Patients with poor contact lens hygiene or trauma with vegetative matter, especially in warmer climates, should raise the suspicion of this condition [21]. Early disease may present with raised epithelial lines, pseudodendrites, epithelial or subepithelial infiltrates, or limbitis [21, 22]. Perineural infiltrates are present in up to 63% of cases. Late-stage findings include ring infiltrates, ulceration, anterior chamber reaction, and scleritis. Diagnosis is made by Giemsa-stained smear, culture on non-nutrient agar with *Escherichia coli*, confocal microscopy, and PCR [23, 24].

Microsporidiosis: This disease is usually associated with immunocompromised individuals who present with superficial punctate keratitis, or immunocompetent individuals in Southeast Asia who present with a suppurative stromal infiltrate but the presentation can vary broadly [25–27]. Light microscopy, histopathologic analysis, and confocal microscopy assist in diagnosis [28].

Peripheral ulcerative keratitis (PUK): This may appear as a curvilinear infiltrate with severe inflammation of the adjacent conjunctiva and sclera that rapidly progresses to thinning and perforation of the peripheral cornea [29]. PUK is frequently associated with collagen vascular diseases and vasculitides including rheumatoid arthritis, granulomatosis with polyangiitis, and systemic lupus erythematosus.

Neurotrophic keratitis: Poor corneal innervation or sensation can lead to epithelial breakdown, stromal thinning, and perforation [30]. The epithelial defect is characterized by smooth, rolled, and elevated edge and is caused by inability of the epithelium to heal due to a lack of tears and growth factors, as well as repeated trauma and underlying inflammation. Predisposing factors include prior herpetic keratitis, trigeminal tumors or ablation, prior ocular surgery, topical anesthetic abuse, or topical medication toxicity.

Vitamin A deficiency: This condition is characterized by xerophthalmia, conjunctival Bitot spots, and conjunctival squamous metaplasia but can also present with peripheral corneal melt or a PUK-like appearance. Clinicians should inquire about a history of malnutrition, malabsorption, or alcoholism [31].

1.4 Diagnosis

While a detailed history and examination can provide clues to the etiology of infection, laboratory diagnosis is recommended to identify the causative organism so that appropriate treatment can be rapidly tailored to the infection.

Cultures and smears are the gold standards for diagnosing the causative organisms and identifying antimicrobial susceptibilities to target therapy for corneal ulcers, especially in those that are severe or vision threatening [32, 33]. The American Academy of Ophthalmology practice guidelines recommend cultures for (1) central, large infiltrates and/or with significant stromal involvement or melt; (2) chronic or unresponsive infections; (3) history of corneal surgeries; (4) lesions with atypical clinical features; and (5) infiltrates with multiple corneal locations [3]. Sampling from the leading edge of infection and direct inoculation into media provide the best yields. Culturing contact lenses and cases may be useful and should be performed where available. Lesions where only deeper stroma is involved may benefit from passage and culture of a suture, or a corneal biopsy [34]. Corneal biopsy is performed using a 3–4 mm skin punch and lamellar dissection at the junction of the infiltrate and unaffected cornea. The button is sent for histopathology and culture can be performed in the bed of the biopsy to get a deeper sample.

Molecular studies using PCR can provide fast results and are highly sensitive, but require suspicion for a specific pathogen and are not widely available [35]. Other diagnostic methods being examined include targeted amplification of ribosomal RNA, alterations in gene expression, and tear proteomics [36, 37].

In vivo confocal microscopy (IVCM) is a useful adjunct to identify fungal and protozoan infections [24, 38]. Fungal elements appear as branching filaments or septae. While highly specific, results are highly dependent on the individual user's experience. Anterior segment optical coherence tomography (AS-OCT) is another potentially useful modality in distinguishing fungal from bacterial and viral infection or in performing corneal endothelial biopsies [39, 40].

1.5 Management of Bacterial Keratitis

Topical therapy with broad-spectrum antibiotics remains the first line of treatment for all infectious corneal ulcers. Ulcers that are large, central, vision threatening, with associated corneal thinning or hypopyon should prompt immediate broad-spectrum fortified antibiotic use. Vancomycin ranging from 1% to 5%, and 1.4% fortified tobramycin dosed hourly or more often initially are the most commonly used broad-spectrum antibiotics. Alternatively, 5% cefazolin and 1.4% gentamicin may be used [41]. Corneal cultures and sensitivities should dictate subsequent antibiotics use.

Fluroquinolone monotherapy is a reasonable strategy for small, peripheral-contact lens–associated corneal infiltrates as they are less toxic, easier to obtain, and have a longer shelf life. Fourth-generation (moxifloxacin and gatifloxacin) fluoroquinolones have better gram-positive and gram-negative coverage than older generations [42]. Atypical mycobacteria, most commonly linked to post-refractive surgery infectious keratitis, are usually treated with either amikacin (40–100 mg/ml) or clarithromycin (10–40 mg/ml) [43]. Oral or intravenous antibiotics are not routinely used in the management of bacterial keratitis unless there is significant involvement of the sclera and limbus.

Unfortunately, resistance of infectious organisms to antibiotics is rapidly becoming a challenge. Methicillin-resistant *Staphylococcus* species are increasing in community-acquired infections, and these bacteria are also resistant in high numbers to erythromycin (over 90%), fluoroquinolones (nearly 60%), and tobramycin (36%). Gram-negative bacteria have a lower incidence of resistance, but the ones that are resistant are often pan-drug resistant [44]. Fortunately, nearly all (99.6%) of gram-positive organisms are sensitive to vancomycin and 97% of gram-negative organisms are sensitive to tobramycin, bolstering the recommendation to use fortified vancomycin and tobramycin in the initial management of severe bacterial keratitis [45].

Management of the severe inflammation associated with bacterial ulcers may help decrease the corneal necrosis and scarring that is the cause of the morbidity associated with this condition. The Steroids in Corneal Ulcers Trial did not demonstrate a significant improvement in outcomes with the use of topical steroids other than in severe central ulcers where it did hasten recovery and resulted in slightly better visual outcomes [46]. Fortunately, it did not demonstrate any harm either except in cases of Nocardia keratitis. If used, they are typically started after 48 hours of antibiotic use in culture proven bacterial ulcers. The use of steroids in ulcers that are not proven to be bacterial, especially in areas with high numbers of fungal infections, is not recommended.

Anti-collagenase agents such as doxycycline and vitamin C given orally are beneficial in aggressive infectious keratitis with significant corneal melting. Increased protease activity causes destruction in the extracellular matrix, and these agents are thought to inhibit these matrix metalloproteinases. However, there is a paucity of controlled trials to confirm their efficacy [47]. Similarly, while povidone iodine was shown to be a very effective antiseptic, it was not shown to be beneficial in infectious keratitis. Anecdotal reports have suggested benefit of treatments such as hyperbaric oxygen and cryotherapy, but there is a lack of controlled studies to confirm their effectiveness.

1.6 Management of Fungal Keratitis

The main drugs for the treatment of fungal disease can be divided into four groups, namely, polyenes, azoles, pyrimidines, and echinocandins. The most commonly used drugs in ophthalmology are polyenes (natamycin and amphotericin B); azoles, including imidazoles such as miconazole and ketoconazole; and triazoles such as voriconazole and posaconazole. Topical 5% natamycin, a polyene, is the first line of treatment for filamentary fungal keratitis but is ineffective against yeast. Topical 1% voriconazole is a popular alternative, but the Mycotic Ulcer Treatment Trial (MUTT I) compared the two drugs and found significant superiority of natamycin over voriconazole and recommended that voriconazole not be used as monotherapy for fungal keratitis. However, it is effective for yeast keratitis [48]. A subsequent trial, MUTT II, similarly demonstrated that concurrent oral voriconazole in addition to topical antifungals had no benefit in the treatment of severe filamentous keratitis, though there was possibly some benefit for severe fusarium keratitis [49]. In addition, it may be beneficial in cases of limbal involvement or penetration into the anterior chamber in deep infections [41]. If used, periodic liver function tests need to be done due to potential liver toxicity. The treatment of choice for yeast-associated infectious keratitis is topical 0.15% amphotericin B. Treatment for fungal keratitis is typically needed for longer periods of time than bacterial keratitis, but less frequent dosing can be used because of the slower replication rate of fungal elements compared to bacteria. Periodic epithelial debridement is controversial as some studies have found it to be beneficial for drug penetration, while others have found it to increase scarring. Steroids are contraindicated in keratomycosis.

Intrastromal and intracameral amphotericin B (5 mg/0.1 mL) or voriconazole (50 mg/mL) have proven to be very effective for deep corneal fungal infections or those that have penetrated into the anterior chamber. Repeating intrastromal and intracameral on a weekly basis may help reduce infiltrate size and fungal load. This method allows for targeted delivery of the medication directly into the corneal stroma and anterior chamber, mitigating the poor penetration of topical fungal medications. On the other hand, subconjunctival antibiotics and antifungals are no longer recommended due to low benefit and high risk. However, they may be used in patients who are poorly compliant or are unable to instill topical drops.

Collagen cross linking (CXL) has been investigated as a treatment for non-responding corneal ulcers. The term "photoactivated chromophore" for infectious keratitis-CXL (PACK-CXL) has been used to identify patients in which 0.1% riboflavin-assisted CXL is performed to treat infectious keratitis using the Dresden protocol (3 mw/cm^2 for 30 min with 0.1% riboflavin). A meta-analysis of PACK-CXL performed by Ting et al. confirmed reduced healing time and morbidity, earlier resolution of the infiltrate, and improved outcomes [50, 51]. The microcidal effectiveness of PACK-CXL has been theorized to be due to the synergistic effects of the two entities. First, UV light effectively damages DNA and RNA molecules, thereby inhibiting replication of bacteria and viruses. Second, riboflavin photoactivation creates reactive oxygen species, which are toxic to the cellular membranes and nucleic acids of microbes [52]. However, PACK-CXL is not recommended for fungal infections due to increased inflammation and risk of corneal perforation [53].

1.7 Surgical Management

Severe cases of infectious keratitis can result in significant corneal thinning and perforation requiring urgent intervention. Surgical interventions in the acute period are needed in approximately 15% of cases and are mostly aimed at reestablishing globe integrity and/or debulking infectious material from the eye. Penetrating keratoplasty is the most commonly performed procedure in these cases and, although it can provide anatomical success, these eyes typically have poor visual outcomes due to complications such as secondary glaucoma, cataract, and graft rejection [54]. Delays in surgery beyond 30 days from onset, diabetes, large grafts, hypopyon, and corneal perforation are prognostic of worse outcomes [55]. In an emergency when fresh donor tissue is not available, glycerol preserved corneas may be successfully used to achieve anatomical integrity [56]. Tectonic deep anterior lamellar keratoplasty (DALK) is a reasonable option to manage descemetoceles and corneal perforations associated with infectious keratitis but carries an increased risk of reinfection possibly due to retention of infectious material in the residual host tissue [57]. Small case series have demonstrated the ability of tectonic Descemet stripping endothelial keratoplasty (DSEK) to help manage infectious keratitis-associated corneal perforations. These cases were successful when other modalities such as corneal gluing, amniotic membrane patching, and bandage contact lens use failed. In one series, optical DALK was performed once the acute episodes subsided. This may be a reasonable modality when anterior lamellar or penetrating keratoplasty are not feasible or considered a higher risk procedure [58].

Cyanoacrylate glue is an excellent alternative for reestablishing globe integrity for patients with corneal thinning or perforation. It is usually a temporizing measure except in small, peripheral ulcers where it may be a definitive treatment. Typically, the glue is used to provide structural strength until the infection can be resolved medically to increase the rates of success of corneal transplantation [59]. However, an additional benefit is the inhibition of inflammation potentially related to the inhibition of migration of polymorphonuclear leukocytes, thereby preventing their collagenolytic and proteolytic effects on the corneal stroma, as well as their bacteriostatic effect [60]. Another option for patching a corneal defect is to use a pedicle conjunctival flap (Fig. 1.5). This can not only help restore corneal mechanical integrity, but its bloody supply can also provide metabolic and serum growth factors to support healing during an acute infection in order to defer PKP until success is more likely [61]. A study of 31 patients with infectious keratitis refractory to medical management, of which over half were fungal, demonstrated that pedunculated corneal flaps were able to restore anatomic integrity and preserve 100% of globes [62].

Amniotic membrane grafts (AMG) are frequently used to aid in healing infectious and non-infectious corneal ulcers. AMG have been found to speed up healing and result in improved uncorrected vision compared to control eyes, with negligible adverse effects [63]. AMGs have been found to promote epithelial healing, decrease inflammation, and promote anti-scarring and anti-angiogenic effects. The mechanism of action, although not completely understood, is thought to be secondary to reduced inflammation due to the presence of anti-inflammatory cytokines such as tissue inhibitor of metalloproteinases in the AMG; the stroma is thought to act as a sink for inflammatory cells [64]. The basement membrane also contains several growth factors that help with epithelial cell migration, adhesion, and differentiation. Several different techniques of applying the AMG have been described including single layer, double layer, a rolled AMG technique, and self-retaining. AMG can also be sutured or glued to the cornea in a multilayer fashion to add volume to the cornea in cases of corneal thinning or perforation. The AMG in these cases incorporates into the host stroma with overlying epithelialization. [65]. An alternative to AMG is an umbilical cord patch, which is also an AM-derived graft but typically much thicker than AMG with a thickness of approximately 400 microns [66].

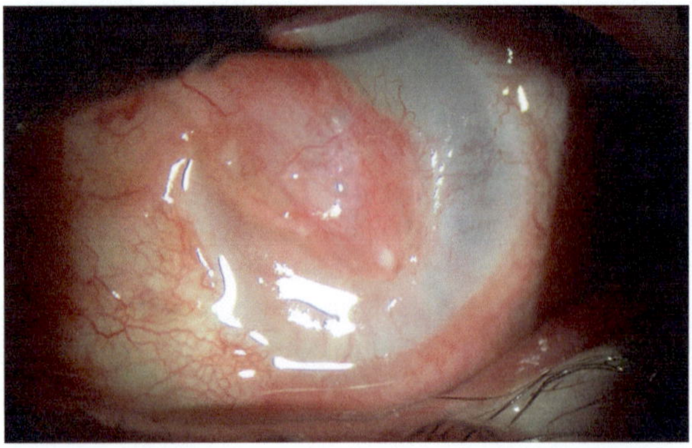

Fig. 1.5 Pedicle conjunctival graft for a nonhealing fungal infection due to Curvularia in a blind eye

Plasma-rich fibrin membranes and autologous platelet rich plasma clot with overlying fibrin membranes are other alternatives that have similar actions and are useful temporizing measures to maintain integrity of the globe and speed up healing [67].

1.8 Future Directions

1.8.1 Diagnostics

Rapid identification of the causative organism can improve outcomes through targeted treatment of the infection. Broad-range 16 s ribosomal RNA PCR and multiplex PCR are tools that can facilitate diagnosis of hard-to-culture organisms and can be used to detect a wide range of organisms simultaneously unlike standard PCR that can only detect a single target at a time [35, 68]. Other techniques that are not diagnostic but can provide clues to the presence of gram-negative bacteria include the use of anterior segment OCT to assess for higher pachymetry and thicker infiltrate, and detection of high levels of cytokines IL-1, IL-6, and IL-8 in the tear film [69]. Deep learning and neural networks are being used for image analysis of photographs and confocal images to aid in diagnosis of infectious keratitis, especially fungal and acanthamoeba keratitis. An intelligent system based on a deep learning algorithm was trained to identify fungal elements on confocal images. A test set of 535 images evaluated by the system correctly identified 515, giving it a sensitivity of 92% and a specificity of 98% [70]. Similarly, a deep learning algorithm was created with a segmentation model for cropping images and application of convolutional neural networks to differentiate between fungal and bacterial keratitis on slit lamp photographs and was found to be superior to the diagnostic performance of ophthalmologists [71].

1.8.2 Management

Novel formulations of antifungal drugs such as water soluble natamycin and lipoidal formulations of amphotericin may help mitigate the problem of poor penetration of antifungal agents into the cornea [72]. Recent studies have demonstrated rose bengal photodynamic antimicrobial therapy as an effective adjunct in eliminating infection and reducing the need for therapeutic penetrating keratoplasty in severe progressive necrotizing infectious keratitis, including fungal keratitis. Rose bengal is photoactivated by a 6 mW/cm^2 green light source and has antimicrobial properties; it has been found to increase collagenase resistance and reinforce corneal integrity [73]. Demand for suitable corneal tissue available for transplantation far outstrips supply in many regions of the world. A novel approach to restoring globe integrity and functional vision in advanced cases of infectious keratitis when human donor tissue is not available includes the use of acellular porcine corneal stroma for anterior lamellar keratoplasty [74]. Finally, scleral contact lenses have been evaluated as a reservoir for antibiotics to provide a depot of medication and improve compliance. A study with 0.5% preservative-free moxifloxacin found promising results with regard to infection resolution and improved healing time even in ulcers that were caused by bacteria with low sensitivity to moxifloxacin [75].

References

1. Jeng BH, Gritz DC, Kumar AB, et al. Epidemiology of ulcerative keratitis in Northern California. ArchOphthalmol. 2010;128(8):1022–8.
2. Garreis F, Gottschalt M, Paulsen FP. Antimicrobial peptides as a major part of the innate immune defense at the ocular surface. Dev Ophthalmol. 2010;45:16–22.
3. Lin A, Rhee MK, Akpek EK, et al. Bacterial Keratitis Preferred Practice Pattern(R). Ophthalmology. 2019;126(1):P1–P55.
4. Stapleton F. Contact lens-related corneal infection in Australia. Clin Exp Optom. 2020;103(4):408–17.
5. Lim M, Goldstein MH, Tuli S, Schultz GS. Growth factor, cytokine and protease interactions during corneal wound healing. OculSurf. 2003;1(2):53–65.
6. Ung L, Acharya NR, Agarwal T, et al. Infectious corneal ulceration: a proposal for neglected tropical disease status. Bull World Health Organ. 2019;97(12):854–6.
7. Ung L, Bispo PJM, Shanbhag SS, Gilmore MS, Chodosh J. The persistent dilemma of microbial keratitis: Global burden, diagnosis, and antimicrobial resistance. Surv Ophthalmol. 2019;64(3):255–71.
8. Stapleton F. The epidemiology of infectious keratitis. Ocul Surf. 2021.
9. Dalmon C, Porco TC, Lietman TM, et al. The clinical differentiation of bacterial and fungal keratitis: a photographic survey. Invest OphthalmolVisSci. 2012;53(4):1787–91.
10. Ung L, Wang Y, Vangel M, et al. Validation of a Comprehensive Clinical Algorithm for the Assessment and Treatment of Microbial Keratitis. Am J Ophthalmol. 2020;214:97–109.
11. Henry CR, Flynn HW Jr, Miller D, Forster RK, Alfonso EC. Infectious keratitis progressing to endophthalmitis: a 15-year study of microbiology, associated factors, and clinical outcomes. Ophthalmology. 2012;119(12):2443–9.
12. Mascarenhas J, Srinivasan M, Chen M, et al. Differentiation of etiologic agents of bacterial keratitis from presentation characteristics. Int Ophthalmol. 2012;32(6):531–8.
13. Ibrahim MM, Vanini R, Ibrahim FM, et al. Epidemiology and medical prediction of microbial keratitis in southeast Brazil. Arq Bras Oftalmol. 2011;74(1):7–12.
14. Brown L, Leck AK, Gichangi M, Burton MJ, Denning DW. The global incidence and diagnosis of fungal keratitis. Lancet Infect Dis. 2021;21(3):e49–57.
15. Mahmoudi S, Masoomi A, Ahmadikia K, et al. Fungal keratitis: An overview of clinical and laboratory aspects. Mycoses. 2018;61(12):916–30.
16. Acharya Y, Acharya B, Karki P. Fungal keratitis: study of increasing trend and common determinants. Nepal J Epidemiol. 2017;7(2):685–93.
17. Ahmadikia K, Aghaei Gharehbolagh S, Fallah B, et al. Distribution, prevalence, and causative agents of fungal keratitis: a systematic review and meta-analysis (1990 to 2020). Front Cell Infect Microbiol. 2021;11:698780.
18. Khurana A, Chanda S, Bhagat P, Aggarwal S, Sharma M, Chauhan L. Clinical characteristics, predisposing factors, and treatment outcome of Curvularia keratitis. Indian J Ophthalmol. 2020;68(10):2088–93.
19. Sun RL, Jones DB, Wilhelmus KR. Clinical characteristics and outcome of Candida keratitis. Am J Ophthalmol. 2007;143(6):1043–5.
20. Wang L, Wang R, Xu C, Zhou H. Pathogenesis of herpes stromal keratitis: immune inflammatory response mediated by inflammatory regulators. Front Immunol. 2020;11(766)
21. Dart JK, Saw VP, Kilvington S. Acanthamoeba keratitis: diagnosis and treatment update 2009. Am J Ophthalmol. 2009;148(4):487–499 e482.

22. Theodore FH, Jakobiec FA, Juechter KB, et al. The diagnostic value of a ring infiltrate in acanthamoebic keratitis. Ophthalmology. 1985;92(11):1471–9.
23. Kheirkhah A, Satitpitakul V, Syed ZA, et al. Factors Influencing the Diagnostic Accuracy of Laser-Scanning In Vivo Confocal Microscopy for Acanthamoeba Keratitis. Cornea. 2018;37(7):818–23.
24. Tu EY, Joslin CE, Sugar J, Booton GC, Shoff ME, Fuerst PA. The relative value of confocal microscopy and superficial corneal scrapings in the diagnosis of Acanthamoeba keratitis. Cornea. 2008;27(7):764–72.
25. Loh RS, Chan CM, Ti SE, Lim L, Chan KS, Tan DT. Emerging prevalence of microsporidial keratitis in Singapore: epidemiology, clinical features, and management. Ophthalmology. 2009;116(12):2348–53.
26. Cali A, Meisler DM, Lowder CY, et al. Corneal microsporidioses: characterization and identification. J Protozool. 1991;38(6):215S–7S.
27. Huang HY, Wu CL, Lin SH, et al. Microsporidial stromal keratitis: characterisation of clinical features, ultrastructural study by electron microscopy and efficacy of different surgical modalities. Br J Ophthalmol. 2020;104(11):1613–20.
28. Malhotra C, Jain AK, Kaur S, Dhingra D, Hemanth V, Sharma SP. In vivo confocal microscopic characteristics of microsporidial keratoconjunctivitis in immunocompetent adults. Br J Ophthalmol. 2017;101(9):1217–22.
29. Gupta Y, Kishore A, Kumari P, et al. Peripheral ulcerative keratitis. Surv Ophthalmol. 2021;66(6):977–98.
30. Jabbour S, Ashton C, Balal S, Kaye A, Ahmad S. The management of neurotrophic keratitis. Curr Opin Ophthalmol. 2021;32(4):362–8.
31. Lata S, Bafna RK, Asif MI, Sachan A. Bilateral liquefactive corneal necrosis: a rare and devastating complication of vitamin A deficiency in the adult. BMJ Case Rep. 2021;14(2)
32. McLeod SD, Kolahdouz-Isfahani A, Rostamian K, Flowers CW, Lee PP, McDonnell PJ. The role of smears, cultures, and antibiotic sensitivity testing in the management of suspected infectious keratitis. Ophthalmology. 1996;103(1):23–8.
33. Rodman RC, Spisak S, Sugar A, Meyer RF, Soong HK, Musch DC. The utility of culturing corneal ulcers in a tertiary referral center versus a general ophthalmology clinic. Ophthalmology. 1997;104(11):1897–901.
34. Egrilmez S, Yildirim-Theveny S. Treatment-Resistant Bacterial Keratitis: Challenges and Solutions. Clin Ophthalmol. 2020;14:287–97.
35. Somerville TF, Corless CE, Sueke H, Neal T, Kaye SB. 16S Ribosomal RNA PCR Versus Conventional Diagnostic Culture in the Investigation of Suspected Bacterial Keratitis. Transl Vis Sci Technol. 2020;9(13):2.
36. Low L, Fuentes-Utrilla P, Hodson J, et al. Evaluation of full-length nanopore 16S sequencing for detection of pathogens in microbial keratitis. PeerJ. 2021;9:e10778.
37. Ung L, Bispo PJM, Doan T, et al. Clinical metagenomics for infectious corneal ulcers: Rags to riches? Ocul Surf. 2020;18(1):1–12.
38. Kheirkhah A, Syed ZA, Satitpitakul V, et al. Sensitivity and specificity of laser-scanning in vivo confocal microscopy for filamentous fungal keratitis: role of observer experience. Am J Ophthalmol. 2017;179:81–9.
39. Takezawa Y, Suzuki T, Shiraishi A. Observation of retrocorneal plaques in patients with infectious keratitis using anterior segment optical coherence tomography. Cornea. 2017;36(10):1237–42.
40. Palioura S, Tsiampali C, Dubovy SR, Yoo SH. Endothelial biopsy for the diagnosis and management of culture-negative retrocorneal fungal keratitis with the assistance of optical coherence tomography imaging. Cornea. 2021;40(9):1193–6.
41. Solanki S, Rathi M, Khanduja S, Dhull CS, Sachdeva S, Phogat J. Recent trends: medical management of infectious keratitis. Oman J Ophthalmol. 2015;8(2):83–5.
42. Thomas PA, Geraldine P. Infectious keratitis. Curr Opin Infect Dis. 2007;20(2):129–41.
43. Gokhale NS. Medical management approach to infectious keratitis. Indian J Ophthalmol. 2008;56(3):215–20.

44. Asbell PA, Sanfilippo CM, Sahm DF, DeCory HH. Trends in antibiotic resistance among ocular microorganisms in the United States From 2009 to 2018. JAMA Ophthalmol. 2020;138(5):439–50.
45. Tam ALC, Cote E, Saldanha M, Lichtinger A, Slomovic AR. Bacterial Keratitis in Toronto: A 16-Year Review of the Microorganisms Isolated and the Resistance Patterns Observed. Cornea. 2017;36(12):1528–34.
46. Srinivasan M, Mascarenhas J, Rajaraman R, et al. Corticosteroids for bacterial keratitis: the Steroids for Corneal Ulcers Trial (SCUT). ArchOphthalmol. 2012;130(2):143–50.
47. Dakhil TAB, Stone DU, Gritz DC. Adjunctive therapies for bacterial keratitis. Middle East Afr J Ophthalmol. 2017;24(1):11–7.
48. Prajna NV, Krishnan T, Mascarenhas J, et al. The mycotic ulcer treatment trial: a randomized trial comparing natamycin vs voriconazole. JAMA Ophthalmol. 2013;131(4):422–9.
49. Prajna NV, Krishnan T, Rajaraman R, et al. Effect of Oral Voriconazole on Fungal Keratitis in the Mycotic Ulcer Treatment Trial II (MUTT II): A Randomized Clinical Trial. JAMA Ophthalmol. 2016;134(12):1365–72.
50. Ting DSJ, Henein C, Said DG, Dua HS. Photoactivated chromophore for infectious keratitis - Corneal cross-linking (PACK-CXL): a systematic review and meta-analysis. Ocul Surf. 2019;17(4):624–34.
51. Li M, Yu T, Gao X, Wu XY. Accelerated corneal collagen cross-linking in clinical management of infectious keratitis. J Int Med Res. 2020;48(6):300060520926411.
52. Tabibian D, Mazzotta C, Hafezi F. PACK-CXL: Corneal cross-linking in infectious keratitis. Eye Vis (Lond). 2016;3:11.
53. Uddaraju M, Mascarenhas J, Das MR, et al. Corneal Cross-linking as an Adjuvant Therapy in the Management of Recalcitrant Deep Stromal Fungal Keratitis: A Randomized Trial. Am J Ophthalmol. 2015;160(1):131–134 e135.
54. Kasim B, Kocluk Y. Long-term outcomes of therapeutic penetrating keratoplasty for microbial keratitis in a tertiary care center in Turkey. Int Ophthalmol. 2020;40(12):3513–9.
55. Zhang Q, Zhao M, Xu M, et al. Outcomes of therapeutic keratoplasty for severe infectious keratitis in Chongqing, a 16-year experience. Infect Drug Resist. 2019;12:2487–93.
56. Niu G, Zhou Q, Huang X, et al. Individualized penetrating keratoplasty using edge-trimmed glycerol-preserved donor corneas for perforated corneal ulcers. BMC Ophthalmol. 2019;19(1):85.
57. Nguyen HT, Pham ND, Mai TQ, et al. Tectonic Deep Anterior Lamellar Keratoplasty to Treat Corneal Perforation and Descemetocele from Microbial Keratitis. Clin Ophthalmol. 2021;15:3549–55.
58. Tourkmani AK, Ansari AS, Hossain PN, Konstantopoulos A, Anderson DF. Tectonic descemet stripping endothelial keratoplasty for the management of corneal perforation: a case series. Cornea. 2020;39(12):1571–5.
59. Singh RB, Zhu S, Yung A, Dohlman TH, Dana R, Yin J. Efficacy of cyanoacrylate tissue adhesive in the management of corneal thinning and perforation due to microbial keratitis. Ocul Surf. 2020;18(4):795–800.
60. Chen WL, Lin CT, Hsieh CY, Tu IH, Chen WY, Hu FR. Comparison of the bacteriostatic effects, corneal cytotoxicity, and the ability to seal corneal incisions among three different tissue adhesives. Cornea. 2007;26(10):1228–34.
61. Stamate AC, Tataru CP, Zemba M. Efficacy of conjunctival flap surgery for deep corneal ulcers. Rom J Ophthalmol. 2021;65(2):171–5.
62. Nizeyimana H, Zhou DD, Liu XF, et al. Clinical efficacy of conjunctival flap surgery in the treatment of refractory fungal keratitis. Exp Ther Med. 2017;14(2):1109–13.
63. Ting DSJ, Henein C, Said DG, Dua HS. Amniotic membrane transplantation for infectious keratitis: a systematic review and meta-analysis. Sci Rep. 2021;11(1):13007.
64. Tuli S, Gray M. Surgical management of corneal infections. Curr Opin Ophthalmol. 2016;27(4):340–7.
65. Berguiga M, Mameletzi E, Nicolas M, Rivier D, Majo F. Long-term follow-up of multilayer amniotic membrane transplantation (MLAMT) for non-traumatic corneal perforations or deep ulcers with descemetocele. Klin Monatsbl Augenheilkd. 2013;230(4):413–8.

66. Xie HT, Zhao D, Liu Y, Zhang MC. Umbilical cord patch transplantation for corneal perforations and descemetoceles. J Ophthalmol. 2017;2017:2767053.
67. Alio JL, Rodriguez AE, Martinez LM, Rio AL. Autologous fibrin membrane combined with solid platelet-rich plasma in the management of perforated corneal ulcers: a pilot study. JAMA Ophthalmol. 2013;131(6):745–51.
68. Tokman HB, Iskeleli G, Dalar ZG, et al. Prevalence and antimicrobial susceptibilities of anaerobic bacteria isolated from perforated corneal ulcers by culture and multiplex PCR: an evaluation in cases with keratitis and endophthalmitis. Clin Lab. 2014;60(11):1879–86.
69. Konstantopoulos A, Cendra MDM, Tsatsos M, Elabiary M, Christodoulides M, Hossain P. Morphological and cytokine profiles as key parameters to distinguish between Gram-negative and Gram-positive bacterial keratitis. Sci Rep. 2020;10(1):20092.
70. Lv J, Zhang K, Chen Q, et al. Deep learning-based automated diagnosis of fungal keratitis with in vivo confocal microscopy images. Ann Transl Med. 2020;8(11):706.
71. Hung N, Shih AK, Lin C, et al. Using slit-lamp images for deep learning-based identification of bacterial and fungal keratitis: model development and validation with different convolutional neural networks. Diagnostics (Basel). 2021;11(7)
72. Saluja G, Sharma N, Agarwal R, et al. Determination of surgical outcomes with a novel formulation of intrastromal natamycin in recalcitrant fungal keratitis: a pilot study. Indian J Ophthalmol. 2021;69(10):2670–4.
73. Naranjo A, Arboleda A, Martinez JD, et al. Rose Bengal photodynamic antimicrobial therapy for patients with progressive infectious keratitis: a pilot clinical study. Am J Ophthalmol. 2019;208:387–96.
74. Li S, Li M, Gu L, et al. Risk factors influencing survival of acellular porcine corneal stroma in infectious keratitis: a prospective clinical study. J Transl Med. 2019;17(1):434.
75. Polania-Baron EJ, Santana-Cruz O, Lichtinger A, Graue-Hernandez EO, Navas A. Treatment of severe infectious keratitis with scleral contact lenses as a reservoir of Moxifloxacin 0.5. Cornea. 2021;40(7):831–6.

Herpes Viral Keratitis

2

Angelica Piccini, Rohan Bir Singh, and Vishal Jhanji

Key Messages

- Herpes keratitis is caused by HSV-1 or VZV and is one of the leading causes of corneal infection.
- Treatment options depend on the affected corneal layer and range from antivirals, corneal debridement, topical corticosteroids, corneal gluing, and antivirals.
- New medical therapies include the development of an HSV vaccine, anti-IL-17 therapeutic antibodies, and nanoparticle ocular immunotherapies.
- Standard surgical interventions when medical therapy fails include keratoplasty, conjunctival graft flaps, amniotic membrane transplantation, tarsorrhaphy, eyelid reconstructive surgery, and corneal neurotization.
- Deep learning may present as a promising avenue to improve rates of early diagnosis of herpes keratitis.

A. Piccini
Massachusetts Eye and Ear, Department of Ophthalmology, Harvard Medical School, Boston, MA, USA

Cooper Medical School of Rowan University, Camden, NJ, USA
e-mail: apiccini@meei.harvard.edu

R. B. Singh
Department of Ophthalmology, Massachusetts Eye and Ear, Harvard Medical School, Boston, MA, USA
e-mail: rohan_singh@meei.harvard.edu

V. Jhanji (✉)
Vision Institute, Department of Ophthalmology, University of Pittsburgh School of Medicine, Pittsburgh, PA, USA
e-mail: jhanjiv@upmc.edu

H. N. Saeed, R. B. Singh (eds.), *Corneal Disorders*, Current Practices in Ophthalmology, https://doi.org/10.1007/978-981-96-5294-5_2

2.1 Introduction

Herpetic eye diseases, caused by herpes simplex virus (HSV) and varicella-zoster virus (VZV), have the potential to cause an array of disorders affecting various ocular tissues, including the cornea. Among the HSV subtypes, herpes simplex virus-1 (HSV-1) is the prevailing cause of ocular infections, while neonatal ocular infections are commonly attributed to herpes simplex virus type 2 (HSV-2) [1].

Herpes keratitis includes herpes simplex virus keratitis and varicella-zoster virus keratitis, which are two of the most common causes of corneal infectious diseases. Herpes keratitis management poses significant challenges for cornea specialists, especially in regard to long-term complications and the emergence of antiviral-resistant strains [2]. McCormick and colleagues estimated that approximately 230,000 individuals had monocular vision impairment associated with HSV keratitis in a year [3]. Another critical aspect pertains to the prognosis and long-term management of herpetic keratitis, primarily due to the high rate of recurrence resulting from viral reactivation.

Herpes keratitis is characterized by the involvement of corneal epithelium, stroma, or endothelium [4]. The clinical presentation of HSV keratitis varies depending on the specific layer of the cornea that is affected. This infection can manifest as epithelial keratitis, stromal keratitis, endotheliitis, or uveitis [5].

Epithelial keratitis caused by HSV-1 can be further classified into three subtypes: punctate, dendritic, and geographic epithelial keratitis [6]. Active punctate epithelial keratitis is characterized by the presence of pinpoint opacities on the corneal surface. Staining of dendritic epithelial keratitis reveals dichotomous, dendriform branching patterns with terminal bulbs on the cornea (Fig. 2.1). Over time, dendritic epithelial keratitis may progress to geographic epithelial keratitis, which involves larger areas of the corneal surface [7].

Interstitial or stromal keratitis is a sterile immune reaction to HSV-1. The clinical presentation of stromal keratitis may manifest as disciform keratitis, characterized

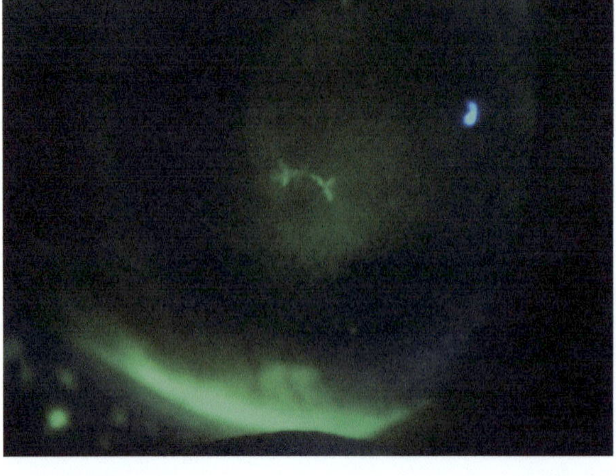

Fig. 2.1 Slit lamp photograph showing dendritic keratitis due to herpes simplex virus

by the formation of circular rings of stromal infiltrate where antibodies interact with antigens [8]. In some cases, stromal keratitis can progress to a diffuse and necrotic form, leading to the development of necrotic corneal lesions and stromal vascularization [9]. Endotheliitis denotes a deeper infection affecting the corneal endothelium, which is accompanied by inflammation. Granulomatous keratic precipitates and overlying stromal edema are typical indicators of endotheliitis [10]. Anterior uveitis refers to an inflammatory reaction occurring in the anterior chamber of the eye. It can range from mild to severe, with severe cases often presenting with a hypopyon [11]. Hypopyon is characterized by the accumulation of white blood cells in the anterior chamber. Additionally, endotheliitis and uveitis may be associated with trabeculitis [10], a condition characterized by inflammation of the trabecular meshwork, as well as elevated intraocular pressure (IOP). These diverse ocular clinical manifestations of herpes simplex virus keratitis can occur individually or coexist in the same patient.

Herpes zoster ophthalmicus (HZO) refers to the ocular complications associated with the reactivation of VZV, commonly known as shingles. This reactivation occurs in the trigeminal ganglion, and when the ophthalmic division of the nerve is involved, it can lead to pathological presentation in the eyes. More than half of HZO patients exhibit corneal changes, particularly varicella-zoster virus keratitis [12]. It is worth noting that on rare occasion, varicella-zoster virus keratitis can also occur simultaneously with varicella (chickenpox) in patients [13].

In its early stages, varicella-zoster virus keratitis is characterized by inflammation triggered by the presence of live VZV in the cornea. Early manifestations may present as punctate epithelial keratitis or plaque-like pseudodendrites. The branched and dendriform appearance of pseudodendrites can sometimes lead to the misdiagnosis of VZV keratitis as dendritic epithelial keratitis secondary to HSV [14]. Therefore, clinicians must be vigilant and recognize the distinct features of VZV lesions, which include microdendritic, peripheral, and stellate pseudodendrites. Late-stage varicella-zoster virus keratitis involves a sterile immune response to nonviable VZV, characterized by corneal mucous plaques, stromal keratitis, endotheliitis, and uveitis.

Several risk factors contribute to the development of herpes keratitis, including lack of varicella immunization, previous varicella or herpes infection, advanced age, immunosuppression, malignancy, chemotherapy, and radiation therapy [14]. Recently, a published report described the first documented case of herpes keratitis with coinfection of both HSV and VZV, likely resulting from systemic immunosuppression [15]. The ophthalmologist must develop an understanding about the potential occurrence of coinfection in immunosuppressed patients as diagnosis and treatment varies by etiology of disease. Recent clinical evidence in the literature has indicated a potential correlation between the utilization of antiglaucoma medications and the likelihood of recurrent HSV and VZV keratitis [16]. Nonetheless, a retrospective cohort study conducted in 2023 reported no discernible association between the administration of topical ocular hypotensive therapies and the recurrence of HSV/HZV keratitis [16].

2.2 Pathogenesis

HSV-1 and VZV infections elicit an innate immune response within the host cells, triggering the secretion of cytokines and various inflammatory mediators. As a consequence, herpes keratitis results in compromised vision due to the ensuing inflammatory processes, ultimately leading to corneal scarring and neovascularization [6].

In infected cornea tissue, HSV-1 replicates in the corneal epithelial cells. HSV-1 is a linear, double-stranded DNA virus with an icosahedral capsid and glycoproteins on the surface [17]. Its glycoproteins gB, gC, gD, gH, and gL are involved in the binding of HSV-1 to heparan sulfate on the surface of the corneal epithelial cells [18], thus facilitating viral fusion to the host cells. HSV-1 binds Toll-like receptors (TLRs) to promote intracellular signaling, leading to infection. Once the HSV-1 infects the corneal epithelium, an innate immune response is triggered, followed by adaptive immune response [19]. Major histocompatibility complex II (MHC-II) on antigen-presenting cells transmits the antigenic information of the HSV-1 virus to T cells, consequently activating them. On activation, T cells generate pro-inflammatory and anti-inflammatory cytokines. Studies have shown that IL-1β, IL-6, IL-10, IL-12, and IFN-γ are the predominant pro-inflammatory cytokines generated following corneal infection with HSV-1 [20]. More recently, IL-17 was observed to play a pro-inflammatory role through the activation of fibroblasts in corneal stroma, further aggravating the inflammatory milieu by contributing to the production of cytokines and factors that induce neutrophil chemotaxis to the corneal tissue [18]. The immune response in the infected corneal tissue is a delayed-type hypersensitivity response to viral antigens that involves mainly T cells, rather than antibodies produced by B cells [21].

After the primary HSV-1 infection of the corneal tissue, the virus remains latent in the trigeminal ganglion and reactivates in episodes of autoimmunity and hypoimmunity [22]. During reactivation, the virus travels along the ophthalmic nerves back to the corneal epithelium, leading to recurrent infection [18] and inflammation. Reactivation can occur in response to ultraviolet light [23], fluctuations in hormone levels [24], psychological stress [25], or other stressors.

2.3 Clinical Presentation

Patients with herpes keratitis present with symptoms of redness, photophobia, tearing, eye pain, and blurred vision. Herpes keratitis can lead to corneal scarring, glaucoma, edema, corneal opacity, corneal perforation, and vision loss. Corneal ulceration and neovascularization [6] are a devastating sequelae of herpes keratitis and can lead to irreversible blindness. Both HSV and VZV keratitis can present with neurotrophic keratopathy and exposure keratopathy [26]. Although any condition disrupting normal corneal innervation can cause neurotrophic keratopathy, herpes keratitis is the most common etiology [27].

Both stromal keratitis and endotheliitis secondary to HSV infection can clinically present with stromal opacity, necessitating the identification of underlying etiology for appropriate treatment. Stromal opacity due to stromal keratitis is associated with corneal neovascularization, which is a sight-threatening condition involving vascularity in the normally avascular cornea. In endotheliitis, viral infection and subsequent inflammation lead to stromal edema and stromal opacity [28]. Stromal keratitis secondary to HSV can be necrotizing or non-necrotizing [29]. Unlike non-necrotizing stromal keratitis, the epithelium is defective in necrotizing stromal keratitis, thus lending an increased risk of stromal melting and corneal perforation.

2.4 Diagnosis

The clinical diagnosis of herpetic keratitis is based on slit lamp eye examination revealing distinctive corneal lesions and a positive history of recurrent herpetic eye disease. Corneal fluorescein staining (Fig. 2.2) is used to examine corneal lesions. PCR tests and viral cultures may be used to test for HSV-1 DNA or live virus. These tests are most sensitive in detecting herpes keratitis with active corneal ulceration, such as in necrotizing herpetic stromal keratitis [30]. PCR tests can also detect viral VZV DNA in skin lesions or tear film. Recently, in a cross-sectional study of 8 patients with HSV keratitis and 12 patients with VZV keratitis, microfluidic real-time PCR performed on tear specimens found that the tests had 100% sensitivity and specificity in detecting HSV and VZV DNA [31]. Tzanck smears on corneal scrapings can also be used to detect the presence of VZV or HSV, but this test is not capable of differentiating the type of virus. Another study evaluated the diagnostic accuracy of tear HSV-sIgA in atypical stromal HSV keratitis. The diagnostic power of tear HSV-sIgA was found to be accurate in all the eyes of all 11 patients [32]. Due

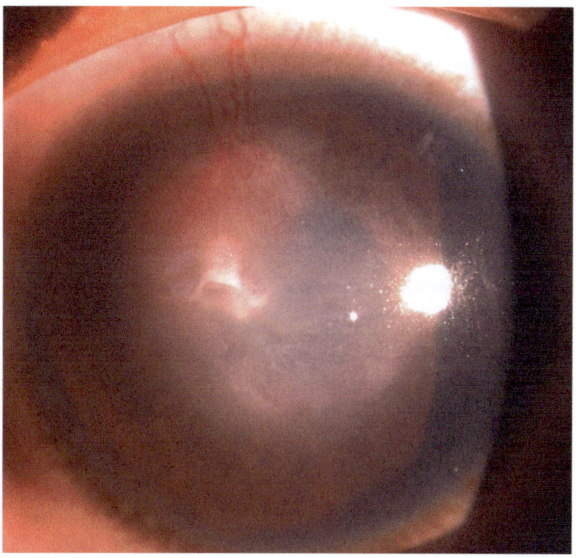

Fig. 2.2 Slit lamp photograph showing deep corneal neovascularization and lipid keratopathy in a patient with active varicella zoster keratitis

to the variable clinical features that may pose a challenge in diagnosing herpetic keratitis, tear HSV-sIgA can potentially become a more widely used tool to assist in the rapid diagnosis of atypical HSV keratitis.

Several other tests are necessary to identify comorbidities. It is recommended to test for reduced corneal sensation because loss of corneal innervation may occur when HSV replicates in the trigeminal ganglion, leading to cell death and increased hyposensitivity. A known prognostic marker for the risk and severity of viral keratitis secondary to herpes zoster involves Hutchinson's sign, which suggests nasociliary nerve involvement when there are painful vesicles or bumps near the tip of the nose of the patient.

Deep learning artificial intelligence algorithms have also been employed to diagnose herpetic keratitis. These may be helpful in areas with scarce resources, where misdiagnosis often leads to increased ocular morbidity. A retrospective study evaluated the effectiveness of a deep learning model called DenseNet to diagnose herpes simplex virus stromal necrotizing keratitis (HSVNK) using photographs from slit lamps biomicroscopy [33]. The study found a diagnostic accuracy of 72% for 285 eyes, with a sensitivity of 69.6% and specificity of 76.5% for detecting HSVNK. While AI-based platforms are still in preclinical stages of development, innovations in this area may serve to aid in the diagnosis of viral keratitis in care centers with limited resources.

2.5 Treatment

The goal of the treatment of herpetic keratitis is to suppress the damaging immune response on the ocular surface and prevent potential viral replication. Appropriate medical treatment for HSV keratitis varies depending on the location and severity of the ocular manifestations. For HSV epithelial keratitis, oral antivirals such as acyclovir 400 mg five times daily, valacyclovir 1 gram three times daily, or famciclovir 500 mg three times daily are included in the standard treatment regimen. Additionally, topical antivirals such as ganciclovir gel or trifluridine drops may also prescribed. Topical trifluridine (Viroptic) 1% nine times daily for 10–14 days has proven efficacious for dendritic and geographic epithelial keratitis [34]. A gentle debridement can be performed to remove the infectious cells, which are less adhesive than normal epithelial corneal cells. Topical corticosteroids are not prescribed due to the risk of recurrence. Cidofovir 0.2%–0.5% and trifluridine 1% are other alternatives for resistant herpes keratitis and may be used alongside epithelial debridement in epithelial keratitis [64].

Stromal keratitis that is secondary to HSV infection is treated with a combination of antiviral prophylaxis and topical corticosteroids since it involves an immune reaction against HSV-1. A systematic review found that herpes stromal keratitis patients who received both acyclovir and prednisolone eye drops had a higher treatment success rate and a longer time to failure compared to patients only given acyclovir [35]. Unlike epithelial keratitis, stromal keratitis involves a delayed hypersensitivity reaction that can be treated with corticosteroids. Therefore, 1%

prednisolone acetate is administered and tapered down in 1–2 weeks along with antiviral treatment. Recurrent HSV keratitis, not involving active viral disease, is known as trophic keratitis, involving a sterile epithelial trophic ulceration. Trophic herpetic keratitis presents with persistent defects in the basement membrane of the corneal epithelium. It can be treated with artificial tear lubricants, bandage contact lenses, and lid closure via tarsorrhaphy.

While standard stromal keratitis, which typically presents with disciform lesions, is treated with steroids, diffuse necrotic stromal keratitis with necrotic corneal lesions and stromal vascularization are treated with antivirals to delay the need of keratoplasty. Additionally, not every recurrent HSV keratitis is a sterile trophic keratitis. The high rate of recurrence of active herpetic stromal keratitis requires systemic oral antivirals to inhibit viral replication. The Herpetic Eye Disease Study showed a decrease in the recurrence of herpetic stromal keratitis from 28% to 14% with the use of oral acyclovir [36].

The management of VZV keratitis includes pain management, gentle debridement of the corneal epithelial lesions, and the use of topical corticosteroids to suppress inflammation. VZV keratitis is a sterile immune reaction to herpes virus in the cornea; therefore, the pseudodendrites do not respond to antivirals. However, oral antivirals such as acyclovir, valacyclovir, or famciclovir are given within 72 hours of symptom onset prophylactically to limit the risk of VZV replication and reduce the duration of viral shedding [37].

The long-term effects of herpes keratitis, including dry eye, meibomian gland dysfunction (MGD), and corneal scarring should also be treated. Ocular lubricants and punctal occlusion, with the insertion of punctal plugs or use of cautery, have been used to address dry eye and MGD. Studies have shown that scleral contact lenses can be effective in addressing irregular astigmatism secondary to corneal scarring and epithelial defects secondary to neurotrophic keratopathy in patients with herpetic keratitis, while supporting the ocular surface [38].

Cyanoacrylate tissue adhesive (CTA) which consists of cyanoacrylic acid with alkyl side chains has been used as a temporary measure for managing small corneal perforations in herpetic keratitis and preventing further corneal melting [39]. The glue is applied for corneal perforations smaller than 3 mm via a pipette, needle, or cannula using a slit lamp and is followed by the placement of a bandage contact lens after the CTA has dried [40]. Studies have shown that CTA inhibits polymorphonuclear leukocyte migration to the area, reducing collagenolytic and proteolytic enzyme loads and stunting the growth of bacterial organisms [41]. The complications of CTA include pro-inflammatory changes at the ocular surface and corneal vascularization.

Fibrin-based corneal glues have also been discussed in recent ophthalmic literature as an alternative to cyanoacrylate glues. Their flexible and noninflammatory properties make fibrin and other blood-based tissue adhesives favorable for corneal perforations [42]. Fibrin glue is less likely than CTA to lead to corneal neovascularization and has been shown to result in more rapid healing of the cornea [43]. However, unlike cyanoacrylate glues, fibrin glues lack bacteriostatic activity and have a very short half-life, making implementation difficult and reducing efficacy [44].

2.6 Surgical Management

While treatment of herpetic keratitis is usually medical, surgical intervention may be necessary to address long-term complications such as scarring, lipid keratopathy, necrotizing keratitis, and severe neurotrophic keratitis [45] (Fig. 2.2). The main pillars of surgical management involve replacing the infected tissue or providing structural support for tissue healing.

Keratoplasty is performed for visual rehabilitation in patients with opacified corneas. When corneal transplantation for severe cases of herpes keratitis cases is performed, clinicians must be vigilant in administering concurrent systemic antiviral therapy to prevent rejection secondary to viral reactivation induced by graft insertion. Keratoplasty can be subdivided into various types, including penetrating keratoplasty (PKP) and lamellar keratoplasty. Penetrating keratoplasty using a tectonic graft is useful for treating perforated corneal ulcers or replacing inflamed corneas unresponsive to treatment. A subtype of lamellar keratoplasty, deep anterior lamellar keratoplasty (DALK), may be performed in cases where endothelium and Descemet's membrane are unaffected.

Rejection rates for PKP are higher in patients with herpetic keratitis compared to PKP in patients with noninflammatory conditions [45]. Non-necrotizing and stromal keratitis with intact epithelium typically heals without scarring when steroids are used [45]. If not treated, stromal keratitis can progress and lead to stromal vascularization, exudation, and vision loss. Patients with significant stromal scarring but intact endothelium are surgically treated with DALK to replace the corneal stroma and preserve the endothelium. DALK results in lower rejection rates than PKP since it preserves the host's corneal endothelium [46, 47]. Although stromal keratitis and non-necrotizing keratitis largely do not require surgery, necrotizing keratitis can lead to corneal ulceration, scarring, and perforation and may warrant surgical intervention [45].

Corneal perforations are typically treated with bandage contact lenses, tissue glue [48], conjunctival flap patches [49], amniotic membrane transplantation [50], and tectonic PKP [51], along with medical therapy. Tectonic PKP is standard for corneal perforations with stromal melting. A study including 43 patients on the outcomes of therapeutic and tectonic penetrating keratoplasty for infectious corneal ulcer perforations reported that corneal integrity was achieved in 97.6% of cases [52].

A long-standing treatment for epithelial defects in the cornea, particularly secondary to neurotrophic keratitis, is amniotic membrane transplantation (AMT) (Fig. 2.3). AMT is useful in providing structural support with collagen and other connective tissue proteins, including laminin and fibronectin [53]. Human amniotic membrane also contains a stromal layer with metalloproteinases, anti-VEGF factors, and interleukin-1 receptor antagonists, helping to suppress inflammation and angiogenesis [54]. The AMT may either cover the entire cornea or be trimmed to

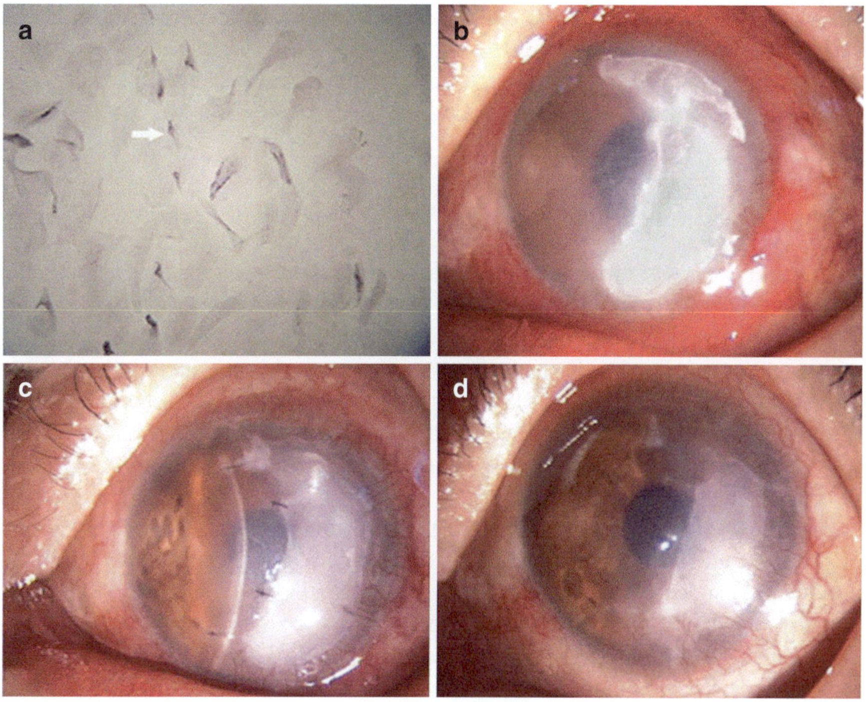

Fig. 2.3 (**a**). Positive purple staining of herpes simplex virus antigen by impression cytology (arrow). (**b**). Temporal corneal ulcer and edematous stroma. (**c**). Presented inferior amniotic membrane graft and dissolved superior amniotic membrane patch. (**d**). Healing of corneal ulcer, thinning and transparent amniotic membrane on postoperative day 20. (Published with permission from Shi et al. [59])

cover a portion of the cornea to provide a scaffold for epithelization and healing [55]. Conjunctival grafts have also been used to treat corneal ulcerations associated with infectious keratitis. These grafts provide growth factors to promote healing, acting like gauze to reduce the risk of stromal necrosis and providing vascularized conjunctival tissue to supply humoral and cellular immunity [56]. There is evidence suggesting improved success and reduced complications with sutured conjunctival grafts by debriding the cornea of necrotic and infected tissue before surgery [57]. Conjunctival grafts have also been utilized to create a superior forniceal conjunctival advancement pedicle (SFCAP) by using a thicker conjunctival flap including Tenon's capsule and a blood vessel. This technique demonstrated better promise in treating perforated corneal ulcers than the thinner traditional conjunctival flaps [58].

In addition to corneal scarring, serious complications of herpes keratitis such as corneal neovascularization, dry eye, and meibomian gland dysfunction that are not improved by standard therapy may merit additional surgical procedures. Recent research suggests that it may be beneficial for patients with vision-threatening corneal neovascularization undergoing corneal transplantation to undergo preoperative treatments like argon laser or cryotherapy before surgery [61]. To address dry eye and gland dysfunction, tarsorrhaphy and eyelid reconstructive surgery may also be performed. Tarsorrhaphy is especially considered in patients with dry eye and a history of neurotrophic keratopathy, exposure keratopathy, previous graft failure, and/or persistent epithelial defect.

2.7 Novel Therapies Under Development

With the discovery of the critical role of IL-17 in the pathogenesis of herpes keratitis, recent studies have shown suppression of delayed-type hypersensitivity response and reduction in the severity of corneal lesions in mouse models with herpes stromal keratitis by using anti-IL-17 antibody [60]. Research teams are also investigating the use of vaccines against HSV to prevent reactivation in patients with latent ocular disease. The HSV vaccination triggers and enhances the CD8+ T cell response in latent infected ganglia to inhibit viral reactivation and consequent inflammation of the cornea [61].

The emergence of antiviral resistance poses a concern for treating herpetic keratitis. Recent studies have shown that mutations in viral thymidylate kinase and DNA polymerase can lead to acyclovir resistance [62]. Nucleoside analog antivirals, specifically guanosine analog antivirals, including acyclovir, penciclovir, and ganciclovir, along with their prodrugs valacyclovir, famciclovir, and valganciclovir all require intracellular activation by phosphorylation to be effective. Thus, mutations in the thymidylate enzymes, including the novel mutation N202K on the *UL23* gene, may pose a threat to their efficacy [63]. Systemic foscarnet may be used to treat acyclovir-resistant herpes keratitis [64]. Foscarnet is a direct viral DNA polymerase inhibitor and therefore does not require activation by thymidylate kinases. However, a mutation in the UL-30 encoded viral DNA-polymerase can cause cross-resistance with the nucleoside analogs and foscarnet [63].

A recent study highlighted the potential application of topical interferon alpha-2a with antivirals in immunosuppressed patients to treat resistant HSV keratitis [65]. Interestingly, several plant-based formulations have recently been found to demonstrate anti-herpetic activity. One study highlighted the antiherpetic activity of extracts from the bark of the *Trichilia catigua* plant [66]. Another study investigated the antiviral potential of a polyphenol-based nutraceutical formulation from the extract of grape pomace. Studies have shown inhibitory activity of this formulation against the early stages of HSV-1 and HSV-2 infection [67].

A preclinical study evaluating the effectiveness of a nanoparticle ocular immunotherapy eye drop using a cat model infected with feline herpesvirus-1 (FHV-1) demonstrated resolution of keratitis and corneal ulcers with the administration of nanoparticles (Fig. 4). Further investigation may provide a potential novel alternative to standard antiviral eye drops, which can cause irritation and take weeks for symptom resolution [68]. The study demonstrated that the liposome-dual Toll-like receptor 3/9 agonist nanoparticles showed suppression of FHIV-1 replication and induction of the type I and II interferon response against viral activity. Since some ocular herpesvirus infections are complicated by coinfection with other pathogens,

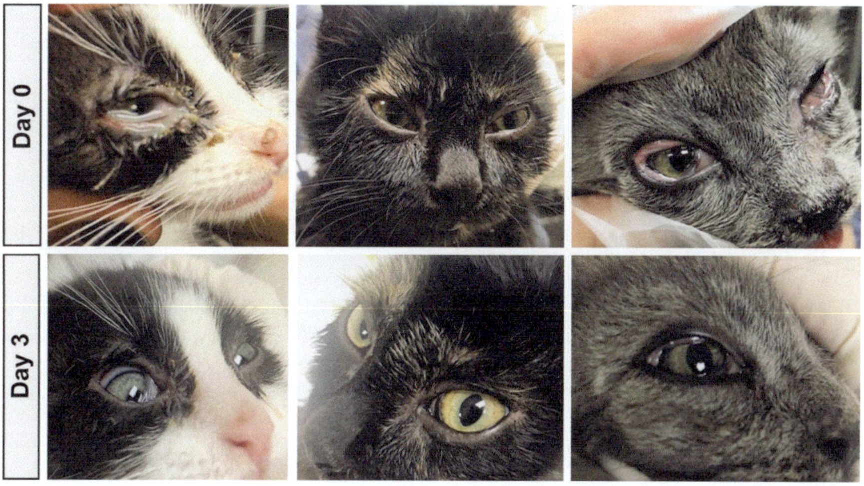

Fig. 2.4 Eyes of feline models with FHV-1 treated with nanoparticle ocular immunotherapy [68] [Open Access CC BY 4.0]

nonspecific effective therapies such as nanoparticle immunotherapy may demonstrate an additional benefit (Fig. 2.4).

Since herpes keratitis results from the reactivation of latent HSV-1 or VZV, nerve cell loss and corneal sensation loss can occur, leading to neurotrophic keratitis. Corneal neurotization is an emerging surgical therapy for treating complications of herpetic keratitis related to loss of corneal sensation [45]. Neurotization involves relocating a healthy nerve to establish the impaired nerve pathway and avoid irreversible damage.

Due to the postoperative complications associated with tectonic penetrating keratoplasty, tectonic lamellar graft patching has been suggested as an alternative procedure to address corneal perforation with stromal melting [69]. Lamellar graft patching may show promise due to the decreased risk of endothelial rejection and damage to intraocular tissues compared to penetrating keratoplasty, in addition to the reduced risk of intraocular pressure elevation and glaucoma progression [70, 71].

References

1. Pepose JS, Keadle TL, Morrison LA. Ocular herpes simplex: changing epidemiology, emerging disease patterns, and the potential of vaccine prevention and therapy. Am J Ophthalmol. 2006;141:547.
2. Azher TN, Yin XT, Tajfirouz D, Huang AJ, Stuart PM. Herpes simplex keratitis: Challenges in diagnosis and clinical management. Clinical Ophthalmol. 2017;11. Preprint at https://doi.org/10.2147/OPTH.S80475
3. McCormick I, et al. Incidence of herpes simplex virus keratitis and other ocular disease: global review and estimates. Ophthalmic Epidemiol. 2022;29:353–62.

4. Lobo AM, Agelidis AM, Shukla D. Pathogenesis of herpes simplex keratitis: The host cell response and ocular surface sequelae to infection and inflammation. Ocular Surface. 2019;17. Preprint at https://doi.org/10.1016/j.jtos.2018.10.002
5. Valerio GS, Lin CC. Ocular manifestations of herpes simplex virus. Curr Opin Ophthalmol. 2019;30:525.
6. Ahmad B, Patel BC. Herpes Simplex Keratitis. StatPearls; 2023.
7. Drancourt M, Boulze Pankert M, Hoffart LC. Keratitis and infections of periorbital structures. Infect Dis. 2017;2:150–157.e2. https://doi.org/10.1016/B978-0-7020-6285-8.00016-2.
8. Koganti R, Yadavalli T, Naqvi RA, Shukla D, Naqvi AR. Pathobiology and treatment of viral keratitis. Exp Eye Res. 2021;205:108483.
9. Kanukollu VM, Patel BC. Herpes simplex ophthalmicus. StatPearls; 2020.
10. Moshirfar M, et al. A review of corneal endotheliitis and endotheliopathy: differential diagnosis, evaluation, and treatment. Ophthalmol Ther. 2019;8:195.
11. Zaidi AA, et al. Hypopyon in patients with uveitis. Ophthalmology. 2010;117:366.
12. Journal O, et al. Medical hypothesis, discovery & innovation eye and periocular skin involvement in herpes zoster infection. Med Hypothesis Discov Innov Ophthalmol. 2015;4
13. Gargouri S, et al. Ocular involvement associated with varicella in adults. J Ophthalmic Inflamm Infect. 2016;6:1–5.
14. Chaloulis SK, Mousteris G, Tsaousis KT. Incidence and risk factors of bilateral herpetic keratitis: 2022 update. Trop Med Infect Dis. 2022;7
15. Matharu KSMAJVKPRKRP. Double trouble: an unusual keratitis case of herpes simplex virus and varicella-zoster virus co-infection. Cornea. 2023;42:1451.
16. He B, et al. Impact of the use of anti-glaucoma medications on the risk of herpetic keratitis recurrence. Int Ophthalmol. 2022;43:1559–64.
17. Jambunathan N, et al. Two sides to every story: Herpes simplex type-1 viral glycoproteins gb, gd, gh/gl, gk, and cellular receptors function as key players in membrane fusion. Viruses. 2021;13. Preprint at https://doi.org/10.3390/v13091849
18. Wang L, Wang R, Xu C, Zhou H. Pathogenesis of herpes stromal keratitis: immune inflammatory response mediated by inflammatory regulators. Front Immunol. 2020;11:766.
19. Koujah L, Suryawanshi RK, Shukla D. Pathological processes activated by herpes simplex virus-1 (HSV-1) infection in the cornea. Cell Mol Life Sci. 2019;76. Preprint at https://doi.org/10.1007/s00018-018-2938-1
20. Azher TN, Yin X-T, Stuart PM. Understanding the role of chemokines and cytokines in experimental models of herpes simplex keratitis; 2017. https://doi.org/10.1155/2017/7261980.
21. Rolinski J, Hus I. Immunological aspects of acute and recurrent herpes simplex keratitis. J Immunol Res. 2014. Preprint at https://doi.org/10.1155/2014/513560;2014
22. Gabhann-Dromgoole JN, et al. Systemic IL-1β production as a consequence of corneal HSV-1 infection-contribution to the development of herpes simplex keratitis. Int J Ophthalmol. 2019;12:1493.
23. Spurney RV, Rosenthal MS. Ultraviolet-induced recurrent herpes simplex virus keratitis. Am J Ophthalmol. 1972;73:609–11.
24. Cherpes TL, Busch JL, Sheridan BS, Harvey SAK, Hendricks RL. Medroxyprogesterone acetate inhibits CD8 + T cell viral specific effector function and induces herpes simplex virus type 1 reactivation.
25. Freeman ML, Sheridan BS, Bonneau RH, Hendricks RL. Psychological stress compromises CD8+ T cell control of latent herpes simplex virus type 1 infections. J Immunol. 2007;179:322.
26. Pérez-Bartolomé F, et al. Post-herpes neurotrophic keratopathy: Aetiopathogenesis, clinical signs and current therapies. Archivos de la Sociedad Espanola de Oftalmologia. 2019;94. Preprint at https://doi.org/10.1016/j.oftal.2019.01.002
27. NaPier E, Camacho M, McDevitt TF, Sweeney AR. Neurotrophic keratopathy: current challenges and future prospects. Ann Med. 2022;54:666–73.
28. Amano S, et al. Herpes simplex virus in the trabeculum of an eye with corneal endotheliitis. Am J Ophthalmol. 1999;127:721–2.

29. Holland EJ, Schwartz GS. Classification of herpes simplex virus keratitis. Cornea. 1999;18:144–54.
30. Fukuda M, Deai T, Higaki S, Hayashi K, Shimomura Y. Presence of a large amount of herpes simplex virus genome in tear fluid of herpetic stromal keratitis and persistent epithelial defect patients. Semin Ophthalmol. 2009;23:217–20. https://doi.org/10.1080/08820530802111366.
31. Hirota A, et al. Rapid detection and diagnosis of herpetic keratitis using quantitative microfluidic polymerase chain reaction system for herpes simplex and varicella-zoster virus DNA: a case series. BMC Ophthalmol. 2023;23:177.
32. Qiu JN, Huang FF, Liu CH, Cao WJ, Zhang CR. Atypical stromal herpes simplex keratitis: clinical features and diagnosis. Jpn J Ophthalmol. 2023;67:43–9.
33. Natarajan R, et al. Advances in the diagnosis of herpes simplex stromal necrotising keratitis: a feasibility study on deep learning approach. Indian J Ophthalmol. 2022;70:3279–83.
34. Wilhelmus KR. Antiviral treatment and other therapeutic interventions for herpes simplex virus epithelial keratitis. Cochrane Database Syst Rev. 2015. Preprint at https://doi.org/10.1002/14651858.CD002898.pub5, 2015
35. Li X, Nayeni M, Malvankar-Mehta MS. Antiviral and anti-inflammatory therapeutic interventions for treating herpes stromal keratitis: a systematic review. Ophthalmic Epidemiol. 2024; https://doi.org/10.1080/09286586.2023.2213324.
36. He T, et al. Acyclovir for the prevention of recurrent herpes simplex virus eye disease Background Long-term treatment with antiviral. New Eng land Journal of Medicine. 300:98.
37. Gnann JW Jr. Antiviral therapy of varicella-zoster virus infections. In: Human herpesviruses: biology, therapy, and immunoprophylaxis; 2007.
38. Hassan OM, Farooq AV, Soin K, Djalilian AR, Hou JH. Management of corneal scarring secondary to herpes zoster keratitis. Cornea. 2017;36:1018–23.
39. Singh RB, et al. Efficacy of cyanoacrylate tissue adhesive in the management of corneal thinning and perforation due to microbial keratitis. Ocular Surface. 2020;18:795–800.
40. Rana M, Savant V. A brief review of techniques used to seal corneal perforation using cyanoacrylate tissue adhesive. Contact Lens and Anterior Eye. 2013;36:156–8.
41. Tuli S, Gray M. Surgical management of corneal infections. Curr Opin Ophthalmol. 2016;27:340–7.
42. Samarawickrama C, et al. Collagen-based fillers as alternatives to cyanoacrylate glue for the sealing of large corneal perforations. Cornea. 2017;37:609–16.
43. Sharma A, et al. Fibrin glue versus N-butyl-2-cyanoacrylate in corneal perforations. Ophthalmology. 2003;110:291–8.
44. Kara S, Arikan S, Ersan I, Taskiran Comez A. Simplified technique for sealing corneal perforations using a fibrin glue-assisted amniotic membrane transplant-plug. Case Rep Ophthalmol Med. 2014;2014:1–3.
45. Coster DJ, Williams KA. The impact of corneal allograft rejection on the long-term outcome of corneal transplantation. Am J Ophthalmol. 2005;140:1112–22.
46. Wang J, Zhao G, Xie L, Chen M, Zhao J. Therapeutic effect of deep anterior lamellar keratoplasty for active or quiescent herpetic stromal keratitis. Graefes Arch Clin Exp Ophthalmol. 2012;250:1187–94.
47. Sarnicola V, Toro P. Deep anterior lamellar keratoplasty in herpes simplex corneal opacities. Cornea. 2010;29:60–4.
48. Yin J. et al, Outcomes of cyanoacrylate tissue adhesive application in corneal thinning and perforation. Cornea. 2019; https://doi.org/10.1097/ICO.0000000000001919.
49. Korah S, Selvin SST, Pradhan ZS, Jacob P, Kuriakose T. Tenons patch graft in the management of large corneal perforations. Cornea. 2016;35:696–9.
50. Grau AE, Durán JA. Treatment of a large corneal perforation with a multilayer of amniotic membrane and TachoSil. Cornea. 2012;31:98–100.
51. Croghan C, Chou CY, Gajree S, Ramaesh K, Anijeet D. Emergency therapeutic penetrating keratoplasty in a tertiary ophthalmic care facility. Eye 2018. 2017;32(*3*):655–7.
52. Doğan C, Arslan OŞ. Outcomes of therapeutic and tectonic penetrating keratoplasty in eyes with perforated infectious corneal ulcer. Turk J Ophthalmol. 2019;49:55–60.

53. Walkden A. Amniotic Membrane Transplantation in Ophthalmology: An Updated Perspective. Clin Ophthalmol. 2020;14:2057.
54. Tseng SCG, et al. How does amniotic membrane work? Ocul Surf. 2004;2:177–87.
55. Lee SH, Tseng SCG. Amniotic membrane transplantation for persistent epithelial defects with ulceration. Am J Ophthalmol. 1997;123:303–12.
56. Gundersen T. Conjunctival flaps in the treatment of corneal disease with reference to a new technique of application. AMA Arch Ophthalmol. 1958;60:880–8.
57. Sun GH, et al. Clinical observation of removal of the necrotic corneal tissue combined with conjunctival flap covering surgery under the guidance of the AS-OCT in treatment of fungal keratitis. Int J Ophthalmol. 2012;5:88–91.
58. Sandinha T, et al. Superior forniceal conjunctival advancement pedicles (SFCAP) in the management of acute and impending corneal perforations. Eye 2006. 2005;20(*1*):84–9.
59. Shi W, Chen M, Xie L. Amniotic membrane transplantation combined with antiviral and steroid therapy for herpes necrotizing stromal keratitis. Ophthalmology. 2007;114:1476.
60. Xia L, et al. Interleukin-17 enhanced immunoinflammatory lesions in a mouse model of recurrent herpetic keratitis. Microbes Infect. 2013;15:126–39.
61. Knickelbein JE, et al. Noncytotoxic lytic granule-mediated CD8+ T cell inhibition of HSV-1 reactivation from neuronal latency. Science (1979). 2008;(322):268–71.
62. Moshirfar M, et al. The impact of antiviral resistance on herpetic keratitis. Eye Contact Lens. 2023;49. Preprint at https://doi.org/10.1097/ICL.0000000000000952
63. De Clerck I, et al. Putting drug resistant epithelial herpes keratitis in the spotlight: a case series. Am J Ophthalmol Case Rep. 2022;25:101268.
64. Choong K, Walker NJ, Apel AJ, Whitby M. Aciclovir-resistant herpes keratitis. Clin Exp Ophthalmol. 2010;38:309–13.
65. Minkovitz JB, Pepose JS. Topical interferon alpha-2A treatment of herpes simplex keratitis resistant to multiple antiviral medications in an immunosuppressed patient. Cornea. 1995;14:326.
66. Ribelato EV, et al. Topical formulations containing Trichilia catigua extract as therapeutic options for a genital and an acyclovir-resistant strain of herpes recurrent infection. Braz J Microbiol. 2023;2023:1–11. https://doi.org/10.1007/S42770-023-01027-W.
67. Zannella C, et al. Antiherpetic Activity of Taurisolo®, a Grape Pomace Polyphenolic Extract. Microorganisms. 2023;11:1346.
68. Lappin M, et al. Nanoparticle ocular immunotherapy for herpesvirus surface eye infections evaluated in cat infection model. PLoS One. 2023;18:e0279462.
69. Ogawa A, et al. Aetiology-specific comparison of long-term outcome of deep anterior lamellar keratoplasty for corneal diseases. Br J Ophthalmol. 2016;100:1176–82.
70. Huang OS, Mehta JS, Htoon HM, Tan DT, Wong TT. Incidence and risk factors of elevated intraocular pressure following deep anterior lamellar keratoplasty. Am J Ophthalmol. 2016;170:153–60.
71. Musa FU, et al. Long-term risk of intraocular pressure elevation and glaucoma escalation after deep anterior lamellar keratoplasty. Clin Experiment Ophthalmol. 2012;40:780–5.

Acanthamoeba Keratitis

3

Catherine Liu and Thomas H. Dohlman

Summary Points

- The incidence of *Acanthamoeba* keratitis is rising, particularly with increased contact lens use worldwide.
- *Acanthamoeba* keratitis can be diagnosed based on clinical presentation, culture data, and confocal microscopy. Making an early diagnosis is critical for optimizing clinical outcomes.
- Mainstays of treatment include frequent topical administration of diamidines and/or biguanides, as well as corneal transplantation in recalcitrant cases. Visual rehabilitation is often in the form of corneal transplantation. Management should be tailored to the presentation and course of each patient.

3.1 Background and Epidemiology

Acanthamoeba keratitis (AK) is a relatively rare but important disease entity with potentially devastating consequences. The first case of AK was described in 1973 [1]. Since then, an increasing number of cases have been reported worldwide [2, 3] with an estimated prevalence of 1–9/100,000 as per the Orphanet database [3]. In the United States, the incidence among contact lens wearers has been estimated to be one to two new cases per one million per year [4], although the actual number of cases may be much higher [5].

Acanthamoeba is a free-living, single-celled amoeba that is found ubiquitously in water, soil, sewage systems, cooling towers, and even heating/ventilation/air conditioning (HVAC) systems [6]. *Acanthamoeba castellanii* is the most common *Acanthamoeba* species associated with keratitis, although *Acanthamoeba*

C. Liu · T. H. Dohlman (✉)
Cornea Service, Massachusetts Eye and Ear, Department of Ophthalmology, Harvard Medical School, Boston, MA, USA
e-mail: catherine_liu@meei.harvard.edu; Thomas_dohlman@meei.harvard.edu

H. N. Saeed, R. B. Singh (eds.), *Corneal Disorders*, Current Practices in Ophthalmology, https://doi.org/10.1007/978-981-96-5294-5_3

polyphaga and *Acanthamoeba hachetti* are also commonly reported as causative organisms [7]. *Acanthamoeba* can exist in one of two forms, trophozoite or cyst. The active form of *Acanthamoeba* is the trophozoite, which replicates by mitosis and is the main infective form [8]. Trophozoites can penetrate Descemet's membrane, although intraocular infections are rare. The *Acanthamoeba* trophozoite has the ability to form a double-walled cyst, usually in response to hostile conditions including nutrient deprivation, desiccation, changes in temperature and pH, and, critically, treatment with topical medications [9, 10]. The cyst form of *Acanthamoeba* is dormant and resistant to environmental challenges, thus making the eradication of *Acanthamoeba* particularly challenging.

In developed countries, the number one risk factor for AK is soft contact lens wear [11–13], with contact lens wearers constituting 85% of all AK patients [14]. Contact lenses cause microtrauma to the corneal epithelium, thus permitting entry to *Acanthamoeba*. In addition, contact lens wear can also induce the production of pathogenic proteases by *Acanthamoeba*, further contributing to disease pathogenesis [15]. In 2006, there was an outbreak of AK cases in the state of Illinois in the United States, prompting a nationwide retrospective survey on AK. Data received from 13 centers with a wide geographic distribution confirmed an increase in AK over a 3-year period, and in 2007, the Centers for Disease Control and Prevention (CDC) found an association between AK and a particular contact lens solution, leading to its commercial recall [6]. Unfortunately, despite the recall, a multicenter follow-up study showed continued record-high levels of AK cases across the United States [5, 16], emphasizing the need for better awareness and understanding of AK diagnosis and management.

Additional risk factors for developing AK include poor contact lens hygiene, swimming and showering while wearing contact lenses, inadequate contact lens disinfection, exposure to contaminated water, and corneal trauma [9]. In non-contact lens wearers, corneal trauma is the most important risk factor for AK [17–19].

3.2 Clinical Features

The clinical course of Acanthamoeba keratitis is often long and protracted [20]. The classic presenting symptom of patients with AK is pain that is out of proportion when compared to clinical signs on slit-lamp examination. Associated symptoms include tearing, redness, photophobia, and decreased vision. The disease is usually unilateral, although bilateral cases can occur in up to 7.5% of cases [21]. Although counterintuitive, a painless presentation should not preclude diagnosis [22] as painless cases have been reported in patients mistakenly diagnosed with HSV, with or without a history of contact lens wear [23, 24].

Early disease usually starts with superficial epithelial keratitis and then progresses more deeply into the stroma (Table 3.1). Tu et al. have defined five levels of severity based on slit-lamp findings: epitheliitis, epitheliitis with radial perineuritis, anterior stromal disease, deep stromal keratitis, and ring infiltrate [25].

Table 3.1 Clinical presentation of *Acanthamoeba* keratitis

Clinical sign	Representative slit-lamp photograph
Epitheliitis	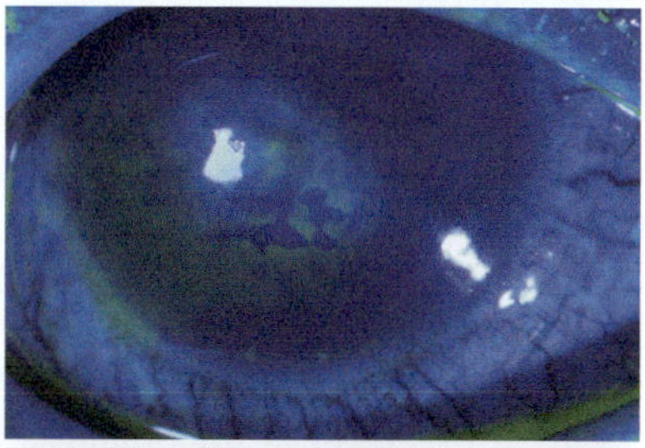
Epitheliitis with radial perineuritis	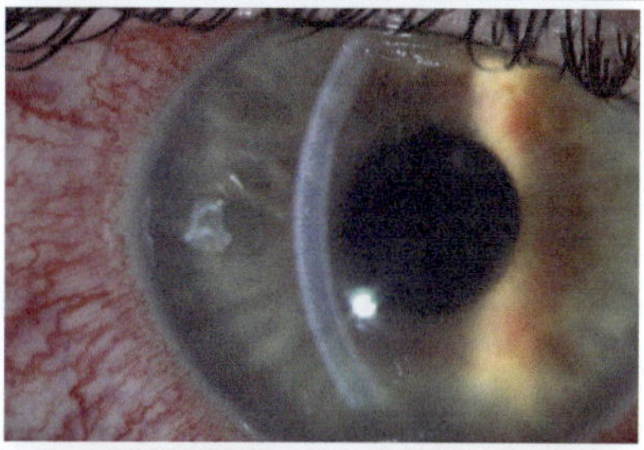
Anterior stromal disease	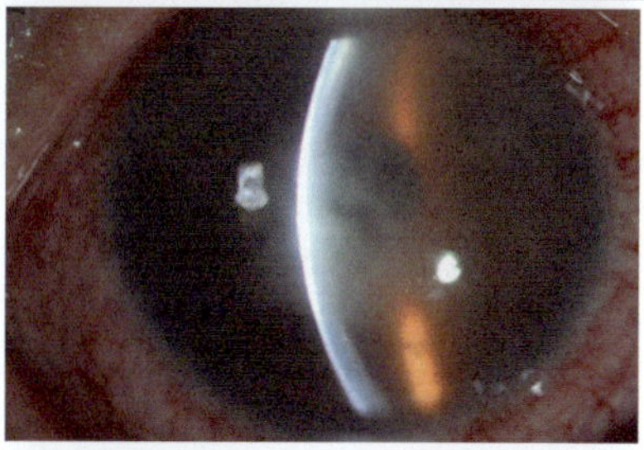
Deep stromal keratitis	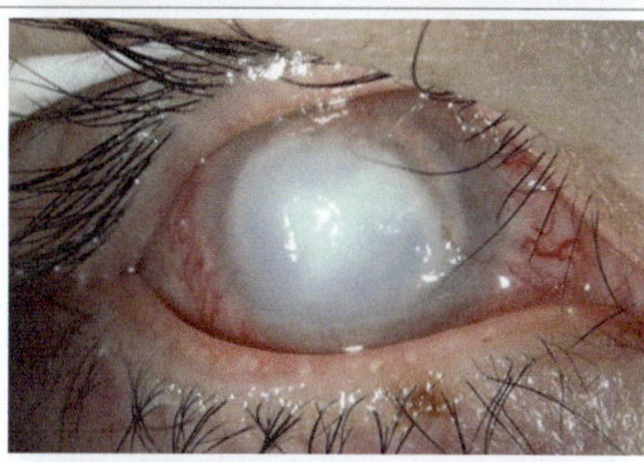
Ring infiltrate	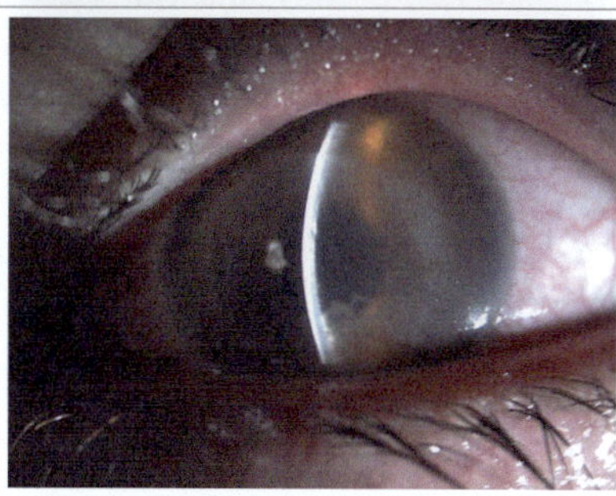

Clinical signs of *Acanthamoeba* keratitis as defined by Tu, Joslin, Sugar, Shoff et al. 2008

Radial perineuritis or keratoneuritis refers to the appearance of inflamed corneal nerves. The finding is most commonly present paracentrally and extends toward the limbus. While radial perineuritis is often associated with AK, it is not pathognomonic, as it has also been described in *Pseudomonas* keratitis, among other disease entities [26]. When the AK disease process involves the stroma, stromal infiltrates may eventually coalesce and form a ring infiltrate [27]. A ring infiltrate is often associated with AK; however, it is not always present, and, like radial perineuritis, it is not specific to AK [28]. Stromal disease can sometimes present with hypopyon and keratic precipitates [29] and in advanced stages of disease, deep stromal involvement can ultimately lead to thinning and perforation [19]. Depth of involvement is important as it can guide management. For example, there may be an adjunctive role for epithelial debridement in cases limited to the epithelium, while cases of impending or actual perforation may require a tectonic intervention such as a corneal transplant.

Clinicians should maintain a high index of suspicion for AK even in the absence of classic clinical signs, especially in contact lens wearers. This is especially true of patients presenting with long, protracted clinical courses and unknown or multiple prior diagnoses. Nonclassical signs of AK include corneal endotheliitis, which has been reported as a potential early sign of AK before epithelial manifestations [27] and extra-corneal manifestations, including limbitis, scleritis, uveitis, and even dacryoadenitis. Endophthalmitis has also been reported [30, 31], and at least one case of chorioretinitis has been confirmed on pathology [32]. In addition, the disease and its treatment can lead to chronic complications, including neurotrophic keratopathy, limbal stem cell dysfunction, cataract, glaucoma, as well as psycho-social changes.

3.3 Diagnosis

Diagnosis of *Acanthamoeba* keratitis is notoriously difficult and requires the visualization of amoeba in stains and/or cultures. Stains include Giemsa or periodic acid-Schiff (PAS), hematoxylin & eosin (H&E), calcofluor white, and acridine orange. Other less commonly used stains include Wright's, lactophenol-cotton blue, silver, and immunoperoxidase [33].

In terms of culture, non-nutrient agar with *Escherichia coli* overlay is most commonly used. *Acanthamoeba* feeds on inactivated *E. coli*, leaving trails that are visible by light microscopy and can be visualized in as little as 24–48 hours after beginning culture in severe infections. The culture plate is monitored daily, and if clinical suspicion is high, treatment should be initiated before formal results become available. In previously treated patients, cultures are often negative or only become positive after prolonged incubation [3, 12]. The sensitivity and specificity for culture have been reported to be 66.7% and 99.9%, respectively [12]; it is important to bear in mind that only up to 53% of patients with clinical AK will have a positive corneal culture [7].

In some centers, polymerase chain reaction (PCR) has been reported to be more sensitive than culture for the detection of *Acanthamoeba* [12, 34]. Furthermore, PCR results can be ready in days, compared to (potentially) weeks for culture, and can provide detailed information. In addition, PCR can distinguish specific genotypes and allows the identification of 15 genotypes (classified as T1-T15), with the T4 genotype being associated with a worse prognosis [35, 36]. Still, some studies suggest that there is no clear advantage of PCR over culture, which may explain why it has not been adopted more widely [37].

In vivo confocal microscopy (IVCM) has become an important ancillary test in the diagnosis of AK. IVCM demonstrates both high sensitivity and specificity when performed by an experienced operator [38, 39]. An experienced operator is important as IVCM is highly user and observer dependent. Sensitivity ranges between 55.8% and 100% and specificity between 77.3% and 100% [38, 40–42]. The diagnosis of AK is made by IVCM in the presence of double-walled cysts, signet rings, and round/oval hyperreflective spots (Fig. 3.1a). Their classic configuration has been described as a "starry sky" appearance (Fig. 3.1b) [43]. Interestingly, the number of cysts has been reported to paradoxically increase after 2 weeks of treatment and then decrease with further medical therapy [44]. Importantly, while visualization of *Acanthamoeba* cysts on IVCM can confirm AK, the absence of cysts on IVCM does not rule out the disease as the field of view is small and the density of cysts can be low [45]. In addition, neither confocal microscopy nor PCR can distinguish between viable and nonviable *Acanthamoeba* cysts [9]. In cases of persistent keratitis, repeat cultures remain the best way to determine whether there is continued *Acanthamoeba* infection or a superimposed infection [9]. If results remain inconclusive after noninvasive diagnostic methods, a corneal biopsy can be helpful for histology and culture [22].

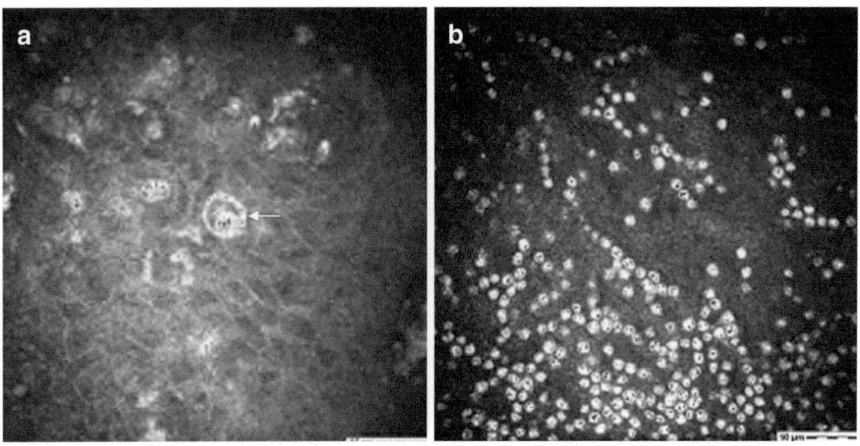

Fig. 3.1 In vivo confocal microscopy (IVCM) images in patients with culture-proven *Acanthamoeba* keratitis depicting (**a**) double-walled cysts and (**b**) a "starry sky" pattern consisting of multiple cysts in linear formation

3.4 Prognosis

The prognosis of AK correlates with the stage of disease at presentation, with early diagnosis being a strong predictor of better outcomes [25, 46, 47]. Other factors affecting prognosis include the severity of disease at diagnosis, depth of corneal involvement, and delay in diagnosis of more than three weeks [22, 39, 43, 48, 49]. Unfortunately, despite being at higher risk of AK, contact lens wearers tend to seek medical advice later in the disease course as they are accustomed to experiencing irritation in the eye [3]. Late diagnosis is also not uncommon in noncontact lens wearers due to a lower index of suspicion. Both of these situations highlight the need for improved disease awareness among both patients and physicians. Disease severity and time to diagnosis predict the duration of treatment, final clinical outcome, quality of life, and eventual need for surgery [50]. In early cases that spare the stroma, the average duration of anti-amoebic therapy is 3–4 months, whereas in cases involving the stroma, the treatment period is prolonged (potentially lasting as long as eight months or more) and is associated with worse outcomes [38, 43, 50, 51]. Severe inflammatory signs such as scleritis and a stromal ring infiltrate also portend poorer outcomes [52]. An important modifiable risk factor is the use of topical steroids, particularly in the context of a delayed diagnosis [52–54]. Steroid use before initiation of anti-amoebic therapy is associated with poorer outcomes, including corneal perforation, need for surgery, longer treatment periods, and worse visual acuity [52].

3.5 Differential Diagnosis

In order to optimize outcomes, it is important to reach an accurate diagnosis of AK in a timely manner. Up to 60% of AK cases are misdiagnosed due to nonspecific early epithelial changes [39]. For example, pseudodendrites can be a part of the presentation in AK and can lead to a diagnosis of herpetic eye disease [13]. Particularly in contact lens wearers, AK should be considered before making a diagnosis of HSV and initiating steroid therapy [55]. The pattern of epitheliopathy in AK is usually multifocal, unlike the contiguous and dendritic pattern in HSV keratitis. Early diagnosis is additionally important as epithelial scraping/debridement may be a beneficial and even therapeutic adjunctive procedure in cases where AK is still limited to the epithelium [56–58]. In contact lens wearers, bacterial keratitis should also be maintained on the differential diagnosis, with *Pseudomonas aeruginosa* being the most common causative organism [59–61].

3.6 Treatment

3.6.1 Medical Therapy

The two main classes of medications used in the treatment of AK are diamidines and biguanides (Table 3.2). In the class of diamidines, propamidine 0.1% and hexamidine 0.1% can be used as eyedrops. Propamidine can also be applied as a 0.15%

Table 3.2 Commonly used medical therapies for *Acanthamoeba* keratitis

Topical therapy				
	Dosing	Mechanism	Killing of trophozoites	Cysticidal
Diamidines	Every 1 hour for 3–5 days, then taper	Disruption of nucleic acid and protein synthesis	✓	✗
Propamidine 0.1%, 0.15% ointment				
Hexamidine 0.1%				
Biguanides	Every 1 hour for 3–5 days, then taper	Increases membrane permeability	✓	✓
Polyhexamethylene biguanide (PHMB) 0.02 to 0.06%				
Chlorhexidine (0.02 to 0.2%)				
Voriconazole 1%	Every 2 hours for 1 week, then taper	Disrupts ergosterol synthesis, induces programmed cell death	✓	✓
Oral therapy				
Antifungals		Disrupts ergosterol synthesis, induces programmed cell death	✓	✓
Imidazoles				
Triazoles				
Voriconazole	200 mg PO BID			
Miltefosine	50 mg PO BID-TID	Anti-protozoal, Inhibits intracellular signaling and cell membrane synthesis and integrity	✓	✓
IV pentamidine	IV 190–400 mg/day for 14 days	Diamidine; increases cytoplasmic permeability	✓	✗

ointment. Diamidines are lethal to the trophozoite form of *Acanthamoeba* but are less effective against mature cysts; hence, they may be most effective at treating early-stage disease when trophozoites are more numerous [7]. Although every clinical situation is different, these topical medications should be given frequently at first, followed by a slow taper. In practice, this often translates to hourly (around the clock) treatment for the first 48 hours, then a taper to hourly during the day only. This intense regimen is then reduced to four times a day through a slow taper over 4–6 weeks. Patients generally require maintenance treatment for six months or longer to completely eliminate cysts [7]. Both diamidines and biguanides can cause significant surface toxicity. In these cases, reducing or stopping the medication and pursuing alternative therapeutic strategies may be considered [7].

In the class of biguanides, polyhexamethylene biguanide (PHMB) 0.02 to 0.06% and chlorhexidine 0.02 to 0.2% are the mainstays of treatment. A key feature of biguanides is their cysticidal activity [22]. Biguanides have been shown to have in vitro and in vivo efficacy against both cysts and trophozoites, whereas other drugs are primarily active against trophozoites. There are no significant differences in treatment effectiveness between PHMB and chlorhexidine [62], and they can be used in combination [63, 64]. Like diamidines, topical biguanides are most commonly used hourly for the first several days of treatment and then tapered over weeks to months, depending on the patient's response. Diamidine- and biguanide-class agents are often used in combination and may even be synergistic [63].

Antifungal therapeutics are another effective option in the treatment of AK. In addition to disrupting ergosterol synthesis to interfere with membrane integrity, voriconazole has also been shown to induce programmed cell death in *Acanthamoeba* in vitro [65]. Antifungal agents that have been used as anti-amoebics include imidazoles such as ketoconazole and miconazole, and triazoles such as voriconazole and posaconazole [66, 67]. In the setting of AK, voriconazole is the best-studied of these medications [68–70]. A recent prospective, double-masked, randomized control study showed that monotherapy with topical voriconazole 1% is effective and comparable to combination treatment with PHMB 0.02% and chlorhexidine 0.02% [71]. Antifungals (oral or topical) can also be used in combination with topical anti-amoebics [72, 73]; agents from different therapeutic classes are often used in combination to treat AK, and treatment regimen is tailored to each patient's clinical course.

3.7 Steroids

The use of topical steroids in AK is controversial. There may be a role for corticosteroids in cases of AK resistant to topical biguanides [22] and challenging cases of AK often have a significant inflammatory component that may benefit from the anti-inflammatory properties of corticosteroid drops [3, 17, 22, 74]. The most common practice is to generally avoid corticosteroids in cases of known or suspected AK. Some centers consider starting steroids after a minimum of 2 weeks of anti-amoebic therapy. Topical corticosteroids may be associated with a delayed diagnosis of *Acanthamoeba* keratitis [52–54], and there is evidence that steroids may increase *Acanthamoeba* pathogenicity [53]. If corticosteroids are given, patients should continue anti-amoebic treatment several weeks after stopping the steroid treatment [3].

3.8 Recalcitrant *Acanthamoeba* Keratitis

Acanthamoeba keratitis is often challenging to treat. This resistance to treatment stems in large part from the ability of the amoeba to encyst [3]. As described above, the cyst form of *Acanthamoeba* is resistant to various stressors, including topical medications, while the trophozoite form is much more readily eliminated. In one multivariable regression analysis, treatment failure was positively correlated with the following factors: older age at presentation, higher stage of disease severity, and topical corticosteroid use [11]. Of note, early referral to a cornea specialist is associated with better clinical outcomes [11].

In cases of recalcitrant AK, options for additional treatment include using higher concentrations of medications and combining multiple agents [75]. As described above, antifungal agents can also be used. Miltefosine, an antiparasitic agent, is effective against various strains of *Acanthamoeba* (Mathers, 2006), and its efficacy was recently described in recalcitrant cases of AK [7]. It is generally a well-tolerated medication but can cause rebound inflammation [76], which can be managed with topical steroids. Intravenous pentamidine, another diamidine-class agent, has also been used in refractory cases of AK and may also be used as an adjunctive therapy before therapeutic keratoplasty [77]. In cases that are not responsive to anti-amoebic therapeutics, bacterial superinfection and concurrent herpetic keratitis should also be considered [22]. A viral, fungal, or bacterial coinfection has been reported in up to 23–55% of AK cases [28, 30].

3.9 Surgical Therapy

Over the years, the role of corneal transplantation in AK has evolved. While aggressive anti-amoebic medical therapy is still encouraged before any consideration of surgical intervention, some reports suggest a role for earlier lamellar and penetrating keratoplasty [47, 78–80]. Surgical options include deep anterior lamellar keratoplasty (DALK) or penetrating keratoplasty (PK). DALK is useful early in the disease when involvement is limited to the anterior stroma [43, 50, 78]. The advantages of DALK over PK include better rates of graft survival and reduced risk of intraocular entry of *Acanthamoeba* at the time of surgery [3, 81]. However, DALK may not be as effective as PK in completely eradicating infection, particularly in late disease or inflamed eyes [43, 50, 78]. More of these cases need to be performed and systematically studied before drawing any conclusions or creating guidelines surrounding DALK in AK.

Full-thickness penetrating keratoplasty (PK) is the preferred surgery in cases of severe and progressive AK as it removes the infectious organism and diseased tissue and prevents intraocular and scleral extension. PK is effective in eliminating the infectious process and preventing recurrences in most cases [14]. It is also indicated for complications related to AK such as corneal perforation, severe corneal abscesses, and visually significant cataract with corneal opacity [9, 22]. In patients who have successfully completed anti-amoebic therapy, optical PK can be performed electively for visual rehabilitation. Visual outcomes after PK in these uninflamed eyes are better than when compared to PK performed in "high-risk" eyes with active infection and inflammation [47].

Complications following PK for *Acanthamoeba* keratitis include disease recurrence, graft failure, cataract, and glaucoma [82]. Disease recurrence following surgery is an overarching concern, with recurrence reported in up to 46% of operated eyes [64]. Recurrence is most likely to happen in the first two weeks after surgery (Nguyen et al., 2010). To minimize the chance of recurrence, it is recommended to remove a 1 mm margin of healthy tissue around the area of the involved cornea (Dart et al., 2009). It is also important to continue anti-amoebic therapy postoperatively, such as PHMB 0.02% six to eight times daily and at least four times a day while steroids are being used [17].

Taken together, several factors need to be considered in the surgical management of AK, including severity and extent of disease, degree of inflammation, and duration of anti-amoebic therapy. Data on the timing of surgery is conflicting, as some studies report better outcomes when surgical intervention is performed earlier, in active and earlier disease, whereas others encourage surgery after reduction of infection and/or inflammation [79, 83]. The need and timing of surgery should thus be determined on a case-by-case basis according to the clinical course.

Amniotic membrane transplantation is an additional adjunctive procedure that can help control inflammation and promote stromal and epithelial healing in patients with AK [84, 85]. Amniotic membrane has anti-inflammatory and pro-regenerative properties that can help restore ocular surface integrity and provide metabolic and mechanical support to the cornea [84]. It may be used in patients with stromal disease and can delay the need for penetrating keratoplasty [86], but it is not curative from an infectious perspective and can only be used in conjunction with anti-amoebic therapies.

3.10 Future Directions

Acanthamoeba keratitis is a relatively rare but important disease whose diagnosis and treatment remain a challenge for ophthalmologists. Currently, diagnostic approaches differ between centers, and while standardization and rigor are needed, the rarity of this condition makes it difficult to conduct meaningful clinical trials. In the future, we might expect more sensitive diagnostic methods in detecting *Acanthamoeba,* whether via PCR a combination of PCR, culture, and/or confocal microscopy [39]. Machine-based learning and image recognition algorithms may help better detect AK in a time-sensitive fashion with high sensitivity and specificity.

With respect to management, biguanides such as PHMB and chlorhexidine are the preferred therapeutics due to their activity against both trophozoites and cysts, and full-thickness penetrating keratoplasty has and will continue to have an important definitive role in the surgical management of advanced AK. Newer therapeutic modalities such as phototherapeutic keratectomy and corneal collagen crosslinking have also been described in case series, but more investigation will be needed to fully determine their efficacy and potential role in the management of AK [38, 87]. Going forward, targeted therapeutic strategies may emerge from our expanding knowledge of microbiology and corneal immunology. As an example, in recent years, basic science investigations have shown interleukin-17A to have a protective effect against AK [9, 88]. There is also potential benefit in combining anti-amoebic therapy with quinolone antibiotics [89]. Although the diagnosis and management of *Acanthamoeba* keratitis may not always be clear-cut, there is currently a general framework to approaching this condition that can be modified on a case-by-case basis, and the future holds promise for additional diagnostic tools and treatment options.

Prepared for Current Practices in Ophthalmology.

Conflicts of Interest None of the authors has any relevant conflicts of interest to disclose.

References

1. Jones DB, Visvesvara GS, Robinson NM. *Acanthamoeba polyphaga* keratitis and Acenthamoeba uveitis associated with fatal meningoencephalitis. Trans Ophthalmol Soc U K. 1975;95(2):221–32.
2. Schaumberg DA, Snow KK, Dana MR. The epidemic of Acanthamoeba keratitis: where do we stand? Cornea. 1998;17(1):3–10.
3. Lorenzo-Morales J, Khan NA, Walochnik J. An update on Acanthamoeba keratitis: diagnosis, pathogenesis and treatment. Parasite Paris Fr. 2015;22:10.
4. Scruggs BA, Quist TS, Salinas JL, Greiner MA. Notes from the field: Acanthamoeba keratitis cases – Iowa, 2002–2017. MMWR Morb Mortal Wkly Rep. 2019;68(19):448–9.
5. Tu EY. Acanthamoeba keratitis: a new normal. Am J Ophthalmol. 2014;158(3):417–9.
6. Centers for Disease Control and Prevention (CDC). Acanthamoeba keratitis multiple states, 2005–2007. MMWR Morb Mortal Wkly Rep. 2007;56(21):532–4.
7. Tu EY. Acanthamoeba and other parasitic corneal infections. In: Cornea. 5th ed. Elsevier; 2021. p. 1976.
8. Illingworth CD, Cook SD. Acanthamoeba keratitis. Surv Ophthalmol. 1998;42(6):493–508.
9. Maycock NJR, Jayaswal R. Update on Acanthamoeba keratitis: diagnosis, treatment, and outcomes. Cornea. 2016;35(5):713–20.
10. Srikanth S, Berk SG. Adaptation of amoebae to cooling tower biocides. Microb Ecol. 1994;27(3):293–301.
11. Randag AC, van Rooij J, van Goor AT, Verkerk S, Wisse RPL, Saelens IEY, et al. The rising incidence of Acanthamoeba keratitis: a 7-year nationwide survey and clinical assessment of risk factors and functional outcomes. PLoS One. 2019;14(9):e0222092.
12. Yera H, Ok V, Lee Koy Kuet F, Dahane N, Ariey F, Hasseine L, et al. PCR and culture for diagnosis of Acanthamoeba keratitis. Br J Ophthalmol. 2020;105:316730.

13. Höllhumer R, Keay L, Watson SL. Acanthamoeba keratitis in Australia: demographics, associated factors, presentation and outcomes: a 15-year case review. Eye Lond Engl. 2020;34(4):725–32.
14. Kumar R, Lloyd D. Recent advances in the treatment of Acanthamoeba keratitis. Clin Infect Dis Off Publ Infect Dis Soc Am. 2002;35(4):434–41.
15. Alizadeh H, Neelam S, Niederkorn JY. Effect of immunization with the mannose-induced Acanthamoeba protein and Acanthamoeba plasminogen activator in mitigating Acanthamoeba keratitis. Invest Ophthalmol Vis Sci. 2007;48(12):5597–604.
16. Yoder JS, Verani J, Heidman N, Hoppe-Bauer J, Alfonso EC, Miller D, et al. Acanthamoeba keratitis: the persistence of cases following a multistate outbreak. Ophthalmic Epidemiol. 2012;19(4):221–5.
17. Garg P, Kalra P, Joseph J. Non-contact lens related Acanthamoeba keratitis. Indian J Ophthalmol. 2017;65(11):1079–86.
18. Sharma S, Garg P, Rao GN. Patient characteristics, diagnosis, and treatment of non-contact lens related Acanthamoeba keratitis. Br J Ophthalmol. 2000;84(10):1103–8.
19. Jiang C, Sun X, Wang Z, Zhang Y. Acanthamoeba keratitis: clinical characteristics and management. Ocul Surf. 2015;13(2):164–8.
20. Claerhout I, Kestelyn P. Acanthamoeba keratitis: a review. Bull Soc Belge Ophtalmol. 1999;274:71–82.
21. Radford CF, Minassian DC, Dart JKG. Acanthamoeba keratitis in England and Wales: incidence, outcome, and risk factors. Br J Ophthalmol. 2002;86(5):536–42.
22. Dart JKG, Saw VPJ, Kilvington S. Acanthamoeba keratitis: diagnosis and treatment update 2009. Am J Ophthalmol. 2009;148(4):487–499.e2.
23. Shukla Kent S, Robert M-C, Tokarewicz AC, Mather R. Painless Acanthamoeba keratitis. Can J Ophthalmol J Can Ophtalmol. 2012;47(4):383–4.
24. Tabin G, Taylor H, Snibson G, Murchison A, Gushchin A, Rogers S. Atypical presentation of Acanthamoeba keratitis. Cornea. 2001;20(7):757–9.
25. Tu EY, Joslin CE, Sugar J, Shoff ME, Booton GC. Prognostic factors affecting visual outcome in Acanthamoeba keratitis. Ophthalmology. 2008;115(11):1998–2003.
26. Feist RM, Sugar J, Tessler H. Radial keratoneuritis in pseudomonas keratitis. Arch Ophthalmol Chic Ill 1960. 1991;109(6):774–5.
27. Lakhani BK, Thajudeen B, Jawaid I, Attzs MS, Maharajan VS. Endotheliitis-a presentation of Acanthamoeba keratitis. Cornea. 2021;40(6):769–73.
28. Szentmáry N, Daas L, Shi L, Laurik KL, Lepper S, Milioti G, et al. Acanthamoeba keratitis – clinical signs, differential diagnosis and treatment. J Curr Ophthalmol. 2019;31(1):16–23.
29. Chew HF, Yildiz EH, Hammersmith KM, Eagle RC, Rapuano CJ, Laibson PR, et al. Clinical outcomes and prognostic factors associated with acanthamoeba keratitis. Cornea. 2011;30(4):435–41.
30. Raghavan A, Baidwal S, Venkatapathy N, Rammohan R. The Acanthamoeba-fungal keratitis study. Am J Ophthalmol. 2019;201:31–6.
31. Davis MJ, Packo KH, Epstein RJ, Grostern RJ, Cohen JA. Acanthamoeba Endophthalmitis following penetrating Keratoplasty for Acanthamoeba keratitis. Arch Ophthalmol. 2010;128(4):505–6.
32. Moshari A, McLean IW, Dodds MT, Damiano RE, McEvoy PL. Chorioretinitis after keratitis caused by Acanthamoeba: case report and review of the literature. Ophthalmology. 2001;108(12):2232–6.
33. Hammersmith KM. Diagnosis and management of Acanthamoeba keratitis. Curr Opin Ophthalmol. 2006;17(4):327–31.
34. Thompson PP, Kowalski RP. A 13-year retrospective review of polymerase chain reaction testing for infectious agents from ocular samples. Ophthalmology. 2011;118(7):1449–53.
35. Di Cave D, Monno R, Bottalico P, Guerriero S, D'Amelio S, D'Orazi C, et al. Acanthamoeba T4 and T15 genotypes associated with keratitis infections in Italy. Eur J Clin Microbiol Infect Dis Off Publ Eur Soc Clin Microbiol. 2009;28(6):607–12.

36. Gatti S, Rama P, Matuska S, Berrilli F, Cavallero A, Carletti S, et al. Isolation and genotyping of Acanthamoeba strains from corneal infections in Italy. J Med Microbiol. 2010;59(Pt 11):1324–30.
37. Kowalski RP, Melan MA, Karenchak LM, Mammen A. Comparison of validated polymerase chain reaction and culture isolation for the routine detection of Acanthamoeba from ocular samples. Eye Contact Lens. 2015;41(6):341–3.
38. Tu EY, Joslin CE, Sugar J, Booton GC, Shoff ME, Fuerst PA. The relative value of confocal microscopy and superficial corneal scrapings in the diagnosis of Acanthamoeba keratitis. Cornea. 2008;27(7):764–72.
39. Goh JWY, Harrison R, Hau S, Alexander CL, Tole DM, Avadhanam VS. Comparison of in vivo confocal microscopy, PCR and culture of corneal scrapes in the diagnosis of Acanthamoeba keratitis. Cornea. 2018;37(4):480–5.
40. Kanavi MR, Javadi M, Yazdani S, Mirdehghanm S. Sensitivity and specificity of confocal scan in the diagnosis of infectious keratitis. Cornea. 2007;26(7):782–6.
41. Vaddavalli PK, Garg P, Sharma S, Sangwan VS, Rao GN, Thomas R. Role of confocal microscopy in the diagnosis of fungal and acanthamoeba keratitis. Ophthalmology. 2011;118(1):29–35.
42. Hau SC, Dart JKG, Vesaluoma M, Parmar DN, Claerhout I, Bibi K, et al. Diagnostic accuracy of microbial keratitis with in vivo scanning laser confocal microscopy. Br J Ophthalmol. 2010;94(8):982–7.
43. Varacalli G, Di Zazzo A, Mori T, Dohlman TH, Spelta S, Coassin M, et al. Challenges in Acanthamoeba keratitis: a review. J Clin Med. 2021;10(5):942.
44. Li S, Bian J, Wang Y, Wang S, Wang X, Shi W. Clinical features and serial changes of Acanthamoeba keratitis: an in vivo confocal microscopy study. Eye Lond Engl. 2020;34(2):327–34.
45. Shiraishi A, Uno T, Oka N, Hara Y, Yamaguchi M, Ohashi Y. In vivo and in vitro laser confocal microscopy to diagnose Acanthamoeba keratitis. Cornea. 2010;29(8):861–5.
46. Bacon AS, Dart JK, Ficker LA, Matheson MM, Wright P. Acanthamoeba keratitis. The value of early diagnosis Ophthalmology. 1993;100(8):1238–43.
47. Robaei D, Carnt N, Minassian DC, Dart JKG. Therapeutic and optical keratoplasty in the management of Acanthamoeba keratitis: risk factors, outcomes, and summary of the literature. Ophthalmology. 2015;122(1):17–24.
48. Tu EY, Joslin CE, Nijm LM, Feder RS, Jain S, Shoff ME. Polymicrobial keratitis: Acanthamoeba and infectious crystalline keratopathy. Am J Ophthalmol. 2009;148(1):13–19.e2.
49. Alfonso-Muñoz EA, Roig-Revert MJ, Fernández-López E, Hernández-Díaz M, Araujo-Miranda R, Peris-Martínez C. A report of 10 patients with Acanthamoeba keratitis. Arch Soc Espanola Oftalmol. 2018;93(10):497–502.
50. Bonini S, Di Zazzo A, Varacalli G, Coassin M. Acanthamoeba keratitis: perspectives for patients. Curr Eye Res. 2021;46(6):771–6.
51. Radford CF, Lehmann OJ, Dart JK. Acanthamoeba keratitis: multicentre survey in England 1992-6. National Acanthamoeba keratitis study group. Br J Ophthalmol. 1998;82(12):1387–92.
52. Carnt N, Robaei D, Minassian DC, Dart JKG. Acanthamoeba keratitis in 194 patients: risk factors for bad outcomes and severe inflammatory complications. Br J Ophthalmol. 2018;102(10):1431–5.
53. Robaei D, Carnt N, Minassian DC, Dart JKG. The impact of topical corticosteroid use before diagnosis on the outcome of Acanthamoeba keratitis. Ophthalmology. 2014;121(7):1383–8.
54. Ross J, Roy SL, Mathers WD, Ritterband DC, Yoder JS, Ayers T, et al. Clinical characteristics of Acanthamoeba keratitis infections in 28 states, 2008 to 2011. Cornea. 2014;33(2):161–8.
55. Lee MJ, Srikumaran D, Zafar S, Salehi M, Liu TS, Woreta FA. Case series: delayed diagnoses of Acanthamoeba keratitis. Am J Ophthalmol Case Rep. 2020;19:100778.
56. Lindquist TD, Sher NA, Doughman DJ. Clinical signs and medical therapy of early Acanthamoeba keratitis. Arch Ophthalmol Chic Ill 1960. 1988;106(1):73–7.
57. Holland GN, Donzis PB. Rapid resolution of early Acanthamoeba keratitis after epithelial debridement. Am J Ophthalmol. 1987;104(1):87–9.

58. Brooks JG, Coster DJ, Badenoch PR. Acanthamoeba keratitis. Resolution after epithelial debridement Cornea. 1994;13(2):186–9.
59. Hoddenbach JG, Boekhoorn SS, Wubbels R, Vreugdenhil W, Van Rooij J, Geerards AJM. Clinical presentation and morbidity of contact lens-associated microbial keratitis: a retrospective study. Graefes Arch Clin Exp Ophthalmol Albrecht Von Graefes Arch Klin Exp Ophthalmol. 2014;252(2):299–306.
60. Saeed A, D'Arcy F, Stack J, Collum LM, Power W, Beatty S. Risk factors, microbiological findings, and clinical outcomes in cases of microbial keratitis admitted to a tertiary referral center in Ireland. Cornea. 2009;28(3):285–92.
61. Stapleton F, Naduvilath T, Keay L, Radford C, Dart J, Edwards K, et al. Risk factors and causative organisms in microbial keratitis in daily disposable contact lens wear. PLoS One. 2017;12(8):e0181343.
62. Alkharashi M, Lindsley K, Law HA, Sikder S. Medical interventions for acanthamoeba keratitis. Cochrane Database Syst Rev. 2015;2015(2):CD010792.
63. Duguid IG, Dart JK, Morlet N, Allan BD, Matheson M, Ficker L, et al. Outcome of acanthamoeba keratitis treated with polyhexamethyl biguanide and propamidine. Ophthalmology. 1997;104(10):1587–92.
64. Kashiwabuchi RT, Freitas DD, Alvarenga LS, Vieira L, Contarini P, Sato E, et al. Corneal graft survival after therapeutic keratoplasty for Acanthamoeba keratitis. Acta Ophthalmol. 2008;86(6):666–9.
65. Martín-Navarro CM, López-Arencibia A, Sifaoui I, Reyes-Batlle M, Valladares B, Martínez-Carretero E, et al. Statins and voriconazole induce programmed cell death in Acanthamoeba castellanii. Antimicrob Agents Chemother. 2015;59(5):2817–24.
66. Iovieno A, Miller D, Ledee DR, Alfonso EC. Cysticidal activity of antifungals against different genotypes of Acanthamoeba. Antimicrob Agents Chemother. 2014;58(9):5626–8.
67. Sharma S, Srinivasan M, George C. Acanthamoeba keratitis in non-contact lens wearers. Arch Ophthalmol Chic Ill 1960. 1990;108(5):676–8.
68. Schuster FL, Guglielmo BJ, Visvesvara GS. In-vitro activity of miltefosine and voriconazole on clinical isolates of free-living amebas: Balamuthia mandrillaris, Acanthamoeba spp., and Naegleria fowleri. J Eukaryot Microbiol. 2006;53(2):121–6.
69. Tu EY, Joslin CE, Shoff ME. Successful treatment of chronic stromal acanthamoeba keratitis with oral voriconazole monotherapy. Cornea. 2010;29(9):1066–8.
70. Bang S, Edell E, Eghrari AO, Gottsch JD. Treatment with voriconazole in 3 eyes with resistant Acanthamoeba keratitis. Am J Ophthalmol. 2010;149(1):66–9.
71. Bagga B, Sharma S, Gour RPS, Mohamed A, Joseph J, Rathi VM, et al. A randomized masked pilot clinical trial to compare the efficacy of topical 1% voriconazole ophthalmic solution as monotherapy with combination therapy of topical 0.02% polyhexamethylene biguanide and 0.02% chlorhexidine in the treatment of Acanthamoeba keratitis. Eye Lond Engl. 2021;35(5):1326–33.
72. Cohen EJ, Parlato CJ, Arentsen JJ, Genvert GI, Eagle RC, Wieland MR, et al. Medical and surgical treatment of Acanthamoeba keratitis. Am J Ophthalmol. 1987;103(5):615–25.
73. Musayeva A, Riedl JC, Schuster AK, Wasielica-Poslednik J, Pfeiffer N, Gericke A. Topical Voriconazole as supplemental treatment for Acanthamoeba keratitis. Cornea. 2020;39(8):986–90.
74. Park DH, Palay DA, Daya SM, Stulting RD, Krachmer JH, Holland EJ. The role of topical corticosteroids in the management of Acanthamoeba keratitis. Cornea. 1997;16(3):277–83.
75. Mathers W. Use of higher medication concentrations in the treatment of acanthamoeba keratitis. Arch Ophthalmol Chic Ill 1960. 2006;124(6):923.
76. Thulasi P, Saeed HN, Rapuano CJ, Hou JH, Appenheimer AB, Chodosh J, et al. Oral Miltefosine as salvage therapy for refractory Acanthamoeba keratitis. Am J Ophthalmol. 2021;223:75–82.
77. Sacher BA, Wagoner MD, Goins KM, Sutphin JE, Greiner MA, Kitzmann AS. Treatment of acanthamoeba keratitis with intravenous pentamidine before therapeutic keratoplasty. Cornea. 2015;34(1):49–53.

78. Sarnicola E, Sarnicola C, Sabatino F, Tosi GM, Perri P, Sarnicola V. Early deep anterior lamellar Keratoplasty (DALK) for Acanthamoeba keratitis poorly responsive to medical treatment. Cornea. 2016;35(1):1–5.
79. Nguyen TH, Weisenthal RW, Florakis GJ, Reidy JJ, Gaster RN, Tom D. Penetrating keratoplasty in active Acanthamoeba keratitis. Cornea. 2010;29(9):1000–4.
80. Laurik KL, Szentmáry N, Daas L, Langenbucher A, Seitz B. Early penetrating Keratoplasty À Chaud may improve outcome in therapy-resistant Acanthamoeba keratitis. Adv Ther. 2019;36(9):2528–40.
81. Parthasarathy A, Tan DT. Deep lamellar keratoplasty for acanthamoeba keratitis. Cornea. 2007;26(8):1021–3.
82. Roozbahani M, Hammersmith KM, Rapuano CJ, Nagra PK, Zhang Q. Therapeutic penetrating keratoplasty for acanthamoeba keratitis: a review of cases, complications and predictive factors. Int Ophthalmol. 2019;39(12):2889–96.
83. Ficker LA, Kirkness C, Wright P. Prognosis for keratoplasty in Acanthamoeba keratitis. Ophthalmology. 1993;100(1):105–10.
84. Abdulhalim B-EH, Wagih MM, Gad AAM, Boghdadi G, Nagy RRS. Amniotic membrane graft to conjunctival flap in treatment of non-viral resistant infectious keratitis: a randomised clinical study. Br J Ophthalmol. 2015;99(1):59–63.
85. Kim JS, Kim JC, Hahn TW, Park WC. Amniotic membrane transplantation in infectious corneal ulcer. Cornea. 2001;20(7):720–6.
86. Bourcier T, Patteau F, Borderie V, Baudrimont M, Rondeau N, Bonnel S, et al. Amniotic membrane transplantation for the treatment severe acanthamoeba keratitis. Can J Ophthalmol J Can Ophtalmol. 2004;39(6):621–31.
87. Kandori M, Inoue T, Shimabukuro M, Hayashi H, Hori Y, Maeda N, et al. Four cases of Acanthamoeba keratitis treated with phototherapeutic keratectomy. Cornea. 2010;29(10):1199–202.
88. Suryawanshi A, Cao Z, Sampson JF, Panjwani N. IL-17A-mediated protection against Acanthamoeba keratitis. J Immunol Baltim Md 1950. 2015;194(2):650–63.
89. Nakagawa H, Hattori T, Koike N, Ehara T, Fujita K, Takahashi H, et al. Investigation of the role of bacteria in the development of Acanthamoeba keratitis. Cornea. 2015;34(10):1308–15.

Neurotrophic Keratopathy

4

Angela Y. Zhu and Asim Ali

4.1 Introduction

Neurotrophic keratopathy (NK) is a rare, neurodegenerative condition in which alterations in corneal nerves lead to impaired sensory and trophic functions, resulting in epithelial breakdown and consequent stromal melting [1]. While it is often interchangeably described by various terms, including neuroparalytic, neuropathic, or neurotrophic keratitis vs. keratopathy, there is overall agreement that the primary etiology is related to an underlying corneal nerve pathology rather than inflammation [2]. The fundamental definition and diagnosis of NK based on the severity of clinical signs/symptoms (Mackie staging) has remained consistent for decades, but improved understanding of corneal repair mechanisms and nerve-mediated trophic factors have allowed for advances in both medical and surgical treatment modalities [3]. Although the mainstay of NK management previously focused on ocular surface protection and prevention of disease progression, there has been a recent shift in the treatment paradigm to targeting the underlying deficiencies in growth factors and corneal nerve function.

A. Y. Zhu
Bascom Palmer Eye Institute, University of Miami Miller School of Medicine, Miami, FL, USA

A. Ali (✉)
Department of Ophthalmology and Vision Sciences, Hospital for Sick Children, Toronto, ON, Canada

Department of Ophthalmology and Visual Sciences, University of Toronto, Toronto, ON, Canada
e-mail: asim.ali@sickkids.ca

H. N. Saeed, R. B. Singh (eds.), *Corneal Disorders*, Current Practices in Ophthalmology, https://doi.org/10.1007/978-981-96-5294-5_4

4.1.1 Epidemiology and Demographics

Though the definition of NK as an orphan disease (ORPHA137596) has not changed, there are limited epidemiological data given a paucity of population-wide information and prior under-recognition of this disease entity [4]. It remains classified as a rare disorder with an estimated prevalence of less than 5/10,000 individuals, but more specific estimates must be extrapolated based on reported incidences of the most common underlying conditions associated with NK [2]. Given a calculated incidence of 1.22/10,000 for herpetic keratitis-associated NK and 0.02/10,000 for postsurgical NK (the two most common causes), the overall population incidence of NK is likely below 1.6/10,000 adults [4]. The prevalence is even lower in the pediatric population as these underlying etiologies are even rarer in children [5]. Further demographic details on the percentage of NK cases caused by other conditions, age or race/ethnicity-specific incidence, or sex predilection have not been reported in the literature.

4.2 Etiology and Pathophysiology

As one of the most sensitive structures in the human body, the cornea relies on its extensive nerve plexi to maintain epithelial integrity and ocular surface health [6]. Any insults along the corneal innervation pathway can disrupt the careful homeostasis between corneal nerves and epithelium, triggering an inflammatory cascade that can potentiate persistent epithelial defects (PEDs) and stromal melting [3]. Loss of corneal sensation also compromises the blink and tear secretion reflex arcs, which further exacerbates the ocular surface and contributes to the development of NK [7].

4.2.1 Anatomy of Corneal Innervation

The cornea is predominantly innervated by sensory nerves from the ophthalmic division of the trigeminal nerve (cranial nerve V1) as well as autonomic nerves. The nasociliary branch of V1 enters the orbit through the superior orbital fissure and gives rise to two to three long ciliary nerves which combine with six short ciliary nerves and penetrate the sclera around the optic nerve to enter the suprachoroidal space, pass anteriorly to supply the iris and ciliary body, and terminate in the limbal plexus [8].

Autonomic innervation primarily consists of sympathetic nerves from the superior cervical ganglion. Some postganglionic fibers then merge directly with long ciliary nerves, while others pass without synapse into the short ciliary nerves and follow the same suprachoroidal trajectory within the globe. Thus, the limbal plexus contains both sensory and autonomic nerves [9].

From the limbal plexus, a mixture of sensory and autonomic nerve bundles enters the cornea radially in the middle third of the stroma, running centrally and anteriorly to penetrate Bowman's layer and emerging in the sub-epithelial plane. Within this plane, numerous neurites divide and re-anastomose to create the subbasal nerve plexus; terminal branches pass anteriorly into the epithelial cell layers providing nerve endings to the corneal surface [10, 11].

4.2.2 Physiology of Corneal Innervation

Corneal nerve physiology encompasses sensory, autonomic, and trophic functions. Sensory innervation reacts to mechanical, chemical, and thermal stimuli via two reflex arcs: the motor reflex arc produces the blink reflex and an autonomous reflex arc which induces tear production and secretion [12]. Thus, a reduction in corneal sensation impairs both of these reflexes with subsequent tear film instability.

Furthermore, a delicate interdependent relationship between the corneal nerves and epithelium is maintained by the expression of trophic factors [13]. Corneal nerves express neuromediators to promote epithelial migration and differentiation; some key mediators include substance P, calcitonin gene–related peptide (CGRP), acetylcholine, noradrenaline, serotonin, neuropeptide Y, and vasointestinal peptide [8, 12]. In turn, corneal epithelial cells release soluble neurotrophic factors that promote neurite extension and survival, notably nerve growth factor (NGF), epidermal growth factor (EGF), ciliary neurotrophic factor (CNTF), and glial-cell-derived neurotrophic factor (GDNF) [14, 15]. The lacrimal gland also plays a role in ocular surface homeostasis, as sensory nerves stimulate autonomous tear production, which contains growth factors (e.g., substance P and NGF) and nutrients [2].

Multiple studies have shown the synergistic action of substance P with EGF and insulin-like growth factor-1 (IGF-1) in promoting corneal epithelial cell migration, which is necessary for wound healing [14, 16]. Loss of sensory innervation has been associated with a significant depletion in the corneolimbal epithelial stem cell population, primarily mediated by NGF and GDNF [17, 18]. Additionally, recent evidence has revealed a complex interaction between the corneal nervous and immune systems, with sensory neuropeptides substance P and CGRP implicated in the neurogenic inflammatory response following tissue injury [19]. Consequently, this T-cell-dependent inflammation seems to promote corneal nerve regeneration, forming a negative feedback loop that keeps both systems mutually in check [20, 21]

4.2.3 Etiologies of NK

Given the interdependent nature of epithelial integrity on corneal nerves, any lasting insult to the corneal sensory innervation can result in NK (Table 4.1). This can

Table 4.1 Different causes of neurotrophic keratopathy based on the type and affected site

Disorder type	Affected anatomical location	Cause
Congenital	Syndromic	Riley-Day syndrome
		Möbius syndrome
		Goldenhar syndrome
		Congenital insensitivity to pain with anhidrosis (CIPA)
		VACTERL syndrome
	Central nervous system	Trigeminal nuclei hypoplasia
	Trigeminal nerve	Familial trigeminal anesthesia

(continued)

Table 4.1 (continued)

Disorder type	Affected anatomical location	Cause
Acquired	Systemic	Diabetes mellitus
		Multiple sclerosis
		Vitamin A/B12 deficiency
		Amyloidosis/disseminated lymphangiomatosis
		Autoimmune polyglandular syndrome
		Disseminated neoplasm
		Leprosy
	Central nervous system	Neoplasm
		Vascular lesion (aneurysm, cerebrovascular accident)
		Wallenberg syndrome
		Post-neurosurgery for: Acoustic neuroma. Trigeminal neuralgia.
		Severe head trauma
		Medication toxicity (neuroleptics, antipsychotics)
	Trigeminal nerve	Ciliary nerve lesion
		Orbital tumor
		Orbital surgery
		Facial trauma
	Ocular nerves	Post-retinal surgery (vitrectomy with endolaser, scleral buckle)
		Post-laser procedure: Panretinal photocoagulation. Laser retinopexy. Diode cyclophotocoagulation.
		Intraocular lymphoma
	Corneal nerves	Infections (herpes simplex, herpes zoster)
		Post-corneal surgery: Laser refractive (LASIK). Keratoplasty. Corneal incisions (e.g., astigmatic keratotomy).
		Chemical and thermal injury
		Contact lens wear
		Topical medication toxicity: Anesthetics. Beta-blockers with benzalkonium chloride (BAK) (e.g., timolol, betaxolol). Trifluridine. Sulfacetamide. Diclofenac.
		Corneal dystrophy (lattice, granular)
Idiopathic	Systemic	Increasing age
		Adie syndrome

include both congenital and acquired conditions, ocular or systemic, that effect permanent damage at any point along the course of cranial nerve V1 from the trigeminal nucleus to the cornea [2]. A recent retrospective epidemiologic study of 354 eyes with NK (age range 6–101, mean 63.1 years) over 8 years found that the most common causes were herpetic eye disease (32.2%), iatrogenic secondary to ocular procedures or medications (31.9%), intracranial tumors and/or surgeries (17.5%), chronic ocular surface disease (17.5%), and diabetes mellitus (10.5%); a multifactorial cause was found in 34.2% [22]. This is consistent with prior retrospective studies [6, 23].

In the pediatric population, acquired causes are rarer, but intracranial tumors remain one of the main etiologies (30.8% in one series) [23, 24]. Congenital causes include both isolated corneal pathology and syndromes associated with trigeminal nerve palsy; a high association with coexisting facial palsy has been reported in this population (69.2% in one series), which can worsen disease presentation and progression [24]. The term "congenital trigeminal anesthesia" encompasses most of these congenital causes, which is subdivided into three types by the Rosenberg classification: [25] Type 1, occurring in isolation, is related to trigeminal nuclei hypoplasia, and is often bilateral [26, 27]; type 2 is associated with ectodermal or mesenchymal maldevelopment, such as Riley-Day, Moebius, and Goldenhar syndromes; type 3 is a combination of corneal anesthesia with a focal brainstem pathology likely secondary to a prenatal vascular event [28]. Another rare cause of congenital corneal anesthesia is congenital insensitivity to pain with anhidrosis (CIPA), a syndrome caused by a mutation in the NGF receptor required for the function of sympathetic and sensory neurons [29–31].

4.2.4 Natural History and Pathophysiology of NK

When corneal sensation is impaired, a sequence of events is initiated that ultimately leads to NK and its consequences (Fig. 4.1). A significant decrease in reflex tear secretion causes the tear film to become irregular and unstable, decreasing its ability to protect against eyelid blink microtrauma [15]. Reduction in neurotrophic mediators impedes epithelial cell maturation and migration, which allows the accumulation of older, less vital epithelial cells centrally that are more easily damaged by eyelid friction [2]. Over time, the ongoing tear film changes and lack of trophic support lead to chronic epithelial instability and damage. This results in spontaneous epithelial defects that are often central and characterized by rolled borders made of pre-exfoliating cells not only unable to adhere to the basement membrane but also unable to be cleared due to inadequate tear production [7]. The local tissue injury triggers an inflammatory reaction; combined with surface dryness and persistent epitheliopathy, the denuded stroma becomes vulnerable to unchecked destruction by matrix metalloproteinases (MMPs) [32]. While this can ultimately lead to stromal melting and perforation, any attempts at healing by protease inhibitors often cause irregular collagen deposition and scar formation, diminishing visual function.

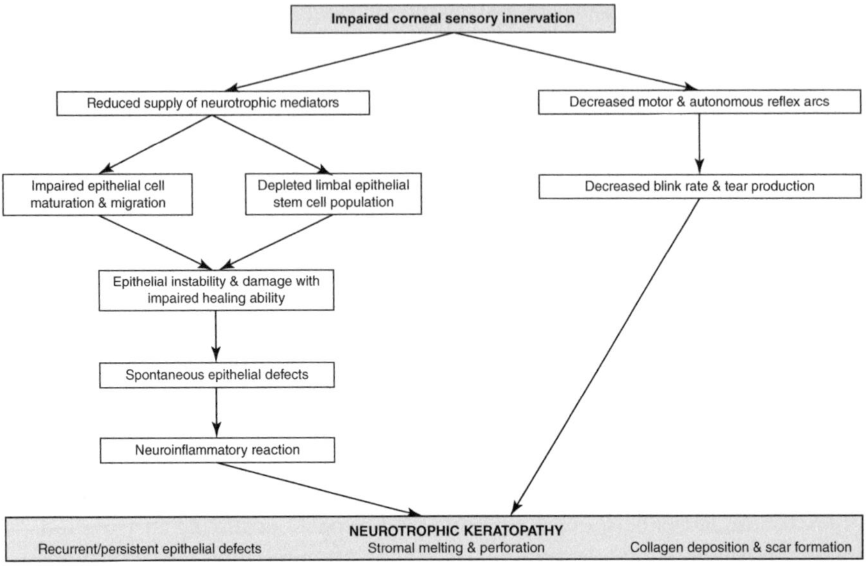

Fig. 4.1 Pathophysiology of neurotrophic keratopathy development. (Adapted from Mastropaqua et al. [15])

Thus, once the corneal nerve damage has been established, the progression of NK becomes a self-perpetuating pathway independent of the underlying conditions that lead to nerve impairment [15].

4.3 Diagnosis and Evaluation

Diagnosis of NK remains clinical despite advances in laboratory testing and imaging, so evaluation should begin with a thorough ocular and systemic review of systems as well as physical examination. Based on a clinical history of conditions associated with trigeminal nerve damage, presence of PEDs or epitheliopathy, and measured corneal hypoesthesia or anesthesia, a presumptive diagnosis of NK can be made. While there may be a discrepancy between clinical findings and symptoms depending on the severity at the time of presentation, the clinician should also maintain a level of suspicion for infectious or immune keratitis as part of the differential diagnosis, as these may masquerade as or superimpose upon a diagnosis of NK [4].

4.3.1 Clinical History and Presentation

A detailed patient history should first be performed to identify known ocular and systemic conditions associated with NK. In particular, the presence of systemic diseases (e.g., diabetes mellitus, neurodegenerative disorders, intracranial tumors and vascular lesions, congenital syndromes), medications and therapy (e.g., neuroleptic drugs, antipsychotics, chemotherapy), neurosurgical interventions, and head/facial trauma should be specifically investigated. Specifically for the ophthalmic history, it is important to elicit information regarding any prior ocular surgeries or laser procedures, current topical medications, and contact lens use (type, fit, and duration of use).

In the early stages, patients often present with dryness, photophobia, and fluctuating blurry vision due to epithelial instability, reduced blink, and impaired quality of vision. These can be worse in the morning or aggravated by air conditioning/fans, air travel, or prolonged screen time, which may explain why most early cases are simply diagnosed as dry eye syndrome [2]. However, NK has the distinctive feature of paradoxical symptomatic alleviation with worsening disease related to sensory dullness from corneal anesthesia. In advanced disease, vision can be severely compromised with central corneal involvement.

4.3.2 Clinical Examination

Clinical examination should first begin with a systemic evaluation to determine a potential underlying etiology for trigeminal nerve damage. Concomitant third, fourth, and/or sixth cranial nerve impairment can imply a cavernous sinus lesion; cranial nerve 7 or 8 palsies may suggest post-neurosurgical damage or acoustic neuroma [6]. Additional detailed neurologic evaluation in conjunction with other specialists (e.g., plastic surgery, neurosurgery, otolaryngology, neurology) may be necessary to fully document anesthesia affecting multiple nerves, as often seen in congenital syndromic etiologies of NK.

The ocular examination should start with evaluating pupillary reactivity and eyelid function for both diagnostic and prognostic value. Pupillary abnormalities may indicate third cranial nerve involvement, sympathetic innervation defects, or rarely Adie syndrome [2]. Lid ptosis may also imply third cranial nerve involvement, while lagophthalmos is often associated with the seventh nerve involvement and can result in superimposed exposure keratopathy [4]. Additional lid features, including malposition (ectropion, entropion), scarring, or lash misdirection, can all be aspects of an underlying cause but can similarly worsen the prognosis of NK due to generalized aggravation of the ocular surface. Though NK is a corneal disease, dilated fundus examination should routinely be performed to assess optic nerve or retina pathology that may be related to the underlying etiology or ocular comorbidities [2].

Slit-lamp examination of the ocular surface should be documented and classified based on Mackie staging (Table 4.2) [33]. The conjunctiva is generally "white and quiet" in NK due to lack of inflammation as a primary driver initially; the presence of significantly inflamed conjunctiva or subconjunctival fibrosis may insinuate superimposed infection or autoimmune disease. Corneal epithelial changes, stromal scarring, and neovascularization should all be carefully noted, as these features may indicate disease severity and prior recurrences, as well as affect the visual prognosis

Table 4.2 Mackie staging of NK with associated symptoms

Stage	Presenting symptoms	Clinical findings
1	Dryness, foreign body sensation	Corneal epithelial hyperplasia and irregularity
	Intermittent blurry vision	Scattered small areas of dried epithelium (Gaule spots)
	Photophobia	Superficial punctate epithelial erosions with subepithelial scarring
		Decreased tear breakup time
		Superficial neovascularization
		Dellen
		Rose bengal staining of the inferior bulbar conjunctiva
2	Persistent blurry vision	Recurrent or persistent corneal epithelial defects with rolled/smooth edges
	Photophobia	Descemet membrane folds
	Minimal/lack of pain	Stromal edema
		Anterior chamber inflammatory reaction with sterile hypopyon (rare)
3	Severely decreased vision	Corneal ulcer with stromal thinning
	Lack of pain	Active stromal lysis with risk of perforation

of potential intervention. The use of vital dyes (e.g., fluorescein, lissamine green, rose bengal) can be useful for assessing tear film and function, corneal epithelial defects, and conjunctival epithelial changes. Since herpetic keratitis remains the most common cause of NK, evidence of anterior chamber inflammation (cell, flare, keratic precipitates) or sectoral iris atrophy combined with corneal neovascularization may help diagnose this association.

4.3.3 Diagnostic Testing and Imaging Modalities

The pathognomonic test for NK involves the evaluation of corneal sensation. This can be measured qualitatively by using a cotton "wisp" or hypertonic (3%) saline drops to gently touch the peripheral and central cornea, then observing the patient's subsequent blink and tearing reflexes as well as a verbalized description of sensation [4, 34]. For more quantitative measurements, esthesiometers can be used to document the level of sensation. The most common instrument is the Cochet-Bonnet esthesiometer, which uses a nylon filament of decreasing length (0–60 mm) to touch different quadrants of the cornea; quantification of corneal sensitivity is documented as the threshold length of filament that elicits a blink reflex or patient response [35]. Noncontact esthesiometers have also been developed, such as the Belmonte gas esthesiometer, which stimulates corneal nerves with a calibrated gas emission. As this device can vary pressure, temperature, and concentration of CO_2 gas discharged from the injection tip, it can theoretically assess all three types of ocular surface neuroreceptors (mechanical, chemical, thermal) with good reproducibility [36].

Structural characterization of corneal nerves in various pathologies has increased in popularity over the last decade. In vivo confocal microscopy (IVCM) allows noninvasive qualitative and quantitative analysis of corneal nerve density, tortuosity, angulation, thickness, and reflectivity [37]. As this method is sensitive enough to visualize minute changes in the stromal and subbasal nerve plexus, it can detect alterations in nerve morphology and density secondary to NK and other diseases [38]. Several studies have shown a decrease in subbasal nerve fiber density on IVCM imaging correlating with decreased corneal sensation in patients with herpes zoster keratitis (HZK), herpes simplex keratitis (HSK), post-laser refractive surgery, diabetic neuropathy, and post-trigeminal ganglionic lesions [37, 39–43]. Of note, the corneal hypoesthesia was only noticed by patients when the measured nerve density was below a certain threshold (~1000 μm/frame by Confoscan), accounting for the discrepancy between perceived corneal sensation and measured nerve fiber density and number in some cases [37, 44]. A few studies have also reported a loss of corneal nerve fibers in the contralateral unaffected eye of infectious keratitis (herpesviral, bacterial, acanthamoeba) patients, supporting the hypothesis that a neurogenic inflammatory response may play a significant role in the disease pathogenesis and similarly affect the contralateral eye [42, 45]. The main limitations of IVCM are its poor repeatability due to the lack of standardized manual segmentation and imaging parameters, variable quality of image acquisition depending on user technique and artifactual influence, and decreased resolution in the presence of concurrent stromal edema, infiltrates, or scarring [46].

In the same way, high-resolution anterior segment optical coherence tomography (AS-OCT) can provide a noninvasive depiction of corneal structure. While some Fourier domain AS-OCT machines have the resolution to demonstrate corneal nerve abnormalities, such as during active infectious keratitis, most instruments do not yet provide the detail to assess architectural changes limited to the nerves [2, 47].

Ancillary testing may be needed to further evaluate for associated underlying or superimposed conditions. If systemic examination reveals concern for intracranial lesion(s) affecting other cranial nerves, urgent neuroimaging should be considered. Impression cytology of the cornea and conjunctival limbus may be a useful adjunctive test to better characterize epithelial changes/conjunctivalization related to other chronic ocular surface diseases, such as dry eye or limbal stem cell deficiency [49]. Likewise, microbial cultures should be performed if there is any suspicion of new infiltrates or inflammation out of proportion to the underlying disease process. These disorders can all be secondary to NK or comorbidities that worsen the disease prognosis.

While some Fourier domain AS-OCT machines has the resolution to demonstrate corneal nerve abnormalities, such as during active infectious keratitis, most instruments do not yet provide the detail to assess architectural changes limited to the nerves [2, 47]. AS-OCT has more utility in depicting the qualitative changes within each corneal layer, such as stromal ulceration and thinning. Since presence of severe

(50%) thinning can have poor prognostic implications and therapeutic outcomes, it has been proposed that the traditional Mackie classification should be edited to include diagnostic use of AS-OCT [48].

4.3.4 Differential Diagnosis

Many ocular surface diseases can mimic the appearance of NK, with impaired corneal sensation being the key distinctive trait. Dry eye disease, blepharitis, exposure keratopathy, limbal stem cell deficiency, chemical injury, toxic and radiation keratopathy, and contact lens related disorders can all have overlapping features with NK; they may also be comorbid or contributory underlying diagnoses that require secondary focused treatment to avoid disease progression.

In advanced stages with the presence of a corneal ulcer, exclusion of infectious, toxic, or immune causes must be performed. The presence of stromal infiltrates and/or associated significant intraocular inflammation requires microbiological evaluation, potential systemic evaluation for immune diseases, and discontinuation of any potential toxic localized treatments.

4.4 Management

Management of NK has long focused on the goals of promoting ocular surface repair, preventing disease progression, and maintaining globe integrity [1]. A stage-based approach is generally recommended, with the early stages treated by conservative modalities and more aggressive surgical interventions being reserved for severe cases. As comorbid ocular surface and eyelid disorders can worsen the progression of NK, they must also be identified and treated concomitantly to optimize the tear film and ocular surface milieu for healing.

4.4.1 Conservative Treatments for Ocular Surface Protection

Nonsurgical therapies aimed at preventing epithelial breakdown and promoting repair are generally first-line treatments of mild NK. The mainstay of conservative management is the discontinuation of potential sources of ocular toxicity (e.g., preservatives) or recurrent mechanical trauma (e.g., eye rubbing), use of frequent preservative-free topical lubricants, and control of concomitant lid disease (e.g., blepharitis, lagophthalmos) [3]. While topical antibiotics are often used prophylactically in cases of epithelial defects, care must be taken to avoid epitheliotoxic compounds, limit dosing (even in preservative-free formulations), and discontinue them if clinical signs indicate early drug toxicity. Punctal plugs can also be considered to enhance the efficacy of topical lubrication, presuming any associated ocular surface inflammation is under control [1].

Hemoderivative eye drops are often considered when commercially available tear supplements are insufficient. These nutritional tear substitutes (serum eye drops) contain growth factors, vitamins, antimicrobials, and proteins involved in wound healing, which all help promote proliferation, migration, and differentiation of corneal epithelial cells [50, 51]. Studies have shown good safety and efficacy of these tear substitutes in healing PEDs secondary to NK, with one prospective study reporting 91% of defects healing within 12 weeks [52]. While autologous serum eye drops (ASEDs) are the most common preparation as they are nonallergenic and biochemically similar to natural tears, patients with systemic autoimmune diseases or who cannot donate blood are poor candidates [53]. Alternative preparations include allogeneic serum eye drops, platelet-rich plasma (PRP) tears, human umbilical cord serum (UCS), and finger-prick autologous blood (FAB). Allogeneic serum drops currently have limited availability in the United States. Both PRP and UCS have higher concentrations of growth factors as well as additional matrix biomaterial scaffolds than ASEDs that allow for increased ocular surface wound healing, with preliminary studies showing slightly superior outcomes in PED closure compared to ASEDs [54–58]. However, these therapies can all be cost-prohibitive with limited ability to access supplies for most patients. FAB has recently been proposed as a potentially cheaper and more convenient option, with a pilot study demonstrating improved wound healing in refractory PEDs [59]. Additional comparative and more controlled studies are necessary for all these modalities to evaluate their long-term efficacy in NK.

Therapeutic contact lenses have long been used as both a temporary and long-term nonsurgical option for corneal protection in chronic ocular surface disease, but their use in NK remains largely anecdotal and unverified by higher levels of evidence. Their rationale for use is straightforward: contact lenses provide a physical barrier between the cornea and eyelids to protect the fragile epithelium from further blink-related microtrauma as well as reduce the risk of corneal desiccation [60]. Soft bandage contact lenses (BCLs) absorb water from the tear film; this hydrated lens material then directly rests on the cornea. Only a few case reports of BCL use in NK have been reported with variable success; it has been proposed that they may be most effective in corneal protection prior to the development of a frank epithelial defect, given the potential risks of microbial keratitis associated with continuous contact lens wear [2, 61]. Scleral contact lenses and prosthetic replacement of the ocular surface ecosystem (PROSE) devices vault over the cornea and limbus but contain a fluid-filled reservoir (liquid bandage) that continually bathes the cornea. Multiple retrospective series have described promising outcomes using scleral lenses and PROSE devices in moderate-severe ocular surface disease (including NK), with the resolution of epithelial defects and significant improvements in visual rehabilitation without high rates of infectious keratitis documented [62–66]. Even in cases of NK with severe corneal thinning or associated with exposure keratopathy, well-fitted scleral lenses have been proposed as a nonsurgical alternative to traditional management options of tarsorrhaphy or patch graft [67–69].

Table 4.3 Targets of medical therapies for neurotrophic keratopathy

Aim	Therapy	Approval status
Ocular surface lubrication and protection	Preservative-free artificial tears and ointments	FDA approved
	Hemoderivative eye drops Autologous and allogeneic serum eye drops (ASEDs). Platelet-rich plasma (PRP). Umbilical cord serum (UCS).	Autologous PRP for NK pending phase 1 trial (NCT04604834). UCS for dry eye pending phase 2 trial (NCT04217785).
Anti-inflammation and prevention of stromal keratolysis	Oral tetracycline	Off-label use
	Ascorbate (vitamin C)	Off-label use
	Topical steroids Prednisolone. Dexamethasone. Medroxyprogesterone.	FDA approved
Epithelial and neural regeneration (growth factors)	Cenegermin (recombinant human nerve growth factor, rhNGF)	FDA approved (January 2019)
	NGF mimetics	Udonitrectag pending phase 2 trial (NCT04276558)
	Thymosin beta 4 (Tβ4)	RGN-259 pending phase 3 trial (NCT03937882)
	Connexin43 inhibitors	Nexagon pending phase 2 trial (NCT04081103)
	AMP cells	ST266 pending phase 2 trial (NCT03687632)
	Ergot derivatives	Preclinical
	Substance P and IGF-1	Preclinical
	Topical insulin	Preclinical
	Coenzyme Q10	Preclinical
	Other neurotrophic factors EGF. CNTF. PEDF. Neuropeptide FF.	Preclinical
Epithelial repair (structural)	Matrix regenerating agents (RGTAs) Cacicol. CALCICOL20.	RGTA-T4020 pending phase 3 trial results (NCT01794312)

4.4.2 Medical Therapies (Table 4.3)

Anti-Inflammatory Therapy

Use of anti-inflammatory drops is critical to minimize the ocular surface inflammatory response and prevent deterioration in NK. Generally, topical preservative-free steroids such as prednisolone, dexamethasone, and medroxyprogesterone 1–2% are used in short courses to prevent progression to stage 3 NK, as care must be taken to limit epitheliotoxicity and steroid-induced glaucoma often associated with higher doses or longer duration treatments [70]. Topical cyclosporine is only approved for primary or secondary dry eye indications, but off-label use in chronic ocular surface inflammatory conditions has been reported [2]. For PEDs at high risk of stromal melting, use of matrix metalloproteinase (MMP) inhibitors, such as oral tetracyclines and topical acetylcysteine, has been widely reported to limit collagenase activity [71, 72]. In conjunction, vitamin C (ascorbate) given systemically or topically provides cofactors for collagen synthesis and helps scavenge reactive oxygen species that perpetuate tissue degradation [2]. In the context of NK, none of these anti-inflammatory therapies have been specifically evaluated for safety and efficacy.

Topical Nerve Growth Factor (NGF)

Cenegermin or recombinant human nerve growth factor (rhNGF) (Oxervate®, Dompé Inc., Italy) is the first FDA-approved medication, specifically PEDs or corneal ulcers due to NK [73]. It is a pro-peptide derived from the bacteria *Escherichia coli* and cleaved to generate mature NGF upon topical instillation in vivo [74]. Early studies using topical NGF laid the groundwork for its approval, starting in 1998 with an open-label study on 12 patients with refractory NK-associated ulcers [75]. After the safety of rhNGF was demonstrated in a phase I trial of 22 healthy volunteers followed by a phase 2 randomized control trial (RCT) of 156 patients, the standard dosing of 20 μg/ml rhNGF six times daily for 8 weeks was determined [76, 77]. A recent, multicenter RCT of 48 patients was conducted in the United States, reporting a significantly higher percentage of patients (65.2%) with complete epithelial defect closure after 8 weeks of treatment compared to vehicle alone (16.7%); only mild adverse effects (commonly localized ocular pain) were described, consistent with prior studies [78]. Interestingly, the primary outcome measure in all of these studies was epithelial healing and not corneal sensation, which did not reach a statistically significant difference between the cenergermin and vehicle-treated (control) groups in any trial [77, 78]. The main limitations of cenegermin therapy are its high cost and poor compound stability causing inconvenience, as patients must refrigerate weekly trays of the medication and draw daily doses in individual syringes.

Since its approval in 2019, the use of cenegermin in the pediatric population has also been highlighted. Multiple case reports have published favorable outcomes with the use of cenegermin for pediatric NK secondary to both congenital and acquired etiologies [79–83]. While the epithelial healing rate may be promising, the overall success of this medication for visual rehabilitation may be limited in this population due to preexisting scarring and amblyopia; higher rates of mild adverse effects have also been reported [84]. Larger, longer-term studies with cost-benefit analysis must be conducted to determine the optimal initiation stage and whether this treatment is suitable for all populations.

Other NGF mimetics have also been studied, as synthetic, small molecule formulations can have more biological stability, penetration, and targeted action for treating NK [85]. A phase 2 clinical trial investigating NGF mimetic Udonitrectag (Recordati Rare Diseases, United States) is currently recruiting (NCT04276558) [53].

Matrix Regenerating Agents (RGTAs)

Matrix regenerating agents (RGTAs) exemplify a new therapeutic strategy for corneal epithelialization in NK [73]. These are polymers engineered to mimic the extracellular matrix, especially the proteoglycan heparan sulfate, which becomes damaged in NK. Exogenous RGTAs provide replacement heparan sulfate to stabilize the stromal matrix, resist further degradation, promote epithelial migration/adhesion, and reduce inflammatory and oxidative stress [86]. Several small clinical studies evaluating two RGTAs, CALCICOL20 (Théa Laboratories, France) and Cacicol (OTR3, France), have shown favorable outcomes in healing refractory PEDs within 1–3 months with good safety profile in NK patients, though recurrences after treatment cessation have been reported [87–91]. A phase 3 clinical trial of RGTA-T4020 (Théa Laboratories, France) was recently completed (NCT01794312), with further studies and analyses pending [53]. Given their potential synergistic mechanism when used in conjunction with other medical treatments (e.g., ASEDs, supplemental growth factors), RGTAs are an extremely promising therapeutic option, but additional controlled trials must first be conducted [92].

Thymosin Beta-4 (Tβ4)

Thymosin beta-4 (Tβ4) is a protein expressed by multiple cell types that have been found to promote corneal epithelial cell migration, decrease MMP expression, and reduce pro-inflammatory cytokines [93]. Its potential in treating neurotrophic epithelial defects was first described in 2010 in a small case series of four patients treated with Tβ4 drops four times daily for 4 weeks [94]. Additional preclinical studies have alluded to a delayed effect due to improved epithelial healing after 30 days of follow-up after treatment cessation [95, 96]. A phase 3 clinical trial (ARISE-3) is currently underway to assess the role of topical 0.1% Tβ4 (RGN-259) in dry eye (NCT03937882), though the parallel trial in NK patients has been halted indefinitely (NCT02600429).

Other Topical Growth Factors

A variety of other medical therapies have also been hypothesized to be beneficial in the treatment of NK, though most are still early in the drug development pipeline (Table 4.3):

1. Connexin43 inhibitors: Connexin43 is a gap junction protein involved in the regulation of apoptosis, with its downregulation correlating to increased wound closure [97]. Application of topical connexin43 antisense oligonucleotide inhibitors has been reported to reduce clinical inflammation and produce complete re-epithelialization in animal and ex vivo models as well as a few in vivo refractory PEDs [98, 99].
2. Substance P and insulin-like growth factor-1 (IGF-1): Topical substance P combined with IGF-1 has demonstrated a synergistic effect in stimulating the proliferation and migration of epithelial cells in multiple animal models [100–102]. Using soluble peptide formulations derived from substance P (FGLM-amide) and IGF-1 (SSSR), small prospective clinical studies have shown complete epi-

thelial defect closure in up to 73% of patients within 4 weeks of treatment initiation [103, 104].

3. Topical insulin: Since receptors are expressed on corneal epithelial cells and keratocytes as well as the lacrimal gland, insulin is known to play a role in corneal wound healing though the mechanism is not well understood [105]. A few clinical case series have described resolution of neurotrophic epithelial defects within 1–4 weeks of topical insulin treatment, as well as a randomized control trial in diabetic patients [106–108].
4. Ergot derivatives: Ergot derivatives such as nicergoline and pergolide are known to induce NGF production within the brain and are used in the treatment of neurological diseases (e.g., stroke, dementia, Parkinson's) [109]. Early animal model studies have shown corneal nerve regeneration with topical and systemic administration of these agents, as well as up to 85% of clinical PEDs in NK patients treated with oral nicergoline in a small prospective study [110, 111].
5. Other growth factors: Multiple other neurotrophic factors are under investigation. EGF has been known to stimulate epithelial and fibroblast proliferation, migration, and differentiation in wound healing [112]. Recombinant human EGF ointment (Easyef ointment, Daewoong Pharmaceutical Co., Ltd., South Korea) was recently tested off-label in 15 patients with PEDs; 80% of patients had a significant reduction in epithelial defect size after 2 months [113]. Other topical preparations of growth factors, including CNTF, pigment epithelial-derived factor (PEDF), and neuropeptide FF, have shown promising increases in neural regeneration and corneal sensitivity in animal models [114].
6. Coenzyme Q10 (CoQ10) and other compounds: Topical CoQ10 has shown potential as adjunctive therapy to promote corneal wound healing due to its role in mitochondrial metabolism, anti-oxidant, and anti-inflammatory effects [115]. The combination of topical CoQ10 with cross-linked hyaluronic acid for increased lubrication has demonstrated encouraging results in dry eye patients [116]. Additional compounds including nanomicelle curcumin, Rho-kinase inhibitors, and liposomal ozonated oil have been described to promote corneal epithelial wound healing and nerve regeneration using in vivo mouse models and a few patients [117–119].
7. Albumin: As the primary protein in serum, albumin has been hypothesized to promote wound healing by suppressing apoptosis [120]. Albumin drops alone have been reported to aid in epithelialization in rat models of epithelial defects and dry eye [121].
8. Amnion-derived multipotent progenitor (AMP) cells: Ever since fetal regenerative wound healing was attributed to the growth factors and cytokines secreted by the placenta, amnion has been a prime source of prospective tissue healing factors. This has been translated to therapeutic potential with ST266 (Noveome Biotherapeutics, United States), a "secretome" matrix of biological factors from amnion-derived multipotent progenitor (AMP) cells. Its neural regenerative properties have been shown in animal models, and it is currently undergoing phase 2 trials for PEDs [122, 123].

9. Amniotic membrane extract eye drops (AMEED): Given the known healing properties of amnion, homogenization and collection of amnion supernatant to generate eye drops (AMEED) has been another prospective therapy for NK. Preliminary studies have shown limbal stem proliferation and epithelial healing secondary to AMEED [124, 125].
10. Adipose tissue–derived stem cells (ADSCs): Topical application of autologous ADSCs have been investigated for epithelial healing due to its abundance, convenient preparation, and multiple differentiation potentials [126]. Recent rat model and preclinical human studies have described successful proliferation and differentiation of corneal epithelial cells in refractory PEDs [126, 127].

These compounds are all predominantly still in preclinical studies, though a few have reached phase 2 clinical trials for epithelial defects not specific to NK (Nexagon connexin43 antisense gel in NCT04081103, ST266 in NCT03687632, Udonitrectag in NCT04276558).

4.4.3 Surgical Interventions

Once NK has exceeded the limits of medical therapy, surgical intervention is generally recommended. Depending on NK severity, the goals of various surgical procedures can be divided into corneal protection, ocular surface and visual rehabilitation, tectonic support to maintain globe integrity, and corneal nerve regeneration. Any surgical interventions are not standalone as the ocular surface must be continually optimized and treated medically even after successful surgical outcomes.

Eyelid Procedures

Partial closure of the eyelids via tarsorrhaphy has long been a cornerstone of NK management, especially if lagophthalmos is present. It is a safe and highly effective procedure for protecting the cornea, with up to a 90.9% success rate in treating epitheliopathy and minimal complications reported in the literature [128]. Temporary tarsorrhaphies can be performed via nonsurgical means, using tape, pressure patching, cyanoacrylate glue, or botulinum toxin injection-induced ptosis to narrow the interpalpebral fissure [129, 130]. Temporary or permanent suture tarsorrhaphies are generally placed laterally but can also be central or medial, depending on the extent and severity of corneal involvement. The predominant technique for a temporary tarsorrhaphy involves passing a double-armed nonabsorbable suture through the inferior and superior eyelids, first through a plastic bolster to protect the eyelid skin, along with the tarsal plate, and exiting through each lid margin grey line; additional absorbable sutures through de-epithelialized upper and lower lid margins to generate permanent scarring are placed in a permanent tarsorrhaphy [131].

Amniotic Membrane Graft (AMG)

Amniotic membrane is a versatile, semitransparent tissue obtained from the placenta that contains stromal and epithelial sides of similar composition to the corneal and conjunctival epithelium [132]. As it is a non-immunogenic tissue containing multiple neurotrophic factors and protease inhibitors to promote corneal re-epithelialization and decrease inflammation, the amniotic membrane is an ideal graft tissue for severe ocular surface diseases [133]. It can be used both as an inlay (graft) that becomes incorporated into the cornea and onlay (patch) that later falls off after promoting epithelial migration under the amniotic membrane epithelium. Fresh cryopreserved and dehydrated (freeze-dried or vacuum-dried) forms can be obtained commercially or from some eye banks. Cryopreserved amniotic membrane generally is kept in sheets that must be sutured, but commercial sutureless products such as ProKera (Bio-Tissue Inc., United States) are available and well tolerated [134]. Commercially available dehydrated amnion has a longer shelf life and usually appears as self-retaining discs that are directly applied to the corneal surface, often with an overlying bandage contact lens.

The use of AMG for the treatment of stages 2 and 3 NK has been widely published [2]. Most studies recommend sutured AMG in one or multiple layers for severe neurotrophic corneal ulcers, with up to 93.3% success rate of epithelialization reported [135, 136]. It has also been used with variable success in cases of deep corneal ulcers with severe thinning/descemetoceles and localized corneal perforations, though there were higher rates of surgical failure compared to traditional management with lamellar or penetrating keratoplasty, necessitating more definitive procedures for management [137, 138].

Conjunctival Flaps

Total conjunctival or Gunderson flaps were first popularized in 1958 as a surgical treatment for nonhealing epithelial defects in end-stage globes [139]. More commonly in NK, partial or pedicled bridge flaps of Tenon's layer and conjunctiva can be performed in cases of severe stromal thinning with concern for impending perforation, which allows the continuous blood supply to the ulcerated area in order to promote epithelialization, halt inflammation, and prevent progression [140]. This procedure has the inherent advantages of being autologous with no need for donor tissue, decreased necessity for postoperative topical immunosuppression, and innate anti-inflammatory effects [141]. However, it is generally reserved for only eyes with poor vision potential due to risks of corneal perforation under the flap, altered globe cosmesis, and difficult reversibility.

Keratoplasty

Indications for keratoplasty in NK can either be for primary tectonic support or definitive visual rehabilitation once neural regeneration and epithelial healing have been restored. For the management of small corneal perforations, cyanoacrylate glue can be attempted to close the defect. Unfortunately for larger or progressive perforations that fail glue, tectonic keratoplasty becomes necessary for globe salvage. However, the prognosis of tectonic keratoplasty in active NK is exceedingly poor due to inferior epithelial wound healing, pro-inflammatory state, and risks of recurrent melting/perforation [142]. Even in cases of keratoplasty for definitive visual rehabilitation, it is generally recommended to combine the procedure with sutured AMG and temporary tarsorrhaphy to enhance epithelialization and survival of the new graft [131].

Corneal Neurotization (CN)
With the initial modern techniques first described in 2009, surgical neurotization of the cornea is a revolutionary procedure that allows reinnervation of the damaged corneal nerves [143]. Two main approaches have been reported: direct neurotization (DCN), in which the normal donor nerve is directly transferred to the anesthetic cornea, and indirect neurotization (ICN), where an interpositional nerve graft is coapted to the normal donor nerve and tunneled into the anesthetic cornea [144]. DCN was first popularized by Terzis et al. using contralateral supraorbital/supratrochlear nerve transfer using a bicoronal incision; since then, a minimally invasive lid crease and endoscopic approaches have been described [145]. Due to the extensiveness of the dissection required by DCN, ICN has gained popularity since 2014, when Elbaz et al. introduced the feasibility of using sural nerve grafts to connect the contralateral supraorbital/supratrochlear donor nerves to the perilimbal area [146]. Since then, ICN using multiple other donor nerves and interpositional acellular nerve allografts have been described [147–149]. A recent multicenter, prospective, comparative study showed no difference in outcomes between DCN and ICN techniques [150].

While most of the initial cases were performed in central etiologies for NK (e.g., intracranial or congenital syndromes), comparable results have been reported in NK secondary to herpetic eye disease, postsurgical trauma, or tumor-related diseases [151]. Most studies report a subjective improvement starting at 6 months postoperatively; objective esthesiometry measures often lag behind and may not improve for 1–2 years postoperatively [152]. The full physiology of corneal nerve regeneration secondary to CN is not well understood, as evidence shows only the corneal nerves regenerate without the normal trigeminal nerve reflex arcs [153, 154]. Other limitations to the procedure include the extensive preoperative planning given complex ocular surfaces and facial syndromes that can limit donor nerve selection or interpositional nerve anatomy, surgical complexity often requiring a multidisciplinary approach (involving plastic surgery, otolaryngology, and/or neurosurgery) with lengthy surgical time, potential intraoperative iatrogenic nerve damage, unknown long-term outcomes with potential disease recurrence, and potential postoperative neurosensory and cosmetic deficits [131, 155].

4.4.4 Stage-Based Approach

Given the spectrum of NK severity, a stage-based approach to management is universally recommended due to the shifting goals of therapy depending on the condition of the ocular surface and degree of corneal anesthesia, supported by modified

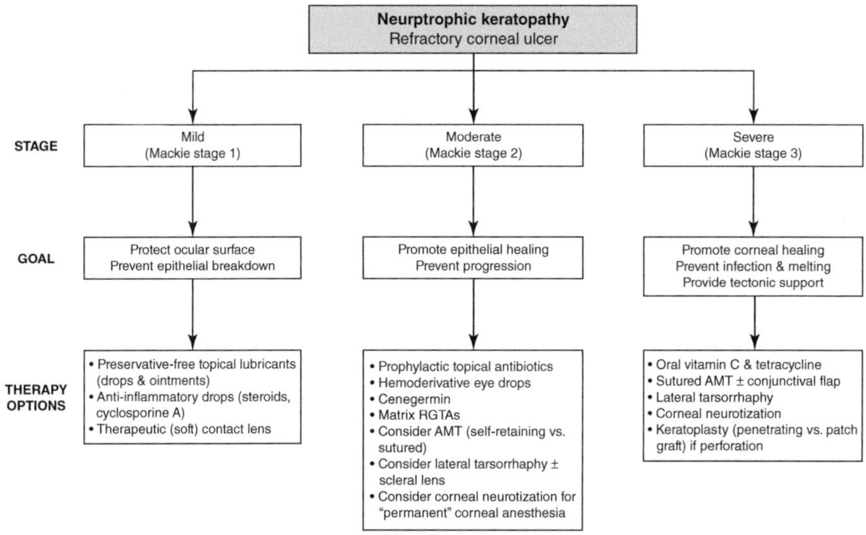

Fig. 4.2 Stage-based approach to the management of neurotrophic keratopathy

Delphi panel expert consensus (Fig. 4.2) [156]. In mild or stage 1 NK, frequent preservative-free lubrication of the ocular surface combined with the optimization of coexisting pathology and reduction of inflammation is generally enough to preserve epithelial integrity. For more moderate to severe NK, additional therapy is often warranted to promote prompt re-epithelialization and prevent stromal breakdown. Newer medical therapies, such as rhNGF and matrix RGTAs, hold the most therapeutic potential to circumvent the necessity of surgical interventions in stage 2 NK. Some minor procedures or nonsurgical alternatives (e.g., scleral lenses, self-retaining amniotic membrane, temporary tarsorrhaphy) may be required adjuvants for more definitive ocular surface protection. A recent meta-analysis showed comparable resolution rates of neurotrophic epithelial defects with rhNGF, ASEDs, AMG, and substance P & IGF-1 supplementation; however, cenegermin currently remains the only therapy supported by level 1 evidence [157].

In stage 3 NK, the goal becomes the prevention of PED complications such as progressive corneal melting, perforation, and devastating infections. Presentation in Mackie stage 3 is a significant risk factor for corneal perforation [158]. While corneal neurotization may have some benefit at an earlier stage and should be considered in patients with "permanent" cornea anesthesia (e.g., in children with congenital conditions), it is often reserved for severe NK given the technical complexity and lengthy recovery of the procedure.

4.5 Future Directions

Despite decades of research on corneal wound healing and neural physiology, NK remains a debilitating disease with a poor prognosis in advanced stages. In the past 10 years, significant progress has been made in the fundamental understanding and cellular mechanisms of the disease, allowing for the development of newer medical and surgical therapies, and FDA approval of cenegermin and corneal neurotization as specific treatments for NK. With the advent of these targeted therapies addressing the underlying corneal anesthesia, the treatment paradigm will likely continue to shift from a stage-based approach to a more directed approach aimed at the causative etiologies. The emphasis will likely be further placed on the prevention of disease formation and progression at an earlier stage.

With new insights into the pathophysiology of NK, there are multiple new medical therapies on the horizon, with additional modalities and approaches to treatment being theorized every year. Further advances in surgical technology and innovation should also facilitate the adoption of surgical neurotization and other curative procedural interventions. As longer-term outcomes of subsequent trials are available for each of these treatments, an improved understanding of the optimal candidates and timing for each therapy should be cultivated. This may further underline the differences in pediatric and adult patients suffering from this disease or in congenital vs. acquired etiologies. Additional research into quality of life outcomes in these individuals will be necessary to tackle the complex psychosocial issues associated with NK. As potential treatment options are rapidly expanding, the ultimate goal will be to devise a patient-specific algorithm for achieving the best possible visual, functional, and anatomical results with each treatment.

Conflicts of Interest The authors report no conflicts of interest. The authors alone are responsible for the content and writing of the chapter.

Funding No funding sources were used to finance this work.

References

1. Jabbour S, Ashton C, Balal S, Kaye A, Ahmad S. The management of neurotrophic keratitis. Curr Opin Ophthalmol. 2021;32(4):362–8.
2. Dua HS, Said DG, Messmer EM, Rolando M, Benitez-Del-Castillo JM, Hossain PN, et al. Neurotrophic keratopathy. Prog Retin Eye Res. 2018;66:107–31.
3. Safi M, Rose-Nussbaumer J. Overview of neurotrophic keratopathy and a stage-based approach to its management. Eye Contact Lens. 2021;47(3):140–3.
4. Sacchetti M, Lambiase A. Diagnosis and management of neurotrophic keratitis. Clin Ophthalmol. 2014;8:571–9.
5. Scelfo C, Mantagos IS. Neurotrophic keratopathy in pediatric patients. Semin Ophthalmol. 2021;36(4):289–95.
6. Bonini S, Rama P, Olzi D, Lambiase A. Neurotrophic keratitis. Eye (Lond). 2003;17(8):989–95.
7. Heigle TJ, Pflugfelder SC. Aqueous tear production in patients with neurotrophic keratitis. Cornea. 1996;15(2):135–8.
8. Muller LJ, Marfurt CF, Kruse F, Tervo TM. Corneal nerves: structure, contents, and function. Exp Eye Res. 2003;76(5):521–42.
9. Marfurt CF, Cox J, Deek S, Dvorscak L. Anatomy of the human corneal innervation. Exp Eye Res. 2010;90(4):478–92.
10. Muller LJ, Vrensen GF, Pels L, Cardozo BN, Willekens B. Architecture of human corneal nerves. Invest Ophthalmol Vis Sci. 1997;38(5):985–94.

11. He J, Bazan NG, Bazan HE. Mapping the entire human corneal nerve architecture. Exp Eye Res. 2010;91(4):513–23.
12. Versura P, Giannaccare G, Pellegrini M, Sebastiani S, Campos EC. Neurotrophic keratitis: current challenges and future prospects. Eye Brain. 2018;10:37–45.
13. Kowtharapu BS, Stahnke T, Wree A, Guthoff RF, Stachs O. Corneal epithelial and neuronal interactions: role in wound healing. Exp Eye Res. 2014;125:53–61.
14. Nishida T. Neurotrophic mediators and corneal wound healing. Ocul Surf. 2005;3(4):194–202.
15. Mastropasqua L, Massaro-Giordano G, Nubile M, Sacchetti M. Understanding the pathogenesis of neurotrophic keratitis: the role of corneal nerves. J Cell Physiol. 2017;232(4):717–24.
16. Blanco-Mezquita T, Martinez-Garcia C, Proenca R, Zieske JD, Bonini S, Lambiase A, et al. Nerve growth factor promotes corneal epithelial migration by enhancing expression of matrix metalloprotease-9. Invest Ophthalmol Vis Sci. 2013;54(6):3880–90.
17. Ueno H, Ferrari G, Hattori T, Saban DR, Katikireddy KR, Chauhan SK, et al. Dependence of corneal stem/progenitor cells on ocular surface innervation. Invest Ophthalmol Vis Sci. 2012;53(2):867–72.
18. Qi H, Chuang EY, Yoon KC, de Paiva CS, Shine HD, Jones DB, et al. Patterned expression of neurotrophic factors and receptors in human limbal and corneal regions. Mol Vis. 2007;13:1934–41.
19. Belmonte C, Acosta MC, Gallar J. Neural basis of sensation in intact and injured corneas. Exp Eye Res. 2004;78(3):513–25.
20. Belmonte C, Nichols JJ, Cox SM, Brock JA, Begley CG, Bereiter DA, et al. TFOS DEWS II pain and sensation report. Ocul Surf. 2017;15(3):404–37.
21. Namavari A, Chaudhary S, Ozturk O, Chang JH, Yco L, Sonawane S, et al. Semaphorin 7a links nerve regeneration and inflammation in the cornea. Invest Ophthalmol Vis Sci. 2012;53(8):4575–85.
22. Saad S, Abdelmassih Y, Saad R, Guindolet D, Khoury SE, Doan S, et al. Neurotrophic keratitis: frequency, etiologies, clinical management and outcomes. Ocul Surf. 2020;18(2):231–6.
23. Mantelli F, Nardella C, Tiberi E, Sacchetti M, Bruscolini A, Lambiase A. Congenital corneal anesthesia and neurotrophic keratitis: diagnosis and management. Biomed Res Int. 2015;2015:805876.
24. Lambley RG, Pereyra-Munoz N, Parulekar M, Mireskandari K, Ali A. Structural and functional outcomes of anaesthetic cornea in children. Br J Ophthalmol. 2015;99(3):418–24.
25. Rosenberg ML. Congenital trigeminal anaesthesia. A review and classification. Brain. 1984;107(Pt 4):1073–82.
26. Morishige N, Morita Y, Yamada N, Nishida T, Sonoda KH. Congenital hypoplastic trigeminal nerve revealed by manifestation of corneal disorders likely caused by neural factor deficiency. Case Rep Ophthalmol. 2014;5(2):181–5.
27. Ohana M, Lipsker D, Chaigne D, Speeg-Schatz C, Sauer A. Unilateral ulceration of the cornea secondary to congenital trigeminal nerve agenesis. Eur J Ophthalmol. 2015;25(4):e35–7.
28. Ramaesh K, Stokes J, Henry E, Dutton GN, Dhillon B. Congenital corneal anesthesia. Surv Ophthalmol. 2007;52(1):50–60.
29. Masri A, Shboul M, Khasawneh A, Jadallah R, ALmustafa A, Escande-Beillard N, et al. Congenital insensitivity to pain with anhidrosis syndrome: a series from Jordan. Clin Neurol Neurosurg. 2020;189:105636.
30. John D, Thomas M, Jacob P. Neurotrophic keratitis and congenital insensitivity to pain with anhidrosis – a case report with 10-year follow-up. Cornea. 2011;30(1):100–2.
31. Jarade EF, El-Sheikh HF, Tabbara KF. Indolent corneal ulcers in a patient with congenital insensitivity to pain with anhidrosis: a case report and literature review. Eur J Ophthalmol. 2002;12(1):60–5.
32. Chotikavanich S, de Paiva CS, Li de Q, Chen JJ, Bian F, Farley WJ, et al. Production and activity of matrix metalloproteinase-9 on the ocular surface increase in dysfunctional tear syndrome. Invest Ophthalmol Vis Sci. 2009;50(7):3203–9.
33. Mackie LA. In: Fraunfelder FT, Roy FH, Grove J, editors. Neuroparalytic keratitis. 4th ed. Philadelphia: W. B. Saunders; 1995.

34. Mandahl A. Hypertonic saline test for ophthalmic nerve impairment. Acta Ophthalmol. 1993;71(4):556–9.
35. Golebiowski B, Papas E, Stapleton F. Assessing the sensory function of the ocular surface: implications of use of a non-contact air jet aesthesiometer versus the Cochet-Bonnet aesthesiometer. Exp Eye Res. 2011;92(5):408–13.
36. Belmonte C, Acosta MC, Schmelz M, Gallar J. Measurement of corneal sensitivity to mechanical and chemical stimulation with a CO2 esthesiometer. Invest Ophthalmol Vis Sci. 1999;40(2):513–9.
37. Cruzat A, Qazi Y, Hamrah P. In vivo confocal microscopy of corneal nerves in health and disease. Ocul Surf. 2017;15(1):15–47.
38. Al-Aqaba MA, Dhillon VK, Mohammed I, Said DG, Dua HS. Corneal nerves in health and disease. Prog Retin Eye Res. 2019;73:100762.
39. Hamrah P, Cruzat A, Dastjerdi MH, Pruss H, Zheng L, Shahatit BM, et al. Unilateral herpes zoster ophthalmicus results in bilateral corneal nerve alteration: an in vivo confocal microscopy study. Ophthalmology. 2013;120(1):40–7.
40. Hamrah P, Cruzat A, Dastjerdi MH, Zheng L, Shahatit BM, Bayhan HA, et al. Corneal sensation and subbasal nerve alterations in patients with herpes simplex keratitis: an in vivo confocal microscopy study. Ophthalmology. 2010;117(10):1930–6.
41. Linna TU, Vesaluoma MH, Perez-Santonja JJ, Petroll WM, Alio JL, Tervo TM. Effect of myopic LASIK on corneal sensitivity and morphology of subbasal nerves. Invest Ophthalmol Vis Sci. 2000;41(2):393–7.
42. Cruzat A, Schrems WA, Schrems-Hoesl LM, Cavalcanti BM, Baniasadi N, Witkin D, et al. Contralateral clinically unaffected eyes of patients with unilateral infectious keratitis demonstrate a sympathetic immune response. Invest Ophthalmol Vis Sci. 2015;56(11):6612–20.
43. Morishige N, Komatsubara T, Chikama T-i, Nishida T. Direct observation of corneal nerve fibres in neurotrophic keratopathy by confocal biomicroscopy. Lancet. 1999;354(9190):1613–4.
44. Cruzat A, Pavan-Langston D, Hamrah P. In vivo confocal microscopy of corneal nerves: analysis and clinical correlation. Semin Ophthalmol. 2010;25(5–6):171–7.
45. Giannaccare G, Pellegrini M, Taroni L, Bernabei F, Bolognesi F, Biglioli F, et al. Longitudinal morphometric analysis of sub-basal nerve plexus in contralateral eyes of patients with unilateral neurotrophic keratitis. Curr Eye Res. 2019;44(10):1047–53.
46. Parissi M, Karanis G, Randjelovic S, Germundsson J, Poletti E, Ruggeri A, et al. Standardized baseline human corneal subbasal nerve density for clinical investigations with laser-scanning in vivo confocal microscopy. Invest Ophthalmol Vis Sci. 2013;54(10):7091–102.
47. Yamazaki N, Kobayashi A, Yokogawa H, Ishibashi Y, Oikawa Y, Tokoro M, et al. In vivo imaging of radial keratoneuritis in patients with Acanthamoeba keratitis by anterior-segment optical coherence tomography. Ophthalmology. 2014;121(11):2153–8.
48. Mastropasqua L, Nubile M, Lanzini M, Calienno R, Dua HS. In vivo microscopic and optical coherence tomography classification of neurotrophic keratopathy. J Cell Physiol. 2019;234(5):6108–15.
49. Sacchetti M, Lambiase A, Cortes M, Sgrulletta R, Bonini S, Merlo D, et al. Clinical and cytological findings in limbal stem cell deficiency. Graefes Arch Clin Exp Ophthalmol. 2005;243(9):870–6.
50. Shtein RM, Shen JF, Kuo AN, Hammersmith KM, Li JY, Weikert MP. Autologous serum-based eye drops for treatment of ocular surface disease: a report by the American academy of ophthalmology. Ophthalmology. 2020;127(1):128–33.
51. Pan Q, Angelina A, Marrone M, Stark WJ, Akpek EK. Autologous serum eye drops for dry eye. Cochrane Database Syst Rev. 2017;2:CD009327.
52. Guadilla AM, Balado P, Baeza A, Merino M. Effectiveness of topical autologous serum treatment in neurotrophic keratopathy. Arch Soc Esp Oftalmol. 2013;88(8):302–6.
53. Ong ES, Jeng BH. Current and future therapies for persistent corneal epithelial defects and neurotrophic keratopathy. Curr Opin Ophthalmol. 2021;32(3):262–7.
54. Erdem E, Yagmur M, Harbiyeli I, Taylan-Sekeroglu H, Ersoz R. Umbilical cord blood serum therapy for the management of persistent corneal epithelial defects. Int J Ophthalmol. 2014;7(5):807–10.

55. Huang CT, Chu HS, Hung KC, Chen LW, Chen MY, Hu FR, et al. The effect of human platelet lysate on corneal nerve regeneration. Br J Ophthalmol. 2021;105(6):884–90.
56. Sanchez-Avila RM, Merayo-Lloves J, Riestra AC, Fernandez-Vega Cueto L, Anitua E, Begona L, et al. Treatment of patients with neurotrophic keratitis stages 2 and 3 with plasma rich in growth factors (PRGF-Endoret) eye-drops. Int Ophthalmol. 2018;38(3):1193–204.
57. Wrobel-Dudzinska D, Alio J, Rodriguez A, Suchodola-Ratajewicz E, Kosior-Jarecka E, Rymgayllo-Jankowska B, et al. Clinical efficacy of platelet-rich plasma in the treatment of neurotrophic corneal ulcer. J Ophthalmol. 2018;2018:3538764.
58. Yoon KC. Use of umbilical cord serum in ophthalmology. Chonnam Med J. 2014;50(3):82–5.
59. Balal S, Nitiahpapand R, Hassan A, Than J, Patel A, Kumar B, et al. Finger-prick autologous blood in the treatment of persistent corneal epithelial defects. Cornea. 2020;39(5):594–7.
60. Witsberger E, Schornack M. Scleral lens use in neurotrophic keratopathy: a review of current concepts and practice. Eye Contact Lens. 2021;47(3):144–8.
61. Reynolds SA, Kabat AG. Therapeutic options for the management of early neurotrophic keratopathy: a case report and review. Optometry. 2006;77(10):503–7.
62. Schornack MM, Pyle J, Patel SV. Scleral lenses in the management of ocular surface disease. Ophthalmology. 2014;121(7):1398–405.
63. Ling JD, Gire A, Pflugfelder SC. PROSE therapy used to minimize corneal trauma in patients with corneal epithelial defects. Am J Ophthalmol. 2013;155(4):615–9. 9.e1-2
64. Cressey A, Jacobs DS, Remington C, Carrasquillo KG. Improvement of chronic corneal opacity in ocular surface disease with prosthetic replacement of the ocular surface ecosystem (PROSE) treatment. Am J Ophthalmol Case Rep. 2018;10:108–13.
65. Kloek CE, Jeng-Miller KW, Jacobs DS, Dunn IF. Prosthetic replacement of the ocular surface ecosystem treatment of ocular surface disease after skull base tumor resection. World Neurosurg. 2018;110:e124–e8.
66. Ciralsky JB, Chapman KO, Rosenblatt MI, Sood P, Fernandez AG, Lee MN, et al. Treatment of refractory persistent corneal epithelial defects: a standardized approach using continuous wear PROSE therapy. Ocul Immunol Inflamm. 2015;23(3):219–24.
67. Weynes, et al. Scleral contact lenses as an alternative to tarsorrhaphy for the long-termmanagement of combined exposure and neurotrophic keratopathy. Cornea. 2013;
68. Grey F, Carley F, Biswas S, Tromans C. Scleral contact lens management of bilateral exposure and neurotrophic keratopathy. Cont Lens Anterior Eye. 2012;35(6):288–91.
69. Gelles JD, Bekerman VP, Greenstein SA, Shafiq M, Hersh PS. Descemetocele management with therapeutic scleral lens wear. Eye Contact Lens. 2021;47(5):314–6.
70. Geerling G, Joussen AM, Daniels JT, Mulholland B, Khaw PT, Dart JK. Matrix metalloproteinases in sterile corneal melts. Ann N Y Acad Sci. 1999;878:571–4.
71. Hahn JN, Kaushik DK, Mishra MK, Wang J, Silva C, Yong VW. Impact of minocycline on extracellular matrix metalloproteinase inducer, a factor implicated in multiple sclerosis immunopathogenesis. J Immunol. 2016;197(10):3850–60.
72. Ogut D, Reel B, Gonen Korkmaz C, Arun MZ, Cilaker Micili S, Ergur BU. Doxycycline down-regulates matrix metalloproteinase expression and inhibits NF-kappaB signaling in LPS-induced PC3 cells. Folia Histochem Cytobiol. 2016;54(4):171–80.
73. Dohlman TH, Singh RB, Dana R. Advances in the medical management of neurotrophic keratitis. Semin Ophthalmol. 2021;36(4):335–40.
74. Sheha H, Tighe S, Hashem O, Hayashida Y. Update on cenegermin eye drops in the treatment of neurotrophic keratitis. Clin Ophthalmol. 2019;13:1973–80.
75. Lambiase A, Rama P, Bonini S, Caprioglio G, Aloe L. Topical treatment with nerve growth factor for corneal neurotrophic ulcers. N Engl J Med. 1998;338(17):1174–80.
76. Ferrari MP, Mantelli F, Sacchetti M, Antonangeli MI, Cattani F, D'Anniballe G, et al. Safety and pharmacokinetics of escalating doses of human recombinant nerve growth factor eye drops in a double-masked, randomized clinical trial. BioDrugs. 2014;28(3):275–83.
77. Bonini S, Lambiase A, Rama P, Sinigaglia F, Allegretti M, Chao W, et al. Phase II randomized, double-masked, vehicle-controlled trial of recombinant human nerve growth factor for neurotrophic keratitis. Ophthalmology. 2018;125(9):1332–43.

78. Pflugfelder SC, Massaro-Giordano M, Perez VL, Hamrah P, Deng SX, Espandar L, et al. Topical recombinant human nerve growth factor (cenegermin) for neurotrophic keratopathy: a multicenter randomized vehicle-controlled pivotal trial. Ophthalmology. 2020;127(1):14–26.
79. Tan MH, Bryars J, Moore J. Use of nerve growth factor to treat congenital neurotrophic corneal ulceration. Cornea. 2006;25(3):352–5.
80. Pedrotti E, Bonetto J, Cozzini T, Fasolo A, Marchini G. Cenegermin in pediatric neurotrophic keratopathy. Cornea. 2019;38(11):1450–2.
81. Leto MG, Toro ME, Indemini PE, Fruttero C, Denina M, Dalmazzo C, et al. Pediatric use of recombinant human nerve growth factor 20 mug/ml eye drops (cenegermin) for bilateral neurotrophic keratopathy in congenital corneal anesthesia. Cornea. 2021;40(2):228–31.
82. Fausto R, Ceccuzzi R, Micheletti E, Clerici R, Riva I, Katsanos A, et al. A case report of pediatric neurotrophic keratopathy in pontine tegmental cap dysplasia treated with cenegermin eye drops. Medicine (Baltimore). 2020;99(30):e20816.
83. Papadopoulos K, Besgen V, Sekundo W. Successful treatment of a pediatric neurotrophic keratopathy with cenegermin. Cornea. 2021;40(4):516–8.
84. Hatcher JB, Soifer M, Morales NG, Farooq AV, Perez VL, Shieh C. Aftermarket effects of cenegermin for neurotrophic keratopathy in pediatric patients. Ocul Surf. 2021;21:52–7.
85. Josephy-Hernandez S, Jmaeff S, Pirvulescu I, Aboulkassim T, Saragovi HU. Neurotrophin receptor agonists and antagonists as therapeutic agents: an evolving paradigm. Neurobiol Dis. 2017;97(Pt B):139–55.
86. Sevik MO, Turhan SA, Toker E. Topical treatment of persistent epithelial defects with a matrix regenerating agent. J Ocul Pharmacol Ther. 2018;34(9):621–7.
87. Aifa A, Gueudry J, Portmann A, Delcampe A, Muraine M. Topical treatment with a new matrix therapy agent (RGTA) for the treatment of corneal neurotrophic ulcers. Invest Ophthalmol Vis Sci. 2012;53(13):8181–5.
88. Guerra M, Marques S, Gil JQ, Campos J, Ramos P, Rosa AM, et al. Neurotrophic keratopathy: therapeutic approach using a novel matrix regenerating agent. J Ocul Pharmacol Ther. 2017;33(9):662–9.
89. Cochener B, Zagnoli C, Hugny-Larroque C, Derrien S. Healing of resistant corneal neurotrophic ulcers using a matrix regenerating agent. J Fr Ophtalmol. 2019;42(2):159–65.
90. Pereira S, Resende R, Coelho P, Sampaio F. Matrix regenerating agent (RGTA) in a neurotrophic corneal ulcer. Cureus. 2020;12(10):e11167.
91. Salazar-Quiñones L, Molero-Senosiáin M, Aguilar-Munoa S, Gegúndez-Fernández JA, Díaz-Valle D, Muñoz-Hernández AM, et al. Management of corneal neurotrophic ulcers with Cacicol®-RGTA (ReGeneraTing agent): a case series. Arch Soc Esp Oftalmol. 2020;95(9):421–8.
92. Gumus K. On the horizon: biologics and nutrients for neurotrophic keratitis. Eye Contact Lens. 2021;47(3):154–6.
93. Sosne G. Thymosin beta 4 and the eye: the journey from bench to bedside. Expert Opin Biol Ther. 2018;18(sup1):99–104.
94. Dunn SP, Heidemann DG, Chow CY, Crockford D, Turjman N, Angel J, et al. Treatment of chronic nonhealing neurotrophic corneal epithelial defects with thymosin beta 4. Arch Ophthalmol. 2010;128(5):636–8.
95. Dunn SP, Heidemann DG, Chow CY, Crockford D, Turjman N, Angel J, et al. Treatment of chronic nonhealing neurotrophic corneal epithelial defects with thymosin beta4. Ann N Y Acad Sci. 2010;1194:199–206.
96. Sosne G, Rimmer D, Kleinman HK, Ousler G. Thymosin beta 4: a potential novel therapy for neurotrophic keratopathy, dry eye, and ocular surface diseases. Vitam Horm. 2016;102:277–306.
97. Qiu C, Coutinho P, Frank S, Franke S, Law LY, Martin P, et al. Targeting connexin43 expression accelerates the rate of wound repair. Curr Biol. 2003;13(19):1697–703.
98. Elbadawy HM, Mirabelli P, Xeroudaki M, Parekh M, Bertolin M, Breda C, et al. Effect of connexin 43 inhibition by the mimetic peptide Gap27 on corneal wound healing, inflammation and neovascularization. Br J Pharmacol. 2016;173(19):2880–93.

99. Ormonde S, Chou CY, Goold L, Petsoglou C, Al-Taie R, Sherwin T, et al. Regulation of connexin43 gap junction protein triggers vascular recovery and healing in human ocular persistent epithelial defect wounds. J Membr Biol. 2012;245(7):381–8.
100. Nagano T, Nakamura M, Nakata K, Yamaguchi T, Takase K, Okahara A, et al. Effects of substance P and IGF-1 in corneal epithelial barrier function and wound healing in a rat model of neurotrophic keratopathy. Invest Ophthalmol Vis Sci. 2003;44(9):3810–5.
101. Nakamura M, Kawahara M, Nakata K, Nishida T. Restoration of corneal epithelial barrier function and wound healing by substance P and IGF-1 in rats with capsaicin-induced neurotrophic keratopathy. Invest Ophthalmol Vis Sci. 2003;44(7):2937–40.
102. Yanai R, Nishida T, Chikama T, Morishige N, Yamada N, Sonoda KH. Potential new modes of treatment of neurotrophic keratopathy. Cornea. 2015;34(Suppl 11):S121–7.
103. Nishida T, Chikama T, Morishige N, Yanai R, Yamada N, Saito J. Persistent epithelial defects due to neurotrophic keratopathy treated with a substance p-derived peptide and insulin-like growth factor 1. Jpn J Ophthalmol. 2007;51(6):442–7.
104. Yamada N, Matsuda R, Morishige N, Yanai R, Chikama TI, Nishida T, et al. Open clinical study of eye-drops containing tetrapeptides derived from substance P and insulin-like growth factor-1 for treatment of persistent corneal epithelial defects associated with neurotrophic keratopathy. Br J Ophthalmol. 2008;92(7):896–900.
105. Tong CM, Iovieno A, Yeung SN. Topical insulin for neurotrophic corneal ulcers. Can J Ophthalmol. 2020;55(5):e170–e2.
106. Wang AL, Weinlander E, Metcalf BM, Barney NP, Gamm DM, Nehls SM, et al. Use of topical insulin to treat refractory neurotrophic corneal ulcers. Cornea. 2017;36(11):1426–8.
107. Galvis V, Nino CA, Tello A, Grice JM, Gomez MA. Topical insulin in neurotrophic keratopathy after resection of acoustic neuroma. Arch Soc Esp Oftalmol. 2019;94(2):100–4.
108. Fai S, Ahem A, Mustapha M, Mohd Noh UK, Bastion MC. Randomized controlled trial of topical insulin for healing corneal epithelial defects induced during vitreoretinal surgery in diabetics. Asia Pac J Ophthalmol (Phila). 2017;6(5):418–24.
109. Kim SY, Yang J, Lee YC. The effects of nicergoline on corneal nerve regeneration in rat corneas after photorefractive keratectomy. Curr Eye Res. 2011;36(1):29–33.
110. Zhang X, Muddana S, Kumar SR, Burton JN, Labroo P, Shea J, et al. Topical pergolide enhance corneal nerve regrowth following induced corneal abrasion. Invest Ophthalmol Vis Sci. 2020;61(1):4.
111. Lee YC, Kim SY. Treatment of neurotrophic keratopathy with nicergoline. Cornea. 2015;34(3):303–7.
112. Daniele S, Gilbard JP, Schepens CL. Treatment of persistent epithelial defects in neurotrophic keratitis with epidermal growth factor: a preliminary open study. Graefes Arch Clin Exp Ophthalmol. 1992;230(4):314–7.
113. Moon HS, Li L, Yoon HJ, Ji YS, Yoon KC. Effect of epidermal growth factor ointment on persistent epithelial defects of the cornea. BMC Ophthalmol. 2020;20(1):147.
114. Sacchetti M, Lambiase A. Neurotrophic factors and corneal nerve regeneration. Neural Regen Res. 2017;12(8):1220–4.
115. Gumus K. Topical coenzyme Q10 eye drops as an adjuvant treatment in challenging refractory corneal ulcers: a case series and literature review. Eye Contact Lens. 2017;43(2):73–80.
116. Postorino EI, Rania L, Aragona E, Mannucci C, Alibrandi A, Calapai G, et al. Efficacy of eyedrops containing cross-linked hyaluronic acid and coenzyme Q10 in treating patients with mild to moderate dry eye. Eur J Ophthalmol. 2018;28(1):25–31.
117. Guo C, Li M, Qi X, Lin G, Cui F, Li F, et al. Intranasal delivery of nanomicelle curcumin promotes corneal epithelial wound healing in streptozotocin-induced diabetic mice. Sci Rep. 2016;6:29753.
118. Mertsch S, Neumann I, Rose C, Schargus M, Geerling G, Schrader S. The effect of Rho Kinase inhibition on corneal nerve regeneration in vitro and in vivo. Ocul Surf. 2021;22:213–23.
119. Passidomo F, Pignatelli F, Addabbo G, Costagliola C. Topical liposomal ozonated oil in complicated corneal disease: a report on three clinical cases. Int Med Case Rep J. 2021;14:327–32.

120. Higuchi A, Ueno R, Shimmura S, Suematsu M, Dogru M, Tsubota K. Albumin rescues ocular epithelial cells from cell death in dry eye. Curr Eye Res. 2007;32(2):83–8.
121. Schargus M, Kohlhaas M, Unterlauft JD. Treatment of severe ocular surface disorders with albumin eye drops. J Ocul Pharmacol Ther. 2015;31(5):291–5.
122. Khan RS, Dine K, Bauman B, Lorentsen M, Lin L, Brown H, et al. Intranasal delivery of a novel amnion cell secretome prevents neuronal damage and preserves function in a mouse multiple sclerosis model. Sci Rep. 2017;7:41768.
123. Grinblat GA, Khan RS, Dine K, Wessel H, Brown L, Shindler KS. RGC neuroprotection following optic nerve trauma mediated by intranasal delivery of amnion cell secretome. Invest Ophthalmol Vis Sci. 2018;59(6):2470–7.
124. Murri MS, Moshirfar M, Birdsong OC, Ronquillo YC, Ding Y, Hoopes PC. Amniotic membrane extract and eye drops: a review of literature and clinical application. Clin Ophthalmol. 2018;12:1105–12.
125. Shayan Asl N, Nejat F, Mohammadi P, Nekoukar A, Hesam S, Ebrahimi M, et al. Amniotic membrane extract eye drop promotes limbal stem cell proliferation and corneal epithelium healing. Cell J. 2019;20(4):459–68.
126. Park GW, Heo J, Kang JY, Yang JW, Kim JS, Kwon KD, et al. Topical cell-free conditioned media harvested from adipose tissue-derived stem cells promote recovery from corneal epithelial defects caused by chemical burns. Sci Rep. 2020;10(1):12448.
127. Bandeira F, Goh TW, Setiawan M, Yam GH, Mehta JS. Cellular therapy of corneal epithelial defect by adipose mesenchymal stem cell-derived epithelial progenitors. Stem Cell Res Ther. 2020;11(1):14.
128. Cosar CB, Cohen EJ, Rapuano CJ, Maus M, Penne RP, Flanagan JC, et al. Tarsorrhaphy: clinical experience from a cornea practice. Cornea. 2001;20(8):787–91.
129. Naik MN, Gangopadhyay N, Fernandes M, Murthy R, Honavar SG. Anterior chemodenervation of levator palpebrae superioris with botulinum toxin type-A (Botox) to induce temporary ptosis for corneal protection. Eye (Lond). 2008;22(9):1132–6.
130. Schilimow A, Wiechens B. Botulinum toxin A induced protective ptosis for the treatment of recurrent epithelial defects in neurotrophic keratopathy. Ophthalmologe. 2017;114(8):745–7.
131. Trinh T, Mimouni M, Santaella G, Cohen E, Chan CC. Surgical management of the ocular surface in neurotrophic keratopathy: amniotic membrane, conjunctival grafts, lid surgery, and neurotization. Eye Contact Lens. 2021;47(3):149–53.
132. Gris O, Wolley-Dod C, Guell JL, Tresserra F, Lerma E, Corcostegui B, et al. Histologic findings after amniotic membrane graft in the human cornea. Ophthalmology. 2002;109(3):508–12.
133. Khokhar S, Natung T, Sony P, Sharma N, Agarwal N, Vajpayee RB. Amniotic membrane transplantation in refractory neurotrophic corneal ulcers: a randomized, controlled clinical trial. Cornea. 2005;24(6):654–60.
134. Suri K, Kosker M, Raber IM, Hammersmith KM, Nagra PK, Ayres BD, et al. Sutureless amniotic membrane ProKera for ocular surface disorders: short-term results. Eye Contact Lens. 2013;39(5):341–7.
135. Chen HJ, Pires RT, Tseng SC. Amniotic membrane transplantation for severe neurotrophic corneal ulcers. Br J Ophthalmol. 2000;84(8):826–33.
136. Park JH, Jeoung JW, Wee WR, Lee JH, Kim MK, Lee JL. Clinical efficacy of amniotic membrane transplantation in the treatment of various ocular surface diseases. Cont Lens Anterior Eye. 2008;31(2):73–80.
137. Solomon A, Meller D, Prabhasawat P, John T, Espana EM, Steuhl KP, et al. Amniotic membrane grafts for nontraumatic corneal perforations, descemetoceles, and deep ulcers. Ophthalmology. 2002;109(4):694–703.
138. Rock T, Bartz-Schmidt KU, Rock D. Management of a neurotrophic deep corneal ulcer with amniotic membrane transplantation in a patient with functional monocular vision: a case report. Medicine (Baltimore). 2017;96(50):e8997.
139. Gundersen T. Conjunctival flaps in the treatment of corneal disease with reference to a new technique of application. AMA Arch Ophthalmol. 1958;60(5):880–8.

140. Zemba M, Stamate AC, Tataru CP, Branisteanu DC, Balta F. Conjunctival flap surgery in the management of ocular surface disease (review). Exp Ther Med. 2020;20(4):3412–6.
141. Alino A. Conjunctival flaps. Ophthalmology. 1998;105(6):1120–3.
142. Margo JA, Jeng BH. Corneal transplantation in the setting of neurotrophic keratopathy – risks and considerations. Curr Ophthalmol Rep. 2017;5(1):14–22.
143. Terzis JK, Dryer MM, Bodner BI. Corneal neurotization: a novel solution to neurotrophic keratopathy. Plast Reconstr Surg. 2009;123(1):112–20.
144. Giannaccare G, Bolognesi F, Pellegrini M, Spena R, Allevi F, Marchetti C, et al. Corneal neurotization: a game-changing surgical procedure for neurotrophic keratopathy. Cornea. 2021;
145. Leyngold I, Weller C, Leyngold M, Tabor M. Endoscopic corneal neurotization: technique and initial experience. Ophthalmic Plast Reconstr Surg. 2018;34(1):82–5.
146. Elbaz U, Bains R, Zuker RM, Borschel GH, Ali A. Restoration of corneal sensation with regional nerve transfers and nerve grafts: a new approach to a difficult problem. JAMA Ophthalmol. 2014;132(11):1289–95.
147. Jowett N, Pineda IR. Corneal neurotisation by great auricular nerve transfer and scleral-corneal tunnel incisions for neurotrophic keratopathy. Br J Ophthalmol. 2019;103(9):1235–8.
148. Liu CY, Arteaga AC, Fung SE, Cortina MS, Leyngold IM, Aakalu VK. Corneal neurotization for neurotrophic keratopathy: review of surgical techniques and outcomes. Ocul Surf. 2021;20:163–72.
149. Weis E, Rubinov A, Al-Ghoul AR, Yau FM. Sural nerve graft for neurotrophic keratitis: early results. Can J Ophthalmol. 2018;53(1):24–9.
150. Fogagnolo P, Giannaccare G, Bolognesi F, Digiuni M, Tranchina L, Rossetti L, et al. Direct versus indirect corneal neurotization for the treatment of neurotrophic keratopahty: a multicenter prospective comparative study. Am J Ophthalmol. 2020;
151. Wolkow N, Habib LA, Yoon MK, Freitag SK. Corneal neurotization: review of a new surgical approach and its developments. Semin Ophthalmol. 2019;34(7–8):473–87.
152. Park JK, Charlson ES, Leyngold I, Kossler AL. Corneal neurotization: a review of pathophysiology and outcomes. Ophthalmic Plast Reconstr Surg. 2020;36(5):431–7.
153. Catapano J, Antonyshyn K, Zhang JJ, Gordon T, Borschel GH. Corneal neurotization improves ocular surface health in a novel rat model of neurotrophic keratopathy and corneal neurotization. Invest Ophthalmol Vis Sci. 2018;59(11):4345–54.
154. Fung SSM, Catapano J, Elbaz U, Zuker RM, Borschel GH, Ali A. In vivo confocal microscopy reveals corneal reinnervation after treatment of neurotrophic keratopathy with corneal neurotization. Cornea. 2018;37(1):109–12.
155. Koaik M, Baig K. Corneal neurotization. Curr Opin Ophthalmol. 2019;30(4):292–8.
156. Dana R, Farid M, Gupta PK, Hamrah P, Karpecki P, McCabe CM, et al. Expert consensus on the identification, diagnosis, and treatment of neurotrophic keratopathy. BMC Ophthalmol. 2021;21(1):327.
157. Di Zazzo A, Coassin M, Varacalli G, Galvagno E, De Vincentis A, Bonini S. Neurotrophic keratopathy: pros and cons of current treatments. Ocul Surf. 2019;17(4):619–23.
158. Trinh T, Santaella G, Mimouni M, Mednick Z, Cohen E, Sorkin N, et al. Assessment of response to multimodal management of neurotrophic corneal disease. Ocul Surf. 2021;19:330–5.

Dry Eye Disease

5

Swati Singh, Anahita Kate, and Sayan Basu

Summary Points

1. Direct assessment of the lacrimal glands, OCT meibography, and tear film biomarkers are the newer diagnostic techniques for dry eye disease (DED).
2. There is renewed interest in minor salivary gland transplantation as a treatment for severe aqueous deficiency DED.
3. Fecal microbial transplant, mesenchymal stem cell therapy, and biomaterials are emerging on the horizon as potential future therapies for DED.

5.1 Introduction

The Dry Eye Workshop (DEWS II) consensus defines dry eye disease (DED) as a multifactorial disease of the ocular surface characterized by a loss of homeostasis of the tear film and accompanied by ocular symptoms in which *tear film instability* and *hyperosmolarity*, *ocular surface inflammation* and *damage*, and *neurosensory*

S. Singh
Prof. Krothapalli Ravindranath Ophthalmic Research Biorepository, L V Prasad Eye Institute, Hyderabad, Telangana, India
e-mail: swatisingh@lvpei.org

A. Kate
Shantilal Shanghvi Cornea Institute, L V Prasad Eye Institute, Vijayawada, Andhra Pradesh, India
e-mail: dranahitakate@lvpei.org

S. Basu (✉)
Prof. Krothapalli Ravindranath Ophthalmic Research Biorepository, L V Prasad Eye Institute, Hyderabad, Telangana, India

Centre for Ocular Regeneration, Prof. Brien Holden Centre for Eye Research (BHERC), L V Prasad Eye Institute, Hyderabad, Telangana, India
e-mail: sayanbasu@lvpei.org

H. N. Saeed, R. B. Singh (eds.), *Corneal Disorders*, Current Practices in Ophthalmology, https://doi.org/10.1007/978-981-96-5294-5_5

abnormalities play etiological roles [1, 2]. The heterogeneous nature and multifactorial etiology of DED make it challenging to restore the disturbed tear film dynamics [2]. The management of DED often includes artificial lubricants, anti-inflammatory drugs like cyclosporine or corticosteroids, and topical and oral therapies targeting meibomian glands. Curative therapies targeting ocular surface inflammation and improving tear or meibum secretion using nanoparticle drug delivery systems are upcoming newer experimental treatment options. The current chapter reviewed the recent literature on severe DED from 2019 to 2022. The diagnosis and management advances described in this chapter include those that were introduced after the 2017 Tear Film and Ocular Surface Society DEWS II report for severe DED.

5.2 Novel Diagnostic Approaches in Dry Eye Disease

5.2.1 Lacrimal Gland Evaluation

The lacrimal gland contributes to the aqueous component of the tear film via secretory ductules opening onto the conjunctiva overlying the palpebral lobe. Traditionally, lacrimal gland activity has been assessed using Schirmer's test, tear film height or area measurement, and tear osmolarity. These techniques are an indirect way of measuring the lacrimal gland function. It is essential to distinguish between aqueous deficient dry eye (ADDE) and evaporative dry eye (EDE) and to detect the presence of ADDE in mixed dry eye. It is also important to recognize the variable lacrimal gland involvement in different forms of ADDE, such as that in Sjogren's syndrome (SS) and cicatrizing ocular surface disorders like Stevens-Johnson syndrome (SJS), as described below.

5.2.1.1 Morphology of the Palpebral Lobe

The palpebral lobes of the lacrimal gland can be visualized with a slit-lamp biomicroscope, and the following parameters can be characterized: their size (exposed area of the gland), shape (convex or flat), and overlying conjunctival appearance (presence of engorged vessels, whitish areas of subepithelial scarring, or symblepharon). The normal palpebral lobe is a convex shaped, raised pinkish lobular structure in the superotemporal fornix with overlying normal conjunctiva, extending up to or beyond the lateral canthus. The lobe looks visibly smaller in patients with SS compared to the palpebral lobe of a normal lacrimal gland [3]. In addition, there can be whitish areas of subepithelial scarring involving the palpebral lobe and inflamed overlying conjunctiva in cases of SS. When compared to palpebral lobes in eyes with SS, those of SJS patients have a higher proportion of lobes with a flat contour, subepithelial scarring with or without symblepharon (Fig. 5.1), and engorged conjunctival vessels [3].

5.2.1.2 Secretory Activity of the Lacrimal Gland

Direct assessment of tear secretion (DATS) from the palpebral lobe can demonstrate significant differences between meibomian gland dysfunction (MGD), ADDE, and

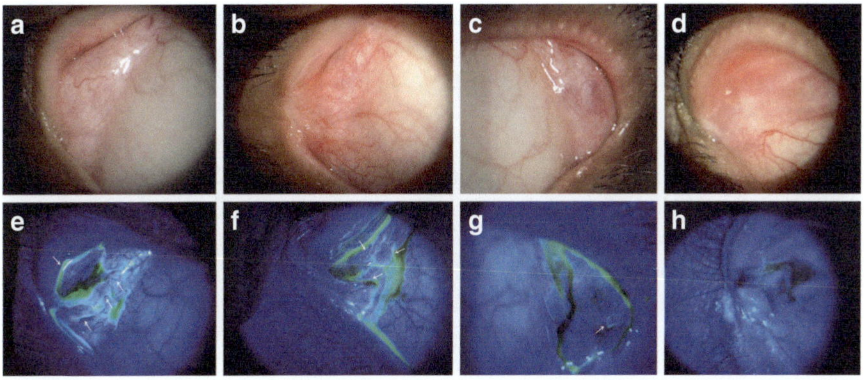

Fig. 5.1 Dynamic assessment of tear secretion in a normal eye and in eyes with evaporative and aqueous deficient dry eye. (**a**) and (**e**) Right palpebral lobe of a young, healthy individual (Schirmer's 27 mm) shows four secretory openings (marked with arrow) with a tear flow rate of 0.91 μl/min. (**b**) and (**f**) Right palpebral lobe of a patient with evaporative dry eye (Schirmer's 24 mm); the lobe is normal appearing and has a tear flow rate of 0.82 μl/min across three secretory openings. (**c**) and (**g**) Left palpebral lobe of a patient with Sjogren's syndrome (Schirmer's 2.0 mm); there is some flattening of the contour and presence of only one secretory opening. (**d**) and (**h**) Right palpebral lobe of a patient with Stevens-Johnson syndrome; there is obliteration of the superotemporal fornix, loss of the normal contour and appearance of the palpebral lobe, and no secretory openings

dry eye in cicatrizing conjunctivitis (CC). DATS was first introduced in 1986 and later quantified by Kim et al. [4, 5]. The technique was further refined by Singh et al., where etiology-based differences in tear flow among various subtypes of DED were analyzed [6].

During DATS, the lacrimal gland's palpebral lobe is exposed by instructing the patient to look inferonasally while the upper eyelid is lifted in the superotemporal direction. Under a slit-lamp biomicroscope, a dry 2% sodium fluorescein ophthalmic strip is applied onto the exposed palpebral lobe. The fluorescein strip should be applied only to the exposed gland area, and the slit-lamp light turned on and focused onto the gland while subjects are looking in the opposite direction to avoid reflex secretion. The washout of fluorescein stain across the applied area is recorded using a slit-lamp mounted camera for a few seconds in eyes with some secretory activity to a maximum of 20 s in eyes with no secretion. An image snapshot is captured at the end of 1 s from the recorded video. One can measure tear flow rate per lobe and ductule (calculated in μL/min), and the time lag between the application of the fluorescein strip and the first appearance of secretory activity (in seconds). Using Image J software, the washout area per ductule (in mm^2/s) is marked from the snapshot captured at 1 s. The total calculated area across all ductules is converted into volume per minute by multiplying it by 10 μm × 60 s as 10 μm is the assumed tear film thickness. Singh et al. found the median number of ductules per lobe to be 4 in normal eyes (range 3–5), 3 in EDE (3–6), 1 in SS (0–3), and 0 in the CC eyes (0–3) [6]. The median tear flow rate per lobe in CC (0.00 μL/min) and SS (0.21 μL/min) was significantly less than that of normal lobes (1.05 μL/min) and EDE (0.99 μL/min).

The tear flow rate differed significantly between SS and CC groups (Fig. 5.1). The maximum time lag occurred in the CC group (median, 20 s), followed by the SS group (median, 1.5 s), whereas the EDE group had a similar time lag (<1 s) to normal glands [6].

5.2.1.3 Minor Salivary Gland Evaluation in a Dry Eye Clinic

As will be described in Sect. 5.3, minor salivary gland transplantation (MSGT) can be employed in severe DED. Evaluation of minor salivary gland secretion can be done in a fashion similar to that of the lacrimal gland.

In a series by Singh et al., the mean salivary flow rate from the lower labial MSGs of normal individuals showed a decade-wise decline (2.7 ± 0.29 μl/min, 2.6 ± 0.39 μl/min, 2.3 ± 0.6 μl/min, 1.9 ± 0.95 μl/min) with a similar trend for the number of secreting MSG openings (38.7, 37.2, 30, 22) [7]. The mean lower labial salivary flow rate in the SS group was 0.5 ± 0.28 μl/min and 2.0 ± 0.95 μl/ min in the SJS group. When compared to normal, SS patients had a significant reduction in the flow rate; however, it was not significant for the SJS group. Also, MSG flow rate and Schirmer's values did not show any correlation in SS or SJS patients [7].

5.2.2 Meibomian Gland Imaging

Meibography has been in use for the past 20 years for imaging structural alterations in the meibomian glands (MG), while in vivo confocal microscopy (IVCM) and optical coherence tomography-meibography (OCT-M) have been recently explored for MG imaging [8]. OCT-M is a customized system with a long coherence swept laser source of a wavelength of 1300 nm and can provide a three-dimensional image of MGs. OCT-M gives a better overview and resolution of dark drop-out areas but has limited availability [8]. IVCM can provide acinar details similar to histological methods, but evaluation needs to be standardized with image analysis software.

5.2.3 Inflammatory Biomarkers in the Tear Film

Tear film biomarkers, which can be used for early DED diagnosis and predicting disease severity, can have different origins: lacrimal gland, meibomian gland, ocular surface, epithelial cells, stromal immune cells, etc. As inflammation is central to DED pathogenesis, numerous biomarkers that have been explored in experimental studies are lactoferrin, lysozyme, epidermal growth factor and aquaporin 5, cytokines such as IL-17, IL-22, IL-6, IL-10, IL-4, IFN-γ, and TNF-α, chemokines like CXCL9, CXCL10, CXCL11, IL-1Ra, CCL5/RANTES, and fractalkine/ CX3CL and matrix metalloproteinases [9]. Commercially, MMP 9 levels (InflammaDry®, Quidel, San Diego, CA, USA) have been used as an indicator for DED severity but is nonspecific and can be elevated in other diseases such as microbial keratitis and acne rosacea [10]. Tests to detect the other markers have not been approved for commercial use in human DED diagnosis and management. SDS-agarose gel electrophoresis of tear proteins (Hyrys-Hydrasys System, Serbia; Evry, France) has been suggested as a potential routine test in the diagnosis and management of DED in high-risk groups such as computer users, contact lens wearers, glaucoma patients, and those undergoing cataract surgery [11]. Identification of specific tear biomarkers in DED is promising but requires standardized reporting and analysis across studies.

5.2.4 Immunological Tests for Sjogren's Syndrome

Recently, three novel autoantibodies (anti-salivary gland protein 1 (SP1), anti-carbonic anhydrase 6 (CA6), and anti-parotid secretory protein (PSP)) have been identified for the early diagnosis of SS in dry eye patients. In a series of 136 patients with dry eye and suspected SS, 41% tested positive for at least one of the above autoantibodies, and anti-CA6 was associated with a severe form of DED [12]. However, multicentric and large population-based studies are needed to determine if these antibodies aid in recognizing SS in its early stage and if they have any prognostic role.

5.3 Novel Interventions in Severe Dry Eye Disease

Thus far, the treatment of DED has been largely palliative, providing symptomatic relief while rarely addressing the underlying cause of DED. The highly differential etiology and pathomechanisms in the spectrum of DED make it difficult to formulate a customized approach to DED management as a whole.

5.3.1 Minor Salivary Gland Transplantation

Patients with severe DED, defined as a Schirmer I value of <2 mm, ocular discomfort that cannot be controlled by conservative means, and patient dependency on frequent lubricant use, are the candidates for minor salivary gland transplantation (MSGT).[13] Such conditions may be observed in the following disorders:

1. Stevens-Johnson syndrome or chronic cicatrizing conjunctivitis.
2. Severe dry eye secondary to chemical injury.
3. Acquired alacrima following excision of lacrimal gland tumor.
4. Congenital alacrima.

MSGT was first performed in 1997 by Murube et al. [13]. The transplantation of MSGs either into the upper or lower conjunctival fornix results in an average improvement of 2 to 4 mm in Schirmer values [14]. MSGT reduces dependency on topical lubricants, but improvement in visual acuity is inconsistent, and outcomes of corneal transplantation following MSGT are unsatisfactory. However, it remains a useful technique in symptomatic relief of dry eye. The technique of performing MSGT is described below.

5.3.1.1 Host Bed Preparation

The conjunctival fornices or palpebral, tarsal, or bulbar conjunctiva can be used as the recipient site for the MSGT. When placed in the upper or lower fornix, Muller's muscle or the lower eyelid retractors are used as a graft anchoring site, respectively. An incision is placed along the tarsal border for a length of 2.5 cm to expose the Muller's muscle or the lower eyelid retractors. The superior bulbar conjunctiva has also been used as a graft anchoring site where the graft is anchored onto the superior rectus muscle. For this, an initial conjunctival incision is made 10 mm superior to the limbus, and the superior rectus is bridled to ensure muscle-to-muscle apposition. This technique claims to retain the submucosal connective tissue niche that might act as a barrier against inflammatory graft infiltration, while muscle-to-muscle apposition may improve graft revascularization.

5.3.1.2 Graft Harvesting

The graft can be harvested from the upper lip, lower lip, or buccal mucosa. The lower labial mucosa is preferred due to ease of manipulation and exposure. Though preoperative evaluation of MSGs is not routinely performed when selecting the donor site, our group developed a simple fluorescein-based technique for evaluating and selecting the area containing MSGs with maximal flow. The published studies usually rely on no history of dry mouth and normal oral mucosa appearance, and sometimes evaluation by oral and maxillofacial surgeon has also been performed. A simple test that can be used in clinics for subjectively measuring MSG flow rates is by applying moistened fluorescein strips over the labial mucosa. The secretory openings of MSGs are visualized as fluorescein washout areas, and the area of maximal washout can be selected for graft harvesting. The usual graft harvest site is slightly lateral to the lip's midline and includes mucosa, submucosa, and glands. Fusiform grafts of 15 mm in length and 5–6 mm in thickness are dissected out [15]. Grafts longer than 20 mm have also been transplanted but have been associated with higher rates of partial necrosis [8, 16].

Sant'Anna et al. demonstrated a technique for symblepharon correction while performing MSGT using the split-thickness labial mucosa from the graft as a conjunctival replacement [17]. The rest of the graft tissue (submucosa with MSGs, without muscle) was then transplanted into the upper fornix. Electrocautery can also be used to reduce bleeding while making full thickness incisions through the labial mucosa down to the muscle. The donor site can be sutured or left to heal via secondary intention; it typically epithelializes in 2–3 weeks.

5.3.1.3 Graft Suturing

The graft is anchored to the adjacent conjunctiva using 8–0 or 7–0 absorbable (e.g., polyglactin) sutures either in a continuous or interlocking manner. Additional quilt sutures apposing the graft to Muller's muscle or the superior rectus or sclera are recommended. A bandage contact lens can be placed to avoid chances of a corneal abrasion from sutures or graft. The graft should start showing signs of vascularization within 1 week and salivary secretion by 2 weeks. The activity of transplanted MSGs can be evaluated with the help of the fluorescein ophthalmic strip, as shown in Fig. 5.2.

5.3.1.4 Outcomes and Complications

The reported mean improvement in tear production following MSGT is 2–3 mm (range, 0–8 mm) [13, 14, 17]. Ocular surface changes in the form of reduction in corneal staining, and neovascularization scores are variable with improvement having been demonstrated in 29–100% of eyes from baseline across studies [14, 17]. Changes in visual acuity are not uniformly reported across studies; however, a few studies have reported improvement in 42–64% of eyes [14]. Complications associated with MSGT are transient labial hypoesthesia (~64%), granuloma formation at the donor site, and graft necrosis [13, 14].

5.3.2 Recent Meta-analysis on Existing Therapies

5.3.2.1 Meibomian Gland Therapies

A Cochrane review on the efficacy of intense pulsed light (IPL) for MGD revealed the available data to be of low or very low quality [18]. The effect of IPL on relieving blocked meibomian glands or on ocular surface staining and tear breakup time values is uncertain, though many studies have reported improvement in subjective symptom scores. Reported complications of IPL therapy are uveitis, iris atrophy, pupillary defects, photophobia, pain, and corneal pigment deposition [18].

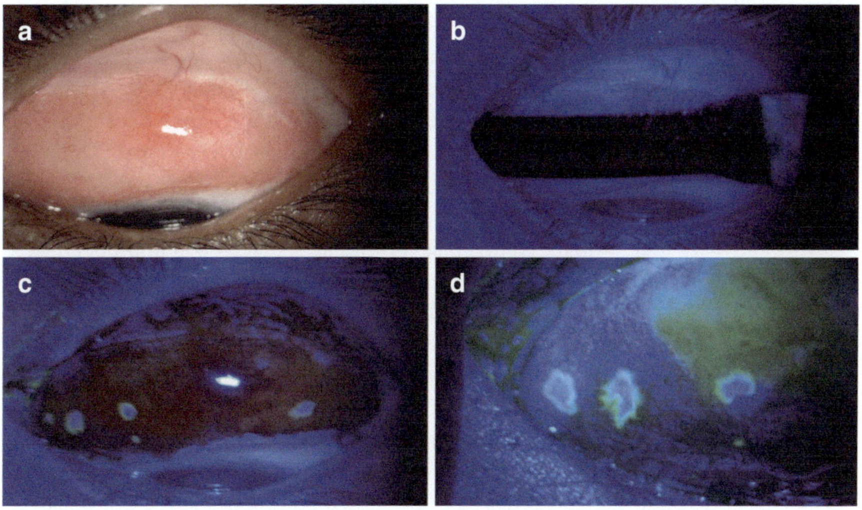

Fig. 5.2 Assessment of secretory activity of transplanted minor salivary gland transplant. (**a**) MSGT into the superior bulbar conjunctiva. (**b**) A moistened fluorescein strip is applied onto the graft surface. (**c**) and (**d**) Three secretory openings can be visualized (Reproduced with permission from Singh S, Basu S. Functional Assessment of Transplanted Minor Salivary Glands. Cornea. 2020;39(8):e21-e22.)

Meta-analysis of thermal pulsation therapy for MGD revealed significant improvements in subjective and objective parameters at 1 month compared to warm compresses alone; however, only the subjective improvements persisted up to 3 months posttreatment [19]. Randomized controlled trials (RCT) are ongoing for evaluating these modalities [20]. Intraductal probing for relieving ductal obstruction in MGD patients has shown benefits in uncontrolled studies, but no improvement was observed in placebo-controlled RCTs [21].

5.3.2.2 Cyclosporin A for Dry Eye Disease

Cyclosporin A 0.05% (CsA) has long been used as an anti-inflammatory therapy for DED. A recently conducted meta-analysis that included 11 RCTs demonstrated CsA to have greater efficacy when compared to lubricants alone. However, the adverse effects were also found to be greater when compared to lubricants [21]. These included burning or stinging sensation in the eyes, ocular pain, itching, redness, and, rarely, blurred vision and swollen eyelids [22, 23]. CsA has also shown some efficacy in MGD with reduction in lid margin inflammation and improved TBUT values [23].

5.3.3 Recent Molecular Therapies

Lifitegrast, an inhibitor of the interaction between intercellular adhesion molecule 1 (ICAM-1) and lymphocyte function–associated antigen 1 (LFA-1), results in T cell activation and migration to target tissues [23]. Lifitegrast ophthalmic solution 5% (XiidraTM, Novartis, USA) was approved in 2016 to treat DED [24] and has shown to provide a significant reduction in ocular staining and dry eye symptomatology after 12 weeks of therapy [25]. The observed ocular adverse effects include eye irritation, dysgeusia, and reduced visual acuity, whereas very rare non-ocular side effects include anaphylactic reactions, bronchospasm, respiratory distress, pharyngeal edema, and utricaria [26]. Although the efficacy of the medication on mild to moderate dry eye disease has been established, its effects on severe DED are unknown [24].

A loteprednol etabonate ophthalmic suspension 0.25% (Eysuvis, Kala Pharmaceuticals) that utilizes Kala Pharmaceuticals' mucus-penetrating particle drug delivery technology has shown promising effects in DED. Animal studies have shown enhanced penetration of loteprednol etabonate into the ocular surface, and the STRIDE 1,2,3 trials have reported a significant reduction in conjunctival hyperemia and improved ocular discomfort within 2 weeks of initiation of the dosage schedule [27].

OTX-101 0.09% (CEQUA, Sun Pharmaceutical Industries, Inc., Cranbury, NJ), a nanomicellar formulation of CsA, achieves better ocular penetration than 0.05% CsA ophthalmic emulsion [28]. An RCT has shown that 84 days of OTX-101 therapy results in a significant reduction in conjunctival and corneal staining with an increase in Schirmer values. The reported side effects are instillation site pain (typically mild in severity) in 24.2%, conjunctival hyperemia in 8.1%, and blepharitis in

1.3% of patients [28]. Other CsA formulations under trial are a 0.1% CsA nonaqueous solution (CyclASol; Novaliq, Heidelberg, Germany) and voclosporin ophthalmic solution 0.2% (Lupkynis; Aurinia Pharmaceuticals Inc. USA). Other molecules under investigation are an siRNA inhibitor, a nonspecific kinase inhibitor, the tear protein lacritin, and TNF inhibitors.

Omega fatty acids in the form of omega-3 (alpha-linolenic acid, eicosapentaenoic acid, and docosahexaenoic acid) and omega-6 supplements have been studied extensively for their effects on DED, especially in the MGD subgroup. A recently conducted meta-analysis of 34 published RCTs concluded that there may be a role for long-chain omega-3 supplementation in managing dry eye disease, but the evidence was uncertain and inconsistent [29]. There was probable evidence for improvement in dry eye symptoms, but the same could not be assessed for outcomes relating to ocular surface staining, Schirmer's test, or TBUT. When omega-3 supplements were withdrawn from patients who were using them for 12 months, no differences in outcomes (OSDI, ocular staining) were observed compared to those who continued using omega-3 supplements [30]. There have been few advancements in the management of MGD, and this is an area of active research.

5.3.4 Cell-Based Therapy

Mesenchymal stem cells (MSCs) have immunomodulatory properties, low immunogenicity, and are easily accessible [31]. These features make them suitable for treating autoimmune DED. The sources of MSCs include the human umbilical cord, adipose tissue, bone marrow, and lacrimal gland [31–33].

A few studies in rabbit autoimmune DED models have demonstrated decreased infiltration of CD3+ or CD4+ cells in the lacrimal gland after MSC injection [32]. The MSCs upregulate regulatory T cells and the production of anti-inflammatory cytokines, which curb the inflammatory cascade in DED. There are very few clinical trials that have evaluated the effect of MSCs in human DED. In vitro experiments have shown an immunomodulatory effect of MSCs on T cells obtained from primary Sjogren's syndrome patients. When these were co-cultured with MSCs, they were upregulated into regulatory T cells, which are anti-inflammatory [32]. Allogeneic adipose–derived and bone marrow–derived MSC therapies have been studied in graft versus host disease patients. Weng et al. found that DED signs and symptoms improved in 54.5% of patients following intravenous injection of human bone marrow–derived MSCs [31]. In another study of aqueous deficient DED, direct transconjunctival injection of allogeneic adipose–derived MSCs in seven patients reduced OSDI scores, tear osmolarity, and corneal staining, and improved tear stability and secretion [33]. Injection of MSCs into the lacrimal gland of aqueous deficient dry eyes might act as a future disease-modifying therapy for severe dry eyes.

5.3.5 Diagnosis and Treatment for Neuropathic Pain in Dry Eye

The concurrent presence of neuropathic pain (NP) with DED should be suspected in cases where the ocular symptoms are disproportionate to the signs. These symptoms are usually very similar to those of DED and include grittiness, burning sensation, and ocular pain, especially in response to light or wind, etc. [34]. The diagnosis of this entity is primarily clinical at this point and can be supported by a few ancillary tests. The Ocular Pain Assessment Survey (OPAS) is a reliable and validated questionnaire aimed at the objective evaluation of corneal pain and its effect on quality of life [35]. It can be used as a baseline measurement to understand the severity of ocular pain and its aggravating factors. It can also be used to monitor the therapeutic effect of various treatment modalities. Since the primary underlying pathology in eyes with NP is damage to corneal nerves due to several inflammatory mediators, an objective assessment of the function of corneal nerves will help support the diagnosis of NP. This can be done via confocal microscopic examination of corneal nerves in addition to evaluation of tear film production, break-up time, and osmolarity, or direct assessment of corneal sensation. The use of the Cochet-Bonnet esthesiometer provides insight into the function of the Aδ mechanoreceptor fibers, while the Belmonte esthesiometer assesses chemical, thermal, and mechanical thresholds and helps evaluate both the Aδ and C fibers [36]. Although there is an overlap of IVCM features of DED and NP in terms of decreased nerve density, branching, and increased dendritiform cell density, the presence of microneuromas is considered to be specific to NP [37].

NP can be caused by pathologic changes in the peripheral nervous system (corneal nerves), central nervous system (spinal cord/brain), or a combination of both [34, 38]. Instillation of topical proparacaine 0.5% helps in delineating these two entities and is essential as the treatment instituted will differ based on the location of the pathology [36]. If the patient experiences complete relief of pain with the instillation of the anesthetic drop, then the involvement is primarily in the peripheral system. These cases are managed with topical anti-inflammatory agents (topical steroids, cyclosporine A, and tacrolimus) to address the inflammatory component and autologous serum tears (AST), which contain several trophic factors that stimulate nerve regeneration. The use of AST is associated with an improvement in signs and symptoms of DED along with an increase in corneal nerve density and resolution of microneuromas on IVCM [36]. The logistics involved in procuring blood for AST and its storage limit its use.

If there is partial or no response to proparacaine, then a central or combined etiology must be suspected. These cases will require a neurology consult for systemic evaluation and for the initiation of oral medications, which is usually done in a stepwise fashion [36, 38, 39]. First-line agents used include tricyclic antidepressants (nortriptyline) and anticonvulsants (carbamazepine), followed by opioid agonists (tramadol) and antagonists (naltrexone). Calcium channel α2δ ligands (gabapentin) are reserved as third-line agents. These medications require close monitoring and dose titration to improve the side effect profile. Both types of NP (peripheral and central) require management of ocular comorbidities such as the DED and MGD, along with lifestyle modifications such as the increased ratio of omega 3:omega 6 fatty acids and regular exercise.

5.4 Future Directions

There is significant research being done targeting severe DED. The ongoing mesenchymal stem cell trials, investigations into gut microbiome alteration, and biomaterial research may produce potential therapies in the future. A few of these therapies are discussed below.

5.4.1 Fecal Microbial Transplant

Gut dysbiosis, i.e., altered fecal flora, has been implicated in immune-mediated DED like SS, where transplantation of healthy fecal flora per rectum in ten individuals resulted in an altered gut microbiome profile at 3 months. Improvement in DED symptoms was reported by 50% of individuals [40]. This potential intervention is still in a preliminary stage, and the optimal route for microbiome transfer is yet to be determined. Also, changes induced in the population of immune cells of the ocular surface following microbiome transfer need to be studied further.

5.4.2 Biomaterials for Dry Eye

An ideal biomaterial for DED treatment is one that increases drug residence duration on the ocular surface without extreme fluctuations in drug concentration and is free of drug-related side effects. Nanostructured ophthalmic products currently marketed for the treatment of DED are Cequa® (Sun Pharma, Mumbai, India), Cyclokat® (preservative-free 0.1% CsA cationic emulsion), Lacrisek® (Vitamin A, Vitamin E liposomal spray), and Artelac Rebalance® (hyaluronic acid, vitamin B12 and viscoelactor eye drops) [40–42]. These nanoformulations have shown good efficacy in mild to moderate DED, but not severe DED. Other biomaterials like hydrogels or drug eluting contact lenses have shown promise in DED animal models; however, trials involving human participants are yet to occur.

5.5 Conclusions

Severe DED is difficult to manage and existing treatment options are palliative. The direct assessment of lacrimal gland in severe DED patients can be a helpful aid in determining the exact etiology of DED. Minor salivary gland transplantation may be useful in severe DED, but topical lubricants are still needed after surgery. Future potential therapies should target reversal of the disease process or regeneration of the lacrimal glands. Trials involving MSCs, bioengineered lacrimal glands, and biomaterials appear promising for DED treatment.

References

1. Craig JP, Nichols KK, Akpek EK, et al. TFOS DEWS II definition and classification report. Ocul Surf. 2017;15:276–83. https://doi.org/10.1016/j.jtos.2017.05.008.
2. Wolffsohn JS, Arita R, Chalmers R, et al. TFOS DEWS II diagnostic methodology report. Ocul Surf. 2017;15:539–74. https://doi.org/10.1016/j.jtos.2017.05.001.
3. Singh S, Shanbhag SS, Basu S. Palpebral lobe of the human lacrimal gland: morphometric analysis in normal versus dry eyes. Br J Ophthalmol. 2021;105:1352–7. https://doi.org/10.1136/bjophthalmol-2020-316929.
4. Bron AJ. Lacrimal streams: the demonstration of human lacrimal fluid secretion and the lacrimal ductules. Br J Ophthalmol. 1986;70:241–5. https://doi.org/10.1136/bjo.70.4.241.
5. Kim EC, Doh SH, Chung SY, et al. Direct visualization of aqueous tear secretion from lacrimal gland. Acta Ophthalmol. 2017;95:e314–22. https://doi.org/10.1111/aos.13335.
6. Singh S, Shanbhag SS, Basu S. Tear secretion from the lacrimal gland: variations in normal versus dry eyes. Br J Ophthalmol. 2021;106:772. https://doi.org/10.1136/bjophthalmol-2020-318159.
7. Singh S, Basu S. A novel diagnostic technique of measuring labial minor salivary gland secretions using sodium fluorescein dye: implications for patients with dry eyes. Semin Ophthalmol. 2021;37:1–6. https://doi.org/10.1080/08820538.2021.1926518.
8. Fineide F, Arita R, Utheim TP. The role of meibography in ocular surface diagnostics: a review. Ocul Surf. 2021;19:133–44. https://doi.org/10.1016/j.jtos.2020.05.004.
9. Roda M, Corazza I, Bacchi Reggiani ML, et al. Dry eye disease and tear cytokine levels–a meta-analysis. Int J Mol Sci. 2020;21:E3111. https://doi.org/10.3390/ijms21093111.
10. Pinto-Fraga J, Enríquez-de-Salamanca A, Calonge M, et al. Severity, therapeutic, and activity tear biomarkers in dry eye disease: an analysis from a phase III clinical trial. Ocul Surf. 2018;16:368–76. https://doi.org/10.1016/j.jtos.2018.05.001.
11. Chiva A. Agarose gel electrophoresis of joint fluid using Hyrys-Hydrasys SEBIA system as a new prognostic tool for periprosthetic osteolysisin revision arthroplasty. J Med Life. 2013;6:249–53.
12. Karakus S, Baer AN, Akpek EK. Clinical correlations of novel autoantibodies in patients with dry eye. J Immunol Res. 2019;2019:7935451. https://doi.org/10.1155/2019/7935451.
13. Geerling G, Raus P, Murube J. Minor salivary gland transplantation. Dev Ophthalmol. 2008;41:243–54. https://doi.org/10.1159/000131093.
14. Vazirani J, Bhalekar S, Amescua G, et al. Minor salivary gland transplantation for severe dry eye disease due to cicatrising conjunctivitis: multicentre long-term outcomes of a modified technique. Br J Ophthalmol. 2020;105:1485. https://doi.org/10.1136/bjophthalmol-2020-316611.
15. Su J-Z, Wang Z, Liu X-J, et al. Use of saliva flow rate measurement in minor salivary glands autotransplantation for treatment of severe dry eye disease. Br J Ophthalmol. 2021;106:902. https://doi.org/10.1136/bjophthalmol-2020-317552.
16. Singh S, Basu S, Geerling G. Salivary gland transplantation for dry eye disease: Indications, techniques, and outcomes. Ocul Surf. 2022. [Ahead of print];26:53.
17. AEBPP S'A, Hazarbassanov RM, de Freitas D, et al. Minor salivary glands and labial mucous membrane graft in the treatment of severe symblepharon and dry eye in patients with Stevens-Johnson syndrome. Br J Ophthalmol. 2012;96:234–9. https://doi.org/10.1136/bjo.2010.199901.
18. Cote S, Zhang AC, Ahmadzai V, et al. Intense pulsed light (IPL) therapy for the treatment of meibomian gland dysfunction. Cochrane Database Syst Rev. 2020;3:CD013559. https://doi.org/10.1002/14651858.CD013559.

19. Pang S-P, Chen Y-T, Tam K-W, et al. Efficacy of vectored thermal pulsation and warm compress treatments in meibomian gland dysfunction: a meta-analysis of randomized controlled trials. Cornea. 2019;38:690–7. https://doi.org/10.1097/ICO.0000000000001907.
20. Sabeti S, Kheirkhah A, Yin J, et al. Management of meibomian gland dysfunction: a review. Surv Ophthalmol. 2020;65:205–17. https://doi.org/10.1016/j.survophthal.2019.08.007.
21. Magno M, Moschowits E, Arita R, et al. Intraductal meibomian gland probing and its efficacy in the treatment of meibomian gland dysfunction. Surv Ophthalmol. 2021;66:612–22. https://doi.org/10.1016/j.survophthal.2020.11.005.
22. Tuan H-I, Chi S-C, Kang Y-N. An updated systematic review with meta-analysis of randomized trials on topical cyclosporin a for dry-eye disease. Drug Des Devel Ther. 2020;14:265–74. https://doi.org/10.2147/DDDT.S207743.
23. Prabhasawat P, Tesavibul N, Mahawong W. A randomized double-masked study of 0.05% cyclosporine ophthalmic emulsion in the treatment of meibomian gland dysfunction. Cornea. 2012;31:1386–93. https://doi.org/10.1097/ICO.0b013e31823cc098.
24. Sheppard JD, Torkildsen GL, Lonsdale JD, et al. Lifitegrast ophthalmic solution 5.0% for treatment of dry eye disease: results of the OPUS-1 phase 3 study. Ophthalmology. 2014;121:475–83. https://doi.org/10.1016/j.ophtha.2013.09.015.
25. Abidi A, Shukla P, Ahmad A. Lifitegrast: a novel drug for treatment of dry eye disease. J Pharmacol Pharmacother. 2016;7:194–8. https://doi.org/10.4103/0976-500X.195920.
26. Tauber J, Karpecki P, Latkany R, et al. Lifitegrast ophthalmic solution 5.0% versus placebo for treatment of dry eye disease: results of the randomized phase III OPUS-2 study. Ophthalmology. 2015;122:2423–31. https://doi.org/10.1016/j.ophtha.2015.08.001.
27. Korenfeld M, Nichols KK, Goldberg D, et al. Safety of KPI-121 ophthalmic suspension 0.25% in patients with dry eye disease: a pooled analysis of 4 multicenter, randomized, vehicle-controlled studies. Cornea. 2021;40:564–70. https://doi.org/10.1097/ICO.0000000000002452.
28. Goldberg DF, Malhotra RP, Schechter BA, et al. A phase 3, randomized, double-masked study of OTX-101 ophthalmic solution 0.09% in the treatment of dry eye disease. Ophthalmology. 2019;126:1230–7. https://doi.org/10.1016/j.ophtha.2019.03.050.
29. Downie LE, Ng SM, Lindsley KB, et al. Omega-3 and omega-6 polyunsaturated fatty acids for dry eye disease. Cochrane Database Syst Rev. 2019;12:CD011016. https://doi.org/10.1002/14651858.CD011016.pub2.
30. Hussain M, Shtein RM, Pistilli M, et al. The dry eye assessment and management (DREAM) extension study – a randomized clinical trial of withdrawal of supplementation with omega-3 fatty acid in patients with dry eye disease. Ocul Surf. 2020;18:47–55. https://doi.org/10.1016/j.jtos.2019.08.002.
31. Weng J, He C, Lai P, et al. Mesenchymal stromal cells treatment attenuates dry eye in patients with chronic graft-versus-host disease. Mol Ther. 2012;20:2347–54. https://doi.org/10.1038/mt.2012.208.
32. Liu Y, Li C, Wang S, et al. Human umbilical cord mesenchymal stem cells confer potent immunosuppressive effects in Sjögren's syndrome by inducing regulatory T cells. Mod Rheumatol. 2021;31:186–96. https://doi.org/10.1080/14397595.2019.1707996.
33. Møller-Hansen M, Larsen A-C, Toft PB, et al. Safety and feasibility of mesenchymal stem cell therapy in patients with aqueous deficient dry eye disease. Ocul Surf. 2021;19:43–52. https://doi.org/10.1016/j.jtos.2020.11.013.
34. Rosenthal P, Borsook D. Ocular neuropathic pain. Br J Ophthalmol. 2016;100:128–34. https://doi.org/10.1136/bjophthalmol-2014-306280.
35. Qazi Y, Hurwitz S, Khan S, et al. Validity and reliability of a novel ocular pain assessment survey (OPAS) in quantifying and monitoring corneal and ocular surface pain. Ophthalmology. 2016;123:1458–68. https://doi.org/10.1016/j.ophtha.2016.03.006.
36. Dieckmann G, Goyal S, Hamrah P. Neuropathic corneal pain: approaches for management. Ophthalmology. 2017;124:S34–47. https://doi.org/10.1016/j.ophtha.2017.08.004.
37. Moein H-R, Akhlaq A, Dieckmann G, et al. Visualization of microneuromas by using in vivo confocal microscopy: an objective biomarker for the diagnosis of neuropathic corneal pain? Ocul Surf. 2020;18:651–6. https://doi.org/10.1016/j.jtos.2020.07.004.

38. Galor A, Moein H-R, Lee C, et al. Neuropathic pain and dry eye. Ocul Surf. 2018;16:31–44. https://doi.org/10.1016/j.jtos.2017.10.001.
39. Galor A, Levitt RC, Felix ER, et al. Neuropathic ocular pain: an important yet underevaluated feature of dry eye. Eye (Lond). 2015;29:301–12. https://doi.org/10.1038/eye.2014.263.
40. Watane A, Cavuoto KM, Rojas M, et al. Fecal microbial transplant in individuals with immune-mediated dry eye. Am J Ophthalmol. 2021;S0002-9394(21):00348–2. https://doi.org/10.1016/j.ajo.2021.06.022.
41. Goldberg DF, Malhotra RP, Schechter BA, Justice A, Weiss SL, Sheppard JD. A phase 3, randomized, double-masked study of OTX-101 ophthalmic solution 0.09% in the treatment of dry eye disease. Ophthalmology. 2019;126:1230. https://doi.org/10.1016/j.ophtha.2019.03.050.
42. Gorantla S, Rapalli VK, Waghule T, Singh PP, Dubey SK, Saha RN, Singhvi G. Nanocarriers for ocular drug delivery: current status and translational opportunity. RSC Adv. 2020;10:27835.

Limbal Stem Cell Deficiency

6

Neeraj S. Chawla, Abdelrahman M. Elhusseiny, and Ali R. Djalilian

6.1 Introduction

The limbus is a highly complex ocular structure located at the junction between the cornea and sclera. The limbal niche is a specialized microenvironment deep in the basal epithelium that houses a distinct population of limbal epithelial stem cells (LESCs). LESCs are unipotent adult stem cells that closely interact with surrounding structures, including a unique extracellular matrix (ECM) and densely innervated and vascularized stroma [1]. These interactions collectively serve to ensure the lifelong maintenance of mature corneal epithelium and barrier integrity between the cornea and conjunctival epithelium—functions vital for the preservation of ocular surface health and vision [2, 3]. Injury to the limbal niche can disturb the LESCs and their normal physiologic function, leading to limbal stem cell deficiency (LSCD) [4].

This chapter serves as an overview of the recent advances in diagnosing and managing LSCD.

N. S. Chawla · A. R. Djalilian (✉)
Department of Ophthalmology and Visual Sciences, Illinois Eye and Ear Infirmary, University of Illinois at Chicago, Chicago, IL, USA
e-mail: nchawla2@uic.edu; adjalili@uic.edu

A. M. Elhusseiny
Department of Ophthalmology and Visual Sciences, Illinois Eye and Ear Infirmary, University of Illinois at Chicago, Chicago, IL, USA

Department of Ophthalmology, Harvey and Bernice Jones Eye Institute, University of Arkansas, Little Rock, AR, USA
e-mail: Amelhusseiny@uams.edu

H. N. Saeed, R. B. Singh (eds.), *Corneal Disorders*, Current Practices in Ophthalmology, https://doi.org/10.1007/978-981-96-5294-5_6

6.2 Anatomy

Nestled within the undulating folds of the palisades of Vogt, the limbal niche is a multicellular microenvironment that supports the healthy function of LESCs [4]. Beyond its ECM and dense neurovascular supply, the limbal niche contains immune cells, signaling molecules, mesenchymal stem cells (MSCs), soluble factors, melanocytes, and other niche cells [1, 5]. LESCs can effectively proliferate, differentiate, and migrate to maintain corneal epithelial homeostasis by interacting with these complex structural and molecular components [4, 6, 7]. Maturation of the corneal epithelium thus occurs along a pathway that extends from the limbus to the central cornea [8].

Unlike other stem cell niches of the human body, the limbal niche can be directly visualized through noninvasive in vivo imaging techniques such as in vivo laser scanning confocal microscopy (IVCM) or anterior segment optical coherence tomography (AS-OCT). These advanced imaging modalities continue to aid in the growing bank of knowledge, diagnostic accuracy, and overall monitoring of LSCD.

6.3 Etiology and Pathophysiology

The dysfunction or absence of LESCs results in LSCD, a disease process characterized by the inability of corneal epithelial regeneration accompanied by secondary conjunctival growth over the cornea. From a pathophysiology standpoint, LSCD involves dysregulated inflammation and impaired wound healing—factors that collectively impair normal limbal niche function [9, 10]. Therefore, it is imperative to identify the underlying cause and degree of LESC failure to develop an effective and targeted treatment plan.

The underlying etiologies of LSCD include genetic deficiencies, autoimmune processes, severe infections, traumatic insults, and other exposure-related causes [11–13]. Globally, severe corneal chemical and thermal injury account for at least two-thirds of LSCD cases that ultimately necessitate stem cell transplantation [12, 14]. Other causes of direct damage include contact lens wear, a history of multiple ocular surgeries involving the limbus, and preservatives such as benzalkonium chloride–containing eye drops [15–17]. In addition, certain medications, such as mitomycin-C (MMC), 5-fluorouracil (5-FU), hydroxyurea, and hydroxycarbamides may also exert toxic effects [18]. The most common genetic cause of LSCD is congenital PAX6-related aniridia. Immune-related causes include Stevens-Johnson syndrome/toxic epidermal necrolysis, mucous membrane pemphigoid, severe atopic and vernal keratoconjunctivitis, and graft-versus-host disease [18–24]. Additional risk factors for developing LSCD include concurrent ocular surface disease, eyelid abnormalities, chemotherapy, tumor cell invasion, and chronic inflammation [11].

6.4 Diagnosis

The diagnosis of LSCD is a multistep process that often includes a careful history, slit-lamp examination with fluorescein staining, cellular sampling and analysis, and anterior segment imaging. Based on the clinical presentation, LSCD can then be categorized into three stages based on corneal and limbal involvement (Table 6.1), as outlined by a global consensus recently devised by an international working group [14]. The accurate staging of LSCD is an important guide for therapeutic management and surgical planning.

6.4.1 Presenting Symptoms

Patients presenting with LSCD often exhibit symptoms related to impaired epithelial wound healing. These may include recurrent ocular discomfort and/or pain, irritation, foreign body sensation, decreased vision, photophobia, excessive tearing, chronic redness, and blepharospasm [14, 25–27]. However, it is important to note that patients may be asymptomatic when the disease is mild or in its early stages.

6.4.2 Physical Examination

Slit-lamp examination with fluorescein staining helps determine if there is an absence of healthy corneal epithelium and/or presence of conjunctival cells on the cornea (conjunctivalization) [11, 14, 26]. Fluorescein staining can aid in the differentiation between the normal and abnormal corneal epithelium and identify the distribution of epithelial cell change, especially when viewing the ocular surface under cobalt blue light. Conjunctival epithelium typically appears thinner, hazy, and irregular, is more permeable than healthy corneal epithelium due to a lack of tight junctions, and may exhibit abnormal delayed staining that lasts longer than 10 min [2, 14]. In early LSCD, these changes are more likely to be observed in the superior cornea. Corneal conjunctivalization may constitute a mixture of metaplastic corneal

Table 6.1 Staging criteria for limbal stem cell deficiency (LSCD) based on clinical presentation [14]

		Subdivision		
Stage	Defining feature	A	B	C
I	Central 5 mm zone of the cornea spared	Under 50% of limbus affected	50% or more of limbus affected (but less than 100%)	100% of limbus affected
II	Central 5 mm zone of the cornea affected	Under 50% of limbus affected	50% or more of limbus affected	–
III	Entire corneal surface affected	–	–	–

and conjunctival epithelium or conjunctival epithelium alone and may include evidence of neovascularization in more severe cases [14].

Fluorescein staining patterns often become more apparent and diffuse as the disease progresses (Fig. 6.1). In milder cases, curve-like punctate or linear granular staining may be observed in the affected sector [11]. With increased corneal conjunctivalization, various findings such as a dull light reflex, irregular, and hazy, opaque epithelial change, superficial vascularization, a peripheral corneal pannus, and loss or flattening of the limbal palisades of Vogt may be observed [14, 26]. However, note that the latter finding is nonspecific since it may also be age related. In severe cases, the abnormal epithelium often spreads spirally, giving rise to an irregular whorl-like epitheliopathy or vortex keratopathy. Additional signs of advanced disease include subepithelial fibrosis or fibrovascular pannus, diffuse corneal stromal scarring, neovascularization, persistent or recurrent epithelial defects, and corneal melting or perforation [11, 14].

6.4.3 Cellular Sampling

The global consensus endorses adjunctive measures in diagnosing LSCD, especially since epithelial changes may be subtle and nonspecific when relying on slit-lamp examination and fluorescein staining alone. Various methods of cellular sampling exist. This includes impression cytology, which harvests cells from the superficial epithelium, or cellular scraping, which also samples cells from deeper epithelial layers. Furthermore, tissue biopsy or surgical tissue excision, though more invasive, can accurately reveal anatomic changes to the ocular surface [14].

Impression cytology—often considered the gold-standard diagnostic test for LSCD—is a minimally invasive and well-established method of cellular sampling [11]. After instilling topical anesthesia, a filter paper composed of nitrocellulose acetate, cellulose acetate, or Biopore (Millipore Corp, Bedford, MA, USA) membrane is placed on the cornea for a few seconds and then removed for analysis [14]. This method can evaluate corneal conjunctivalization by detecting the presence of goblet cell markers. In addition, impression cytology can also monitor the restoration of the normal corneal phenotype following limbal transplantation [14].

The number of harvested cells and overall sensitivity of impression cytology depends on numerous factors. This includes filter pore size, sampling material, amount of pressure applied on the filter, and degree of conjunctivalization, since the retrieval of conjunctival cells is typically easier than that of corneal epithelial cells [11, 14].

Fig. 6.1 Slit-lamp examination in eyes presenting varying degrees of limbal stem cell deficiency (LSCD). (**a**) Healthy eye under bright light (left) and blue cobalt filter (right). (**b**) Mild LSCD, with unremarkable findings under bright light (left), but with superior linear granular fluorescein staining (right). (**c**) Moderate LSCD, showing a sectoral irregular epithelial reflex with opacification (left) and well-demarcated fluorescein staining that involves the visual axis (right). (**d**) Severe LSCD, with diffuse epithelial opacification and corneal haze (left) and diffuse irregular whorl-like fluorescein staining (right). (*Illustration with permission from Bonnet* et al. [11])

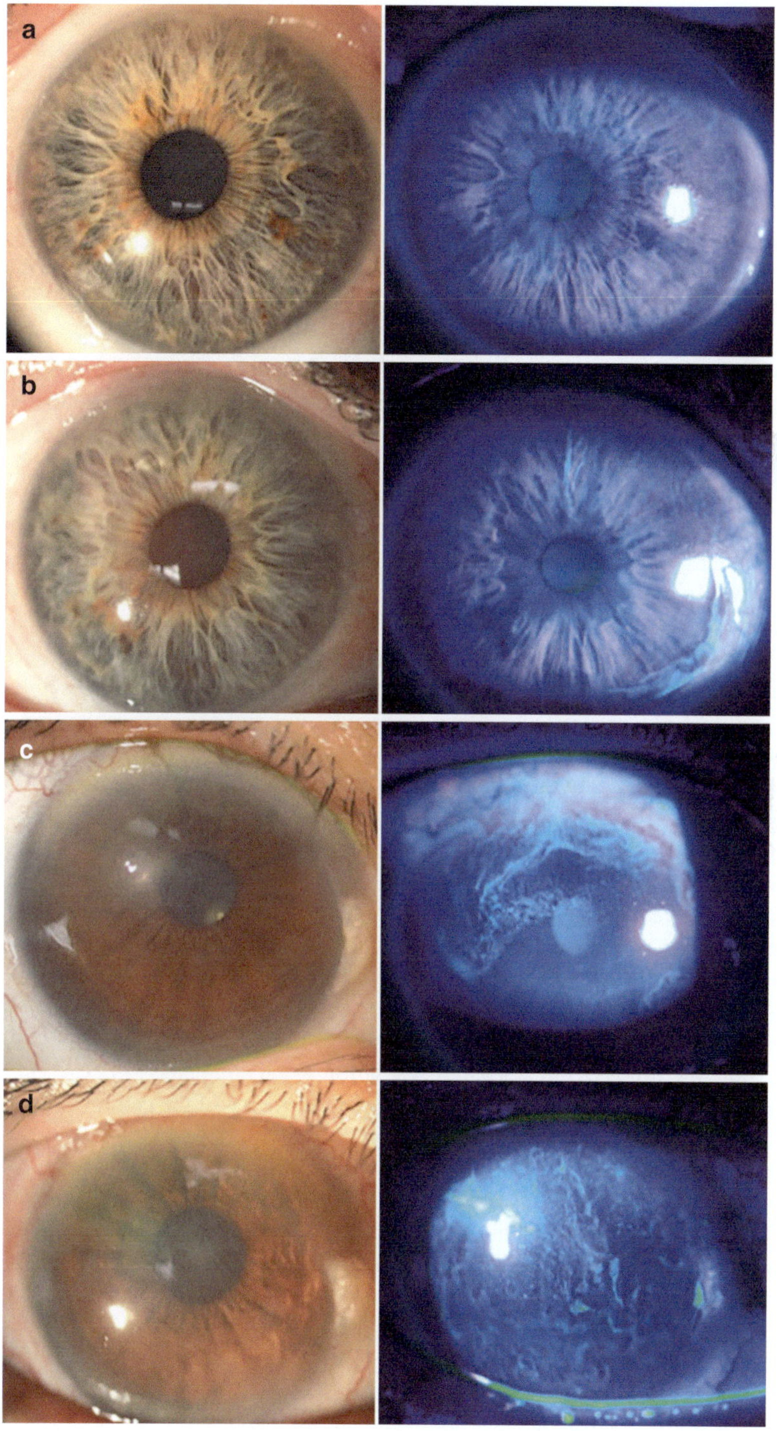
a
b
c
d

Additionally, the location and size of sampling is especially important when the LSCD is sectoral rather than diffuse [11]. Due to these potential sources of sampling bias, impression cytology does not aid in the quantitative staging of LSCD.

Samples from impression cytology or cellular scraping are traditionally stained with either periodic acid-Schiff stain or hematoxylin and eosin. These conventional histochemistry techniques help detect the presence of goblet cells on the cornea [11]. Though this finding can confirm the diagnosis of LSCD, a negative result does not rule out LSCD since goblet cells may be absent when a concurrent ocular surface condition, such as keratinization, is also present [14]. For these reasons, immunohistochemistry is now commonly performed instead since it can detect intracellular conjunctival cell proteins, such as cytokeratins and other secreted proteins normally expressed in conjunctival epithelial cells and goblet cells [11, 14]. Finally, reverse transcription-polymerase chain reaction (RT-PCR) is a highly sensitive method of detecting specific conjunctival markers that is starting to gain recognition [14].

6.4.4 Diagnostic Imaging

Advanced in vivo imaging techniques, including IVCM, AS-OCT, and AS-OCT angiography (AS-OCTA), are especially useful in the staging of LSCD. They are also recognized as diagnostic adjuncts that do not require the removal of corneal epithelium for analysis, unlike cellular sampling techniques. If imaging is not available and LSCD is suspected, referral to a well-equipped eye care center should be considered.

IVCM is a technique that shares a high degree of concordance with impression cytology in diagnosing LSCD [14, 26]. IVCM distinguishes between the presence of corneal, conjunctival, and limbal epithelium based on cellular morphology and can also detect the presence of goblet cells. Additionally, IVCM can identify microstructural limbal changes typical of LSCD, such as epithelial thinning and reduced subbasal nerve plexus and basal cell density [28]. Through these many functions, not only is IVCM useful in diagnosing and staging LSCD, but it can also help monitor disease progression and treatment response [11, 14, 28].

AS-OCT is an alternative imaging technique that provides a larger field of view (including the limbus), but at a lower resolution when compared to IVCM. In addition, AS-OCT provides three-dimensional measurements of the central corneal and limbal epithelial thickness [29]. This is useful since LSCD eyes typically exhibit a significant reduction of limbal epithelium thickness and a greater degree of variability in central corneal thickness. AS-OCT can also measure pannus depth and detect the loss of stromal undulations and loss of clear transition between corneal and conjunctival epithelium [29, 30]. Furthermore, AS-OCT helps diagnose LSCD when other complex ocular surface diseases are present, such as squamous neoplasia [14, 29].

AS-OCT angiography (AS-OCTA) provides direct volumetric analysis of corneal microvasculature. It works by detecting changes in signals produced by red blood cell motion through sequential scans at the same site [29]. AS-OCTA can determine the degree of vascular extension over the cornea and vascular thickness from the most superficial to the deepest corneal vessel [29, 30]. However, it is important to note that corneal neovascularization does not always reliably quantify disease severity since this can be a nonspecific ocular surface finding [11].

6.5 Management

The current therapeutic approach for LSCD consists of two overarching goals: (1) directly repopulate LESCs and (2) restore the limbal niche over the long term (Fig. 6.2) [25]. Management strategy depends on the underlying cause(s), laterality and severity of disease, the quantity of functioning residual LESCs, clinical disease course, patient preferences, and available resources for treatment. The decision-making process should also include consideration of fibrovascular pannus and the extent of corneal stromal scarring. In 2019, Deng et al. published the first global consensus for the stepwise medical and surgical management of LSCD [31].

Treatment often begins with optimizing the ocular surface, which includes controlling comorbidities and emphasizing avoidance of contributive factors such as contact lens wear or preservative-containing eye drops. Management of comorbid conditions includes adequate immunosuppression for autoimmune disease and chronic inflammatory processes as well as aggressive lubrication, punctal occlusion, and autologous serum tears for dry eye disease and exposure keratopathy. In severe concurrent dry eyes, surgical procedures such as tarsorrhaphy or canthoplasty can further optimize the ocular surface [31].

Like many other ocular pathologies, the initial treatment approach for LSCD is largely conservative, especially in milder cases (stages I and IIA). This may include

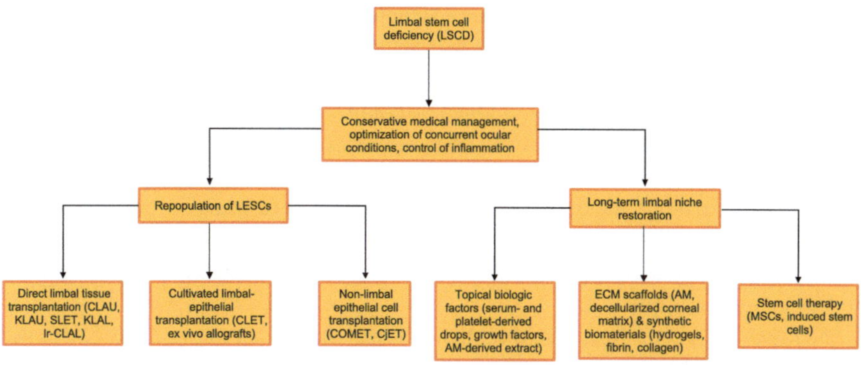

Fig. 6.2 Schematic summarizing current and prospective therapeutic approaches against limbal stem cell deficiency. Abbreviations: *LSCD* limbal stem cell disease, *LESC* limbal epithelial stem cell, *CLAU* conjunctival limbal autograft, *KLAU* keratolimbal autograft, *SLET* simple limbal epithelial transplantation, *KLAL* keratolimbal allograft, *lr-CLAL* living-related conjunctival limbal allograft, *CLET* cultivated limbal epithelial transplantation, *COMET* cultivated oral mucosal epithelial transplantation, *CjET* conjunctival epithelial transplantation, *AM* amniotic membrane, *ECM* extracellular matrix, *MSC* a mesenchymal stem cell

anti-inflammatory and immunomodulatory agents, biologically derived growth factors, and topical medications that promote corneal epithelialization [31, 32]. This approach is also crucial in stabilizing advanced cases (stages IIB and III) while patients await surgery.

When medical treatment fails, clinicians should consider using large-diameter fluid-filled scleral lens devices before surgery [11]. For milder cases that affect visual acuity, superficial keratectomy with amniotic membrane may be considered [11]. Furthermore, sectoral interventions such as sequential sector conjunctival epitheliectomy (SSCE) should be considered in patients with partial LSCD, especially when the conjunctival epithelium extends into the visual axis [33].

Surgical intervention for advanced LSCD typically aims to restore the stem cell population through direct tissue transplantation. They are characterized by the source of stem cells (autologous vs. allogeneic), type of graft used (limbal vs. non-limbal), degree of corneal conjunctivalization, and possible use of ex vivo cultures for stem cell expansion [31]. Any active inflammation should be adequately addressed before transplantation, typically with a topical steroid or cyclosporine, as an inflamed eye is associated with a significantly poorer postoperative prognosis. Additionally, a general health evaluation including complete blood workup, kidney and liver function tests, and blood sugar levels should be completed before proceeding with surgery [33–35]. Current surgical approaches for both unilateral and bilateral LSCD and other advanced therapeutic strategies are discussed in the following sections.

6.5.1 Limbal Epithelial Cell Transplants

6.5.1.1 Unilateral LSCD

Autologous limbal epithelial transplants, which rely on an intact and healthy limbal tissue bed in the contralateral eye, are the surgical treatment of choice for unilateral LSCD. Autologous grafts exhibit significantly higher retention and lower complication rates when compared to their allogeneic counterparts [34] [35]. A meta-analysis of 2202 eyes from 40 studies showed improvement of the ocular surface in approximately 85% of cases undergoing autologous transplantation, whether direct or cultivated. On the other hand, allogeneic transplantation resulted in 58% and 63% success rates for direct and cultivated grafts, respectively [35]. Regardless of the source of the graft, a 360° peritomy of the recipient eye is typically performed prior to transplantation [33].

Kenyon and Tseng first described the conjunctival limbal autograft (CLAU) for unilateral total LSCD in 1989 [36], a lasting procedure that has since been shown to successfully restore the corneal epithelium in approximately 75% of cases [37]. It involves obtaining and placing two trapezoid-shaped grafts of 2 clock hours each from the limbus and adjacent rim of conjunctiva from the patient's healthy contralateral eye (Fig. 6.3) [33, 36]. This procedure carries minimal to no risk of rejection and does not require postoperative immunosuppression.

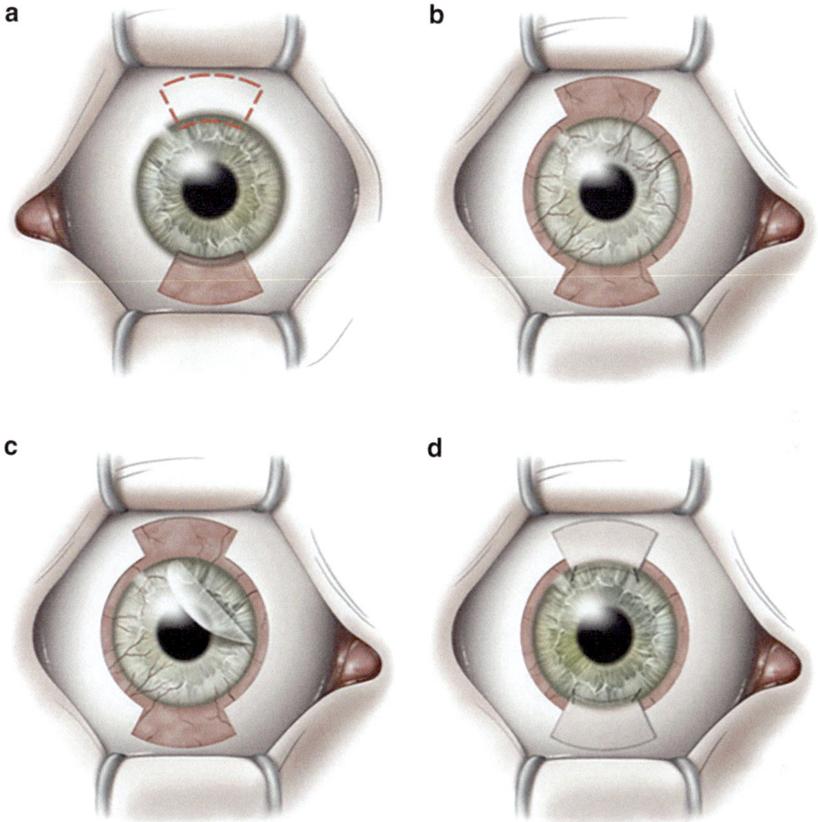

Fig. 6.3 Conjunctival limbal autograft (CLAU) surgery schematic. (**a**) Marking and harvesting donor graft tissue at the 12 and 6 o'clock positions. (**b**) Recipient bed preparation, including 360° peritomy and conjunctival resection at the 12 and 6 o'clock positions. (**c**) Superficial keratectomy of recipient cornea. (**d**) CLAU graft placement. (*Illustration with permission from Niparugs* et al. [33])

With advancements in culture techniques, other methods of autologous transplantation have since become available. Cultivated limbal epithelial transplantation (CLET) involves extracting a small, 2 mm^2 graft from the patient's healthy eye and cultivating corneal epithelial cells in vitro, which can then be transplanted on the recipient bed via amniotic membrane or fibrin gel carriers [38–40]. Simple limbal epithelial transplantation (SLET) is another recently introduced and technically easier-to-perform alternative to CLET that similarly requires less donor limbal tissue [41–43]. It involves extracting a small, 1-clock-hour limbal tissue block from the healthy eye, dividing it into smaller pieces, and transplanting it over an amniotic membrane with fibrin glue to the recipient bed (Fig. 6.4) [33, 43]. A multicenter study of 68 SLET eyes across three countries revealed ocular surface improvement in approximately 84% of cases at a median follow-up of 12 months [42]. Clinical

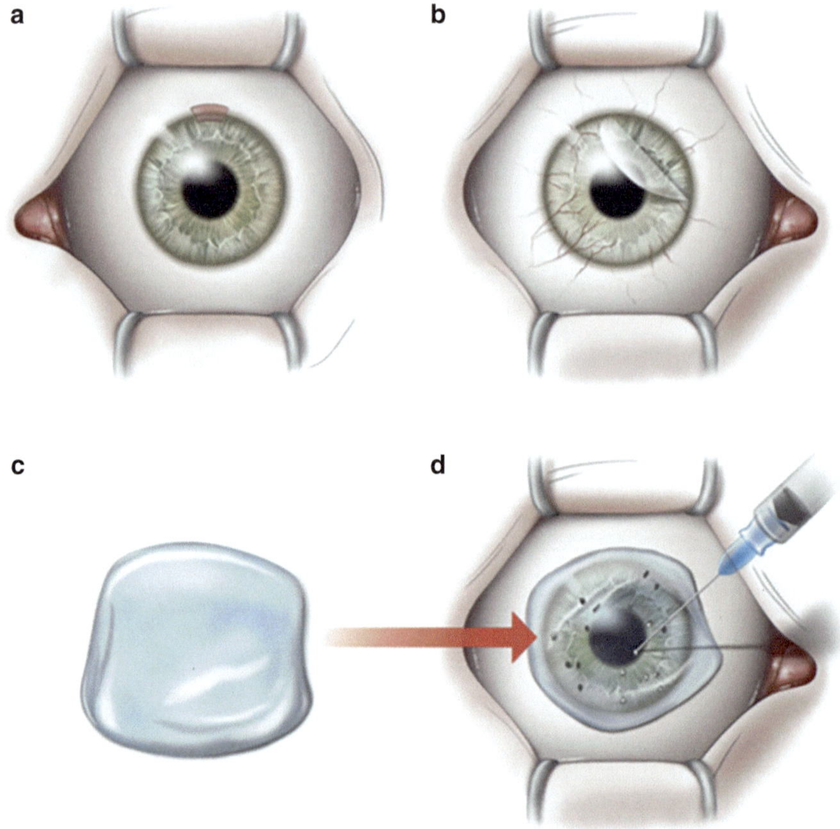

Fig. 6.4 Simple limbal epithelial transplant (SLET) surgery schematic. (**a**) Marking and harvesting of small-donor limbal graft tissue. (**b**) Superficial keratectomy of recipient cornea. (**c**) Amniotic membrane placement on recipient cornea. (**d**) Division of limbal graft tissue into smaller pieces, with the peripheral placement of six to eight pieces and paracentral placement of two to three pieces using tissue glue. (*Illustration with permission from Niparugs* et al. [33])

trials have also reported a 76% success rate for CLET and SLET in LSCD eyes resulting from ocular chemical burns [42, 44].

6.5.1.2 Bilateral LSCD

Allogeneic transplantation—including living-related conjunctival limbal allografts (lr-CLAL), cadaveric keratolimbal allografts (KLAL), and ex vivo–cultivated LESC allografts—represents the mainstay surgical approach for advanced bilateral LSCD [31]. These patients require allogeneic tissue grafts since their own ocular tissue is nonviable. Overall, success rates for allogeneic limbal grafts range anywhere from 33% to 77% depending on the underlying cause of LSCD [4].

Lr-CLAL utilizes healthy limbal and conjunctival tissue from the patient's living relative. After the allograft is harvested from the donor's eye in a conservative manner, the graft is gently placed on glove paper and kept wet before transferring to the recipient's eye. Transplantation of the allograft can be secured with fibrin glue or 10-0 nylon interrupted sutures [33]. On the other hand, KLAL is preferred in cases that primarily affect the limbus but with minimal conjunctival involvement [31]. The success of KLAL depends on the quantity of healthy LESCs that can be transferred to the recipient, which is why younger donors under the age of 50 are often preferred. In addition, this procedure requires the adjacent placement of three KLAL graft segments onto the recipient bed to reduce the chances of postoperative conjunctival invasion (Fig. 6.5) [33]. For unilateral or bilateral cases with severe conjunctival involvement requiring additional reconstruction, the "Cincinnati procedure"—which combines KLAL and lr-CLAL to restore a 360° limbus—may be considered. However, this approach carries a particularly high risk of graft rejection [45].

Allogeneic transplants require lifetime systemic immunosuppression to prevent graft rejection and ensure long-term donor cell survival [4, 31, 33]. A multidisciplinary approach is ideal for immunosuppressive management, possibly coordinating with an organ transplant specialist. Though rapid-acting and commonplace, corticosteroids are associated with a myriad of ophthalmic and systemic side effects. Therefore, a combination of short-term steroids and long-term immunosuppressants, including an antimetabolite (e.g., mycophenolate) and a calcineurin blocker (e.g., tacrolimus or cyclosporine), is currently recommended [31]. Keratoprostheses, which are not discussed here, are alternative options for bilateral LSCD that do not necessitate systemic immunosuppression.

6.5.2 Non-limbal Epithelial Cell Transplants

Given the risk of immune rejection and shortage of available allogeneic grafts, alternative options such as non-limbal autologous epithelial grafts have been investigated. Cultivated oral mucosal epithelial transplantation (COMET), which was first described in 2004 by Nishida et al., has been shown to improve ocular surface

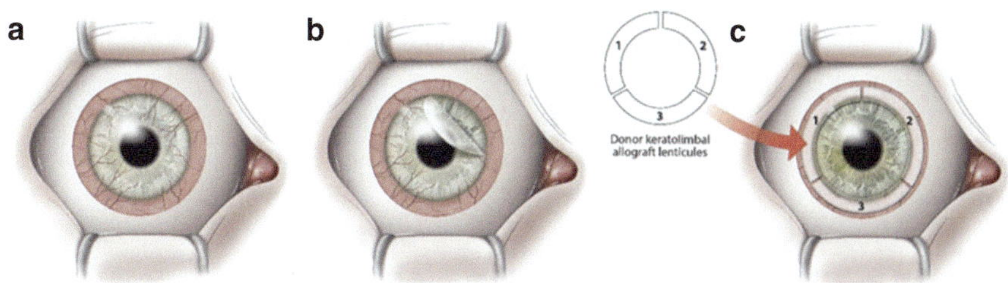

Fig. 6.5 Keratolimbal allograft (KLAL) surgery schematic. (**a**) 360° conjunctival peritomy and tenectomy of recipient bed. (**b**) Removal of abnormal corneal epithelium and fibrovascular pannus via blunt and sharp superficial dissection. (**c**) Creation of donor KLAL lenticules using two cadaver corneoscleral rims with subsequent adjacent placement of KLAL lenticules on the recipient limbus. (*Illustration with permission from Niparugs* et al. [33])

stability in 72% of cases [46]. However, COMET may produce suboptimal visual outcomes due to the thick and opaque nature of the oral mucosal epithelium and the increased risk of postsurgical peripheral corneal neovascularization [47, 48]. Randomized trials comparing COMET to allogeneic LESC transplantation also remain lacking [11]. Another option is ex vivo–cultivated conjunctival epithelial transplantation (CjET), first described in 2013; it exhibited an 86% success rate at an average follow-up of 18.5 months [49]. However, preliminary data suggest that mucosal and conjunctival epithelial tissue lack the ideal characteristics and functionality of corneal epithelial cells [4].

Overall, the role of non-limbal epithelial cell transplants for limbal niche regeneration is a relatively novel avenue of exploration that requires more robust clinical evidence before widespread implementation can be expected.

6.5.3 Stem Cell Therapy

Stem cell therapy using cultured cells was first applied to LESCs in 2006 [50, 51]. Since then, induced pluripotent stem cells (iPSCs), embryonic stem cells (ESCs), and MSCs that is discussed in the next section, have been introduced as options for regenerating corneal epithelium–like cells [52, 53]. However, randomized controlled trials and human clinical data are necessary to address the safety, costs, and efficacy of these emerging therapies.

6.5.4 Mesenchymal Stem Cells

Mesenchymal (MSCs) are multipotent stromal cells found in various tissues, including the corneal limbus, bone marrow, and fat [54, 55]. MSCs may be a potential therapeutic adjunct in restoring the defective limbal niche [4].

Studies have shown that MSCs are capable of producing an ECM in three-dimensional culture systems. In addition, they exhibit immunomodulatory properties by secreting anti-inflammatory and growth factors [56, 57]. Ocular burn models have revealed that the topical or subconjunctival administration of limbus-derived MSCs may decrease corneal opacification and neovascularization [58]. Additionally, in vitro cultivated limbal MSCs have been shown to promote corneal epithelialization [59]. Recently, a clinical trial comparing allogeneic bone marrow MSC transplantation with CLET has revealed promising safety and efficacy profiles. However, sufficient data regarding the benefits of MSCs for LSCD remain limited [60, 61].

6.5.5 Extracellular Matrix Scaffolds

The uniquely organized extracellular matrix is vital to LESC function and ocular surface homeostasis. Therefore, bioengineered ECM scaffolds have been explored as potential donor cell carriers for ocular surface repair and reconstruction.

Amniotic membrane, which is comprised of a thick basement membrane and a stromal matrix free of blood vessels and nerves, is a popular and widely studied ECM scaffold. In addition to promoting the proliferation, differentiation, migration, and adhesion of epithelial cells, amniotic membrane exhibits anti-inflammatory, anti-angiogenic, antimicrobial, and anti-fibrotic properties that render it a useful tool for tissue engineering, ex vivo cell expansion, and cell delivery [62–65]. Amniotic membrane can be used in ocular surface reconstruction in multiple ways: as a temporary biologic overlay that protects and facilitates the epithelial healing process, as a permanent inlay to help fill in a tissue defect, or as a combined overlay and inlay for more severe and deeper-penetrating ocular surface disorders [31]. Downsides include its lack of transparency, low tensile strength, risk of infectious disease transmission, and rapid digestion following transplantation that diminish its long-term utility [4, 62].

A range of other natural and synthetic biomaterials that contain structural proteins and healing factors have been proposed as possible platforms for the delivery of cultivated LESCs [4]. These include decellularized corneal matrix, hydrogels, fibrin, collagen, siloxane hydrogen contact lenses, and silk fibroin [66–69]. Additionally, three-dimensional LESC niche models produced through bioprinting technology are being explored [11, 13]. Overall, bioengineered scaffolds are a promising therapy that may add therapeutic benefit for LSCD as they gradually become more commonplace [25].

6.5.6 Biological Factors

The local delivery of exogenous biological factors is a noninvasive approach that augments limbal niche restoration. Potential sources include hemoderivatives, soluble recombinant growth factors, and amniotic membrane extract [50].

Autologous serum-derived eye drops (ASE) have been found to improve ocular surface health in graft-versus-host disease, keratoconjunctivitis, dry eye disease, and Sjogren's disease [70]. Similar to human tears, these drops are rich in various growth factors and cytokines, fibronectin, and vitamin A—nutrients and epitheliotrophic factors essential for the physiologic maintenance of the ocular surface [71]. The concentration of serum in ASEs ranges anywhere from 20% to 100% [31]. However, drawbacks include the risk of infection with extended use, imperfect stability, and the current lack of standardized manufacturing protocols. Furthermore, platelet-derived preparations such as platelet releasate, plasma rich in growth factors, and platelet-rich plasma have exhibited comparable reconstructive abilities as ASE based on preliminary studies [72].

Certain soluble growth factors possess anti-inflammatory, and neuroprotective properties that have been shown to enhance corneal healing and promote LESC function. Examples include pigment epithelium–derived factor and nerve growth factor [73, 74]. Additionally, cocktails containing cryopreserved amniotic membrane derivatives and umbilical cord components may aid in the cultivation of LESCs [75]. Though amniotic membrane–containing local therapies are not yet regulated by the US FDA, several products have been approved for distribution, and clinical trials are underway [76].

Although the long-term efficacy of biological factors remains largely unknown, preliminary small-trial data suggest that they hold valuable properties that will likely enable their widespread incorporation into topical formulations as part of the LSCD treatment strategy [71–76].

6.6 Future Directions

Randomized controlled clinical trials are essential in advancing the clinical understanding and management approach for LSCD. Since long-term graft survival data are starting to reveal the limits of current surgical techniques, there is an increasingly acknowledged premise that reconstruction of a healthy limbal niche is just as important as surgical transplantation and stem cell repopulation [77]. Therefore, current investigations are exploring methods of enhancing surgical techniques and outcomes while taking into consideration the efficacy of various locally delivered formulations that could help restore the limbal niche [50, 51, 77, 78].

Important knowledge gaps that should guide these investigations include the following [77]:

- The underlying mechanisms and degree by which various types of grafts improve clinical outcomes in LSCD versus other ocular surface pathologies.
- The real-world utility of ex vivo LESC expansion when compared with more traditional methods of grafting.
- Supplemental strategies that will maximize long-term maintenance of a healthy limbal niche.

Multiple stem cell based therapeutics using autologous and non-autologous sources, as well as topical bioactive therapies are under development for limbal stem cell deficiency such as those derived from oral mucosa and conjunctiva, LESC regeneration via stem cell sources including but not limited to HLA-matched iPSCs, MSCs, ESCs, and other reprogrammed differentiated cell lineages, topical biological factors, and extracellular matrix scaffolds for improved grafts survival, and secretome-derived preparations [54, 59, 78]. Other emerging treatments include tissue-engineered stem cell niche grafts, small molecules that promote LESCs proliferation, and extracellular vesicles derived from corneal stromal stem cells [11].

6.7 Conclusion

Limbal stem cell deficiency is a rare sight-threatening disease of the cornea with several underlying causes. Since the clinical presentation of LSCD may greatly vary, accurate diagnosis and staging require a thorough eye examination that ideally incorporates modern noninvasive imaging modalities. Currently, ophthalmologists can offer patients multiple avenues of medical and surgical intervention with the overarching goals of restoring the limbal niche and preserving long-term ocular surface health.

In this chapter, we discussed a wide range of current and prospective therapeutic approaches for LSCD. Though medical treatment may suffice for milder cases, surgery is often indicated for advanced disease. Unilateral LSCD has been successfully treated with autografts, including CLAU, CLET, and SLET. Bilateral LSCD typically relies on allogeneic transplantation such as KLAL or lr-CLAL, with subsequent systemic immunosuppression. The continued refinement of existing practices and clinical execution of non-epithelial-based interventions that span from bioengineered stem cell derivatives to topical immunomodulatory agents will only improve long-term visual outcomes in this patient population.

Acknowledgments None.

Disclosure None.

Funding None.

References

1. Figueiredo FC, Glanville JM, Arber M, Carr E, Rydevik G, Hogg J, et al. A systematic review of cellular therapies for the treatment of limbal stem cell deficiency affecting one or both eyes. Ocul Surf. 2021;20(3):48–61.
2. Dziasko MA, Daniels JT. Anatomical features and cell-cell interactions in the human limbal epithelial stem cell niche. Ocul Surf. 2016;14(3):322–30.
3. Cotsarelis G, Cheng SZ, Dong G, Sun TT, Lavker RM. Existence of slow-cycling limbal epithelial basal cells that can be preferentially stimulated to proliferate: implications on epithelial stem cells. Cell. 1989;57:201–9.
4. Yazdanpanah G, Haq Z, Kang K, Jabbehdari S, Rosenblatt MI, Djalilian AR. Strategies for reconstructing the limbal stem cell niche. Ocul Surf. 2019;17(2):230–40.
5. Scadden DT. Nice neighborhood: emerging concepts of the stem cell niche. Cell. 2014;157(1):41–50.
6. Lane SW, Williams DA, Watt FM. Modulating the stem cell niche for tissue regeneration. Nat Biotechnol. 2014;32:795–803.
7. Seyed-Safi AG, Daniels JT. The limbus: structure and function. Exp Eye Res. 2020;197
8. Thoft RA, Friend J. The X, Y, Z hypothesis of corneal epithelial maintenance. Invest Ophthalmol Vis Sci. 1983;24(10):1442–3.
9. Liu CY, Kao WY. Corneal epithelial wound healing. Prog Mol Biol Transl Sci. 2015;134:61–71.
10. Chang JH, Putra I, Huang YH, Chang M, Han K, Zhong W, et al. Limited versus total epithelial debridement ocular surface injury: live fluorescence imaging of hemangiogenesis and lymphangiogenesis in Prox1-GFP/Flk1::Myr-mCherry mice. Biochim Biophys Acta. 2016;1860(10):2148–56.
11. Bonnet C, Roberts JS, Deng SX. Limbal stem cell diseases. Exp Eye Res. 2021;205
12. Vazirani J, Nair D, Shanbhag S, Wurity S, Ranjan A, Sangwan V. Limbal stem cell deficiency – demography and underlying causes. Am J Ophthalmol. 2018;188:99–103.

13. Prabhasawat P, Ekpo P, Uiprasertkul M, Chotikavanich S, Tesavibul N, Pornpanich K, et al. Long-term result of autologous cultivated oral mucosal epithelial transplantation for severe ocular surface disease. Cell Tissue Bank. 2016;17(3):491–503.
14. Deng SX, Borderie V, Chan CC, Dana R, Figuieredo FC, Gomes JAP, et al. Global consensus on the definition, classification, diagnosis and staging of limbal stem cell deficiency. Cornea. 2019;38(3):364–75.
15. Kang BS, Kim MK, Wee WR, Oh JY. Infectious keratitis in limbal stem cell deficiency: Stevens– Johnson syndrome versus chemical burn. Cornea. 2016;35(1):51–5.
16. Rossen J, Amram A, Milani B, Park D, Harthan J, Joslin C, et al. Contact lens-induced limbal stem cell deficiency. Ocul Surf. 2016;14(4):419–34.
17. Shimazaki J, Satake Y, Higa K, Yamaguchi T, Noma H, Tsubota K. Long-term outcomes of cultivated cell sheet transplantation for treating total limbal stem cell deficiency. Ocul Surf. 2020;18(4):663–71.
18. Haagdorens M, Van Acker SI, Van Gerwen V, Dhubhghaill SN, Koppen C, Tassignon MJ, et al. Limbal stem cell deficiency: current treatment options and emerging therapies. Stem Cells Int. 2016;2016:9798374.
19. Khoo LW, Attzs M, Srinivasan S, Roberts F. Limbal stem cell deficiency secondary to diffuse non-necrotizing anterior scleritis: a clinicopathological report. Cornea. 2018;37(9):1175–7.
20. Pérez RL, Pérez-Simón JA, Caballero-Velazquez T, Flores T, Carrancio S, Herrero C, et al. Limbus damage in ocular graft-versus-host disease. Biol Blood Marrow Transplant. 2011;17(2):270–3.
21. Feizi S, Javadi MA, Alemzadeh-Ansari M, Arabi A, Shahraki T, Kheirkhah A. Management of corneal complications in vernal keratoconjunctivitis: a review. Ocul Surf. 2021;19:282–9.
22. Jabbehdari S, Starnes TW, Kurji KH, Eslani KH, Cortina MS, Holland EJ, et al. Management of advanced ocular surface disease in patients with severe atopic keratoconjunctivitis. Ocul Surf. 2019;17(2):303–9.
23. Singh S, Jakati S, Shanbhag SS, Elhusseiny AM, Djalilian AR, Basu S. Lid margin keratinization in Stevens-Johnson syndrome: review of pathophysiology and histopathology. Ocul Surf. 2021;21:299–305.
24. Yazdanpanah G, Bohm KJ, Hassan OM, et al. Management of congenital aniridia-associated keratopathy: long-term outcomes from a tertiary referral center. Am J Ophthalmol. 2020;210:8–18.
25. Kang KB, Rosenblatt MI, Djalilian AR. Novel approaches for restoring the function of the limbal stem cell niche. In: Foundations of corneal disease. Springer; 2020. p. 241–7.
26. Le Q, Xu J, Deng SX. The diagnosis of limbal stem cell deficiency. Ocul Surf. 2018;16(1):58–69.
27. Chan CC, Holland EJ. Severe limbal stem cell deficiency from contact lens wear: patient clinical features. Am J Ophthalmol. 2013;155(3):544–9.
28. Chuephanich P, Supiyaphun C, Aravena C, Bozkurt TK, Yu F, Deng SX. Characterization of corneal subbasal nerve plexus in limbal stem cell deficiency. Cornea. 2017;36(3):347–52.
29. Binotti WW, Nosé RM, Koseoglu ND, Dieckmann GM, Kenyon K, Hamrah P. The utility of anterior segment optical coherence tomography angiography for the assessment of limbal stem cell deficiency. Ocul Surf. 2021;19:94–103.
30. Bizheva K, Tan B, MacLellan B, Hosseinaee Z, Mason E, Hileeto D, et al. In-vivo imaging of the palisades of Vogt and the limbal crypts with sub-micrometer axial resolution optical coherence tomography. Biomed Opt Express. 2017;8(9):4141–51.
31. Deng SX, Kruse F, Gomes JAP, Chan CC, Daya S, Dana R, et al. Global consensus on the management of limbal stem cell deficiency. Cornea. 2020;39(10):1291–302.
32. Soleimani M, Naderan M. Management strategies of ocular chemical burns: current perspectives. Clin Ophthalmol. 2020;14:2687–99.
33. Niparugs M, Nonpassopon M, Shareef F, Elhusseiny AM, Djalilian AR. Ocular surface transplantation and amniotic membrane surgery. In: Albert and Jackobiec's principles and practice of ophthalmology: volume 2. 4th ed; 2021.
34. Le Q, Chauhan T, Yung M, Tseng CH, Deng SX. Outcomes of limbal stem cell transplant: a meta-analysis. JAMA Ophthalmol. 2020;138(6):660–70.

35. Le Q, Chauhan T, Deng SX. Diagnostic criteria for limbal stem cell deficiency before surgical intervention–a systemic literature review and analysis. Surv Ophthalmol. 2020;65(1):32–40.
36. Keivyon KR, Tseng SC. Limbal autograft transplantation for ocular surface disorders. Ophthalmology. 1989;96(5):709–23.
37. Shanbhag SS, Nikpoor N, Donthineni PR, Singh V, Chodosh J, Basu S. Autologous limbal stem cell transplantation: a systematic review of clinical outcomes with different surgical techniques. Br J Ophthalmol. 2020;104(2):247–53.
38. Sasamoto Y, Sasamoto N, Tran J, Mishra A, Ksander BR, Frank MH, et al. Investigation of factors associated with ABCB5-positive limbal stem cell isolation yields from human donors. Ocul Surf. 2020;18(1):114–20.
39. Eslani M, Cheung AY, Kurji K, Pierson K, Sarnicola E, Holland EJ. Long-term outcomes of conjunctival limbal autograft in patients with unilateral total limbal stem cell deficiency. Ocul Surf. 2019;17(4):670–4.
40. Tananuvat N, Bumroongkit K, Tocharusa C, Sevatee U, Kongkaew A, Ausayakhun S. Limbal stem cell and oral mucosal epithelial transplantation from ex vivo cultivation in LSCD-induced rabbits: histology and immunologic study of the transplant epithelial sheet. Int Ophthalmol. 2017;37(6):1289–98.
41. Sangwan VS, Basu S, MacNeil S, Balasubramanian D. Simple limbal epithelial transplantation (SLET): a novel surgical technique for the treatment of unilateral limbal stem cell deficiency. Br J Ophthalmol. 2012;96(7):931–4.
42. Vazirani J, Ali MH, Sharma N, Gupta N, Mittal V, Atallah M, et al. Autologous simple limbal epithelial transplantation for unilateral limbal stem cell deficiency: multicentre results. Br J Ophthalmol. 2016;100(10):1416–20.
43. Basu S, Sureka SP, Shanbhag SS, Kethiri AR, Singh V, Sangwan VS. Simple limbal epithelial transplantation: long-term clinical outcomes in 125 cases of unilateral chronic ocular surface burns. Ophthalmology. 2016;123(5):1000–10.
44. Rama P, Matuska S, Paganoni G, Spinelli A, De Luca M, Pellegrini G. Limbal stem-cell therapy and long-term corneal regeneration. N Engl J Med. 2010;363(2):147–55.
45. Chan CC, Biber JM, Holland EJ. The modified Cincinnati procedure: combined conjunctival limbal autografts and keratolimbal allografts for severe unilateral ocular surface failure. Cornea. 2012;31(11):1264–72.
46. Nakamura T, Endo KI, Cooper LJ, Fullwood NJ, Tanifuji N, Tsuzuki M, et al. The successful culture and autologous transplantation of rabbit oral mucosal epithelial cells on amniotic membrane. Invest Ophthalmol Vis Sci. 2003;44(1):106–16.
47. Kolli S, Ahmad S, Mudhar HS, Meeny A, Lako M, Figueiredo FC. Successful application of ex vivo expanded human autologous oral mucosal epithelium for the treatment of total bilateral limbal stem cell deficiency. Stem Cells. 2014;32(8):2135–46.
48. Kiritoshi S, Oie Y, Nampei K, Sato S, Morota M, Nishida K. Anterior segment optical coherence tomography angiography in patients following cultivated oral mucosal epithelial transplantation. Am J Ophthalmol. 2019;208:242–50.
49. Ricardo JRS, Cristovam PC, Filho PAN, Farias CC, de Araujo AL, Loureiro RR, et al. Transplantation of conjunctival epithelial cells cultivated ex vivo in patients with total limbal stem cell deficiency. Cornea. 2013;32(3):221–8.
50. Yazdanpanah G, Jabbehdari S, Djalilian AR. Emerging approaches for ocular surface regeneration. Curr Ophthalmol Rep. 2019;7(1):1–10.
51. De Luca M, Pellegrini G, Green H. Regeneration of squamous epithelia from stem cells of cultured grafts. Regen Med. 2006;1(1):45–57.
52. Ahmad S, Stewart R, Yung S, Kolli S, Armstrong L, Stojkovic M, et al. Differentiation of human embryonic stem cells into corneal epithelial-like cells by in vitro replication of the corneal epithelial stem cell niche. Stem Cells. 2007;25(5):1145–55.
53. Shalom-Feuerstein R, Serror L, De La Forest Divonne S, Petit I, Aberdam E, Camargo L, et al. Pluripotent stem cell model reveals essential roles for miR-450b-5p and miR-184 in embryonic corneal lineage specification. Stem Cells. 2012;30(5):898–909.

54. Mansoor H, Ong HS, Riau AK, Stanzel TP, Mehta JS, Yam GHF. Current trends and future perspective of mesenchymal stem cells and exosomes in corneal diseases. Int J Mol Sci. 2019;20(12):2853.
55. Putra I, Shen X, Anwar KN, Rabiee B, Samaeekia R, Almazyad E, et al. Preclinical evaluation of the safety and efficacy of cryopreserved bone marrow mesenchymal stromal cells for corneal repair. Transl Vis Sci Technol. 2021;10(10):3.
56. Wang M, Yuan Q, Xie L. Mesenchymal stem cell-based immunomodulation: properties and clinical application. Stem Cells Int. 2018:3057624.
57. Dehghani S, Rasoulianboroujeni M, Ghasemi H, Keshel SH, Nozarian Z, Hashemian MN, et al. 3D-printed membrane as an alternative to amniotic membrane for ocular surface/conjunctival defect reconstruction: an in vitro & in vivo study. Biomaterials. 2018;174:95–112.
58. Acar U, Pinarli FA, Acar DE, Beyazyildiz E, Sobaci G, Ozgermen BB, et al. Effect of allogeneic limbal mesenchymal stem cell therapy in corneal healing: role of administration route. Ophthalmic Res. 2015;53(2):82–9.
59. Eslani M, Putra I, Shen X, Hamouie J, Tadepalli A, Anwar KN, et al. Cornea-derived mesenchymal stromal cells therapeutically modulate macrophage immunophenotype and angiogenic function. Stem Cells. 2018;36(5):775–84.
60. Calonge M, Pérez I, Galindo S, Nieto-Miguel T, López-Paniagua M, Fernández I, et al. A proof-of-concept clinical trial using mesenchymal stem cells for the treatment of corneal epithelial stem cell deficiency. Transl Res. 2019;206:18–40.
61. Liang L, Luo X, Zhang J, Su W, Zhu W, Xie Y, et al. Safety and feasibility of subconjunctival injection of mesenchymal stem cells for acute severe ocular burns: a single arm study. Ocul Surf. 2021;22:103–9.
62. Rahman I, Said D, Maharajan V, Dua H. Amniotic membrane in ophthalmology: indications and limitations. Eye. 2009;23(10):1954–61.
63. Tabatabaei SA, Soleimani M, Behrouz MJ, Torkashvand A, Anvari P, Yaseri M. A randomized clinical trial to evaluate the usefulness of amniotic membrane transplantation in bacterial keratitis healing. Ocul Surf. 2017;15(2):218–26.
64. Malhotra C, Jain AK. Human amniotic membrane transplantation: different modalities of its use in ophthalmology. World J Transplant. 2014;4(2):111–21.
65. Elhusseiny AM, Gise R, Scelfo C, Mantagos IS. Amniotic membrane transplantation in a 2-month-old infant with toxic epidermal necrolysis. Am J Ophthalmol Case Rep. 2021;21:101017.
66. Nguyen KN, Bobba S, Richardson A, Park M, Watson SL, Wakefield D, et al. Native and synthetic scaffolds for limbal epithelial stem cell transplantation. Acta Biomater. 2018;65:21–35.
67. Levis HJ, Brown RA, Daniels JT. Plastic compressed collagen as a biomimetic substrate for human limbal epithelial cell culture. Biomaterials. 2010;31(30):7726–37.
68. Brown KD, Low S, Mariappan I, Abberton KM, Short R, Zhang H, et al. Plasma polymer-coated contact lenses for the culture and transfer of corneal epithelial cells in the treatment of limbal stem cell deficiency. Tissue Eng Part A. 2014;20(3–4):646–55.
69. Kang KB, Lawrence BD, Gao XR, Luo Y, Zhou Q, Liu A, et al. Micro-and nanoscale topographies on silk regulate gene expression of human corneal epithelial cells. Invest Ophthalmol Vis Sci. 2017;58(14):6388–98.
70. Azari AA, Rapuano CJ. Autologous serum eye drops for the treatment of ocular surface disease. Eye Contact Lens. 2015;41(3):133–40.
71. Akcam HT, Unlu M, Karaca EE, Yazici H, Aydin B, Hondur AM. Autologous serum eye-drops and enhanced epithelial healing time after photorefractive keratectomy. Clin Exp Optom. 2018;101(1):34–7.
72. Freire V, Andollo N, Etxebarria J, Hernaez-Moya R, Duran JA, Morales MC. Corneal wound healing promoted by 3 blood derivatives: an in vitro and in vivo comparative study. Cornea. 2014;33(6):614–20.
73. Ho TC, Chen SL, Wu JY, Ho MY, Chen LJ, Hsieh JW, et al. PEDF promotes self-renewal of limbal stem cell and accelerates corneal epithelial wound healing. Stem Cells. 2013;31(9):1775–84.

74. Lambiase A, Sacchetti M, Bonini S. Nerve growth factor therapy for corneal disease. Curr Opin Ophthalmol. 2012 Jul;23(4):296–302.
75. Baradaran-Rafii A, Asl NS, Ebrahimi M, Jabbehdari S, Bamdad S, Roshandel D, et al. The role of amniotic membrane extract eye drop (AMEED) in in vivo cultivation of limbal stem cells. Ocul Surf. 2018;16(1):146–53.
76. Murri MS, Moshirfar M, Birdsong OC, Ronquillo YC, Ding Y, Hoopes PC. Amniotic membrane extract and eye drops: a review of literature and clinical application. Clin Ophthalmol. 2018;12:1105–12.
77. Ghareeb AE, Lako M, Figueiredo FC. Recent advances in stem cell therapy for limbal stem cell deficiency: a narrative review. Ophthalmol Ther. 2020;9(4):809–31.
78. Sasamoto Y, Ksander BR, Frank MH, Frank NY. Repairing the corneal epithelium using limbal stem cells or alternative cell-based therapies. Expert Opin Biol Ther. 2018;18(5):505–13.

End-Stage Corneal Disease and Keratoprosthesis

7

Ankit Anil Harwani, Shweta Agarwal, Bhaskar Srinivasan, and Geetha Iyer

Key Points

- Keratoprosthesis (KPro) is the last resort for bilateral end-stage corneal and ocular surface disorders.
- Because of the potential for severe complications, this procedure requires meticulous planning, execution, compliance, and follow-up.
- There are various types of KPro available. As important as appropriate patient selection is for KPro implantation, appropriate KPro selection is equally important.
- Understanding perioperative care, the nuances of surgical techniques, and identification and management of complications are all crucial for a successful outcome.

7.1 Introduction

Keratoprosthesis (KPro) implantation involves the replacement of a damaged cornea with an artificial optical prosthesis. It is considered the last resort for visual rehabilitation in bilateral end-stage corneal and ocular surface disease and is reserved for eyes not amenable to conventional penetrating keratoplasty. These

A. A. Harwani · S. Agarwal
CJ Shah Cornea Services, Dr G Sitalakshmi Memorial Clinic for Ocular Surface Disorders, Sankara Nethralaya, Chennai, Tamil Nadu, India
e-mail: draah@snmail.org; drsb@snmail.org

B. Srinivasan · G. Iyer (✉)
CJ Shah Cornea Services, Dr G Sitalakshmi Memorial Clinic for Ocular Surface Disorders, Sankara Nethralaya, Chennai, Tamil Nadu, India

CODE Eye Care, Institute of Excellence for Cornea, Ocular Surface and Dry Eye, Chennai, India

H. N. Saeed, R. B. Singh (eds.), *Corneal Disorders*, Current Practices in Ophthalmology, https://doi.org/10.1007/978-981-96-5294-5_7

include eyes with repeated graft failures, limbal stem cell deficiency, cicatrizing ocular surface disease with or without severe dryness, and/or ocular surface keratinization [1].

7.2 End-Stage Ocular Surface Disease

End-stage ocular surface disease (OSD) can progress to bilateral blindness. Eyes with OSD are categorized as high risk not only for penetrating keratoplasty but also for limbal stem cell transplantation (LSCT) [2, 3]. Generally, the bilaterality of the condition precludes the use of limbal tissue from the contralateral eye, necessitating a high-risk allograft with systemic immunosuppression. In these eyes, surgical decision-making is required in weighing the benefits and drawbacks of LSCT vs KPro. This decision-making is based on several patient and surgeon factors. OSD with severe dryness, surface keratinization, and severe forniceal shortening despite reconstructive attempts requires KPro for visual rehabilitation [3, 4].

OSDs and pathology that can lead to corneal blindness include:

- Stevens-Johnson syndrome (SJS).
- Ocular cicatricial pemphigoid (OCP).
- Chemical injuries.
- Limbal stem cell deficiency.
- Severe dry eye.
- Ocular surface keratinization.

7.3 Keratoprosthesis

Artificial corneal transplantation using a glass lens was first described in 1789 by a French surgeon, Pillier de Quengsy [5, 6]. However, due to limitations in knowledge about anesthesia, antibiotics, and asepsis at the time, his outcomes were disheartening, and the idea was abandoned for many years. Much later, in the mid-nineteenth century, discovery of the biocompatibility of polymethylmethacrylate (PMMA) served as an impetus for further developments in the field of KPro. Experiments to use this inert material for KPros soon began, and a two-part "core-skirt" skeleton for KPro was developed [7, 8]. However, early and late postoperative complications, primarily due to the lack of permanent bio-integration, were still a significant concern [6, 9, 10]. In the last half-century, many modifications and improvements in KPro design and material, preoperative prognostications, postoperative regimens, and follow-up commitment have improved the success rate of KPro and reduced complication rates; however, the search for the ideal KPro continues [9, 11, 12].

This chapter gives a comprehensive review of the current trends in KPro, focusing on the types, surgical techniques, challenges, postoperative management, and outcomes.

7.4 Types of Keratoprostheses and Their Indications

KPros can be grouped in a variety of ways, including based on their fixation method in the eye as collar-stud (e.g., Boston KPro), intracorneal (e.g., Alphacor), or epicorneal (e.g., osteodonto KPro); or on the material of the skirt (haptic) that carries the optic as biocompatible (e.g., Boston), bio-integrated (e.g., Pintucci), or biological (e.g., osteodonto KPro) [13].

However, more commonly, they are grouped as type 1 and 2 based on the level of ocular disease they cater to: type 1 may be performed in moist eyes and type 2 in dry, keratinized eyes. Each type has its variants depending on the material used to assemble the KPro complex (Fig. 7.1). The various types and materials used are listed in Table 7.1.

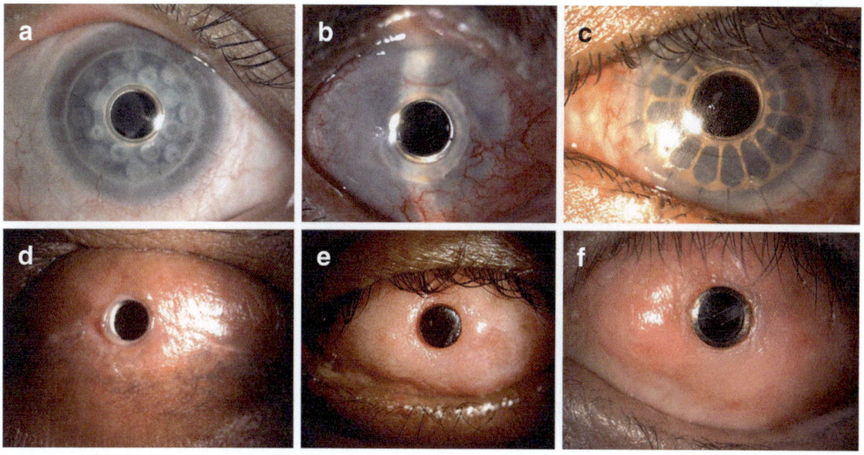

Fig. 7.1 Final appearance of different types of KPro devices postimplantation. (**a**) Type 1 Boston KPro for silicone oil–induced keratopathy in a monocular patient with chronic hypotony post-retinal detachment surgery 12 years prior. Patient is maintaining a best corrected visual acuity of 20/120 at 10 years of follow-up post-KPro. A faint retroprosthetic membrane not affecting vision is noted. (**b**) Auro KPro—Implanted following ocular surface reconstructive procedures in an eye post-alkali chemical injury. Patient is maintaining 20/80 vision at 7 years of follow-up. (**c**) Lucia KPro in a 28-year-old male post acid injury maintaining 20/30 vision at two and a half years of follow-up. (**d**) Type 2 Boston KPro in a patient with SJS and bilateral end-stage keratinized ocular surface. Patient is maintaining 20/40 vision at 5 years of follow-up. (**e**) MOOKP in a patient with SJS, maintaining 20/20 vision at 15 years of follow-up. (**f**) Lux KPro demonstrating a titanium sleeve around the optic in a patient with SJS, maintaining a visual acuity of 20/40 at 3 years of follow-up

Table 7.1 Optic, Support, and Cover Tissue Characteristics Across Keratoprosthesis Types

Type	Variants	Optic	Skirt/support	Anterior cover tissue
Type 1	Boston type 1 and its variants (Lucia, Auro KPro) [10, 14, 15]	PMMA	PMMA/titanium (biocompatible) + corneal allograft	Bandage contact lens
Type 2	Boston type 2 [10]	PMMA	PMMA/titanium (biocompatible) + corneal allograft	Eyelid skin
	Osteo-odonto [16]	PMMA	Human canine tooth (biological)	Buccal mucosa
	Osteo [17]	PMMA	Tibia bone (biological)	Buccal mucosa
	Lux [18]	PMMA	Titanium (biocompatible) + corneal allograft	Buccal mucosa
	LVP [19]	PMMA	PMMA/titanium (biocompatible) + corneal allograft	Buccal mucosa
	Pintucci [20]	PMMA	Dacron mesh (bio-integrated)	Buccal mucosa
	Seoul type [21]	PMMA	Expanded polytetrafluoroethylene or polyurethane (bio-integrated)	Amniotic membrane
	Titanium skirt KPros [22–24]	Threaded PMMA	Titanium ring with flanges (biocompatible)	Buccal mucosa or corneal allograft

7.5 Type 1 Keratoprosthesis

Type 1 KPros, due to their ease of availability, relatively simple implantation technique, lower complications rates, and reduced dependence on ancillary specialties, have become the most commonly implanted KPros worldwide [25, 26]. Type 1 KPros are indicated in eyes that are wet and do not have any eyelid abnormalities or an underlying immunological disorder [27]. Eyes with multiple failed grafts and silicone oil are considered to have a better prognosis after KPro than eyes with chemical injury. The Boston type 1 KPro is the prototype and mainstream type 1 KPro used [28] (Fig. 7.2).

7.5.1 Boston Keratoprosthesis Type 1

The Boston KPro was introduced in the 1970s by Dr. Claes Dohlman and received FDA approval in 1992 [29, 30]. The initial collar-button design consisted of four parts: a front plate, allograft corneal skirt, backplate, and locking ring. The front plate has a central 3.5–3.7 mm optical cylinder, which protrudes through the allograft corneal button. The power of the Boston KPro is determined by the axial length of the patient's eye, lens status (pseudophakic/aphakic), and front radius of curvature of the optical cylinder. For pseudophakic patients, a single, standard

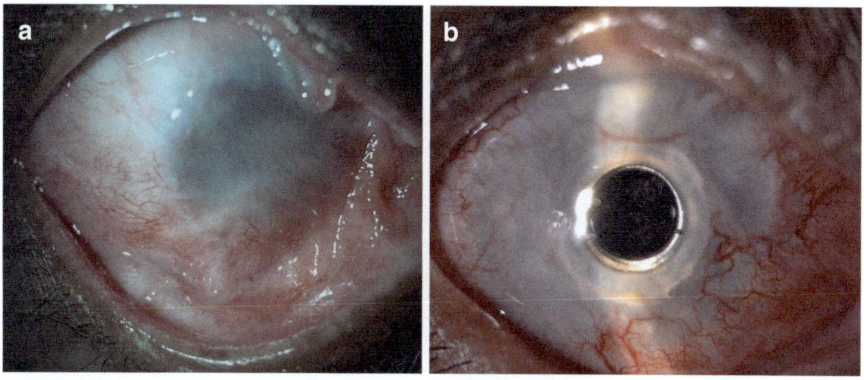

Fig. 7.2 (**a**) A moist eye post-bilateral alkali chemical injury. The inferonasal fornix was further reconstructed using amniotic membrane grafting on the bulbar surface and oral mucosal graft over the palpebral surface. Following fornix reconstruction, Auro KPro was implanted in the eye for visual rehabilitation. (**b**) Maintaining best corrected visual acuity of 20/80 at 7 years of follow-up

power Boston KPro is available, and for aphakic patients, a customized power KPro is available depending on the axial length (ranging from 16 to 31 mm axial length in 1 mm increments). The backplate initially was a solid PMMA structure, but due to a high incidence of sterile melt of the corneal allograft, it was replaced by a fenestrated version having holes to provide nutrition to the corneal allograft. It is available in two diameters, 8.5 mm (16 holes) and 7 mm (8 holes). A titanium version was introduced in 2005 as a thinner, lightweight alternative to PMMA that is more resistant to corrosion and can be colored for improved cosmesis. The locking ring, which was used to lock the whole KPro assembly in place, underwent a series of modifications from being threaded to threadless, until 2014, when it was replaced by a click-on backplate system, eliminating the need for any locking ring for stability [30].

As the light entering the eyes of patients with a KPro has to pass through a 3.5–3.7 mm wide cylinder, the postoperative visual field of the patient, in the absence of glaucoma or another visual-field-limiting disease, is approximately 95° [31].

7.5.2 Auro KPro

In developing countries, cost is often a limiting factor in obtaining and performing the Boston type 1 KPro. In 2011, the Boston type 1 KPro design was shared with an Indian manufacturer (AuroLab, Madurai, India), and an alternative to the Boston KPro was developed. The Indian version, named Auro KPro, is similar to the Boston type 1 KPro, except that it has a PMMA backplate, and comes in only one size (i.e., 8.5 mm). This device is available in pseudophakic or aphakic powers with axial lengths ranging from 15 to 30 mm and is available for use in India only [32].

7.5.3 Lucia KPro

The Lucia modifications to the Boston KPro were another attempt to reduce the cost of KPro for resource-poor countries. The Lucia KPro received FDA approval in 2019 and consists of a titanium backplate anodized to a brown or blue color with 16 petaloid radial holes, providing a better cosmetic appearance. The backplate is available in only one diameter of 7.75 mm, rendering it suitable for all eyeball sizes. The front plate is designed in only two powers, one for pseudophakic eyes and one for aphakic eyes, presuming an axial length of 23.5 mm [14].

7.6 Type 2 Keratoprosthesis

Type 2 KPros are primarily indicated for eyes with cicatrizing conjunctival disorders, and dry or keratinized ocular surfaces with or without an underlying immunological disorder and with or without associated eyelid abnormalities [28]. The various devices that belong to this category and their detailed design are described as follows.

7.6.1 Boston Type 2 KPro

The Boston type 2 KPro is similar in design to its type 1 counterpart but has a 2 mm long anterior nub that traverses the lid and provides a visual field of approximately 90°, slightly less than that of the type 1 [31]. The backplate is made of titanium and is a click-on version, thus eliminating the need for an extra locking ring. Patients with dry, keratinized surfaces or underlying immunological disorders, or those in whom osteo-odonto keratoprosthesis (OOKP) is not being considered, are candidates for the Boston type 2 KPro, provided the patient has a normal eyelid structure [33–35].

7.6.2 Osteo-odonto Keratoprosthesis (OOKP)

A tooth root-alveolar bone complex was first used as a biological skirt for better integration of a type 2 KPro by Strampelli in 1963 [16]. Falcinelli made several modifications to the technique, and this version is currently known as the modified osteo-odonto keratoprosthesis (MOOKP) [36]. The canine tooth, being single-rooted, is usually used for the alveodental lamina skirt preparation. The whole assembly is covered with a buccal mucus membrane graft (MMG), which provides physical strength and nutritional support to the alveodental complex. The MOOKP provides an enduring option in patients with severe dryness and absent lids or blink. The central cylinder originally had an anterior diameter of 3.85 mm, a posterior diameter of 4.09 mm, and a length of approximately 8 mm. This design provided a visual field of 40°, which increased to 65°after further modifications [37].

7.6.3 Osteo Keratoprosthesis (OKP)

In patients in whom the canine teeth are missing or are not healthy, the patient's tibial bone may be used and was first used by Temprano in 1985 as a carrier for the optic cylinder [17]. The assembly and surgical steps are similar to that for the MOOKP other than the tibial bone lamina being used to make the skirt of the device rather than a tooth.

7.6.4 Lux Keratoprosthesis (LKP)

This device is an alternative to MOOKP and the Boston type 2 KPro for patients with inadequate lid skin and unhealthy or absent canine teeth. It consists of a PMMA cylinder with a titanium sleeve for better biocompatibility and a titanium backplate, with a corneal allograft sandwiched in between, similar to the Boston KPros. The complete assembly is sutured to the host cornea and then covered with an MMG. A central opening is created for the optic like in the MOOKP. Thus, it has the advantages of both the conventional type 2 KPros without the limiting factors of tooth or lid skin and is less bulky [18].However, the cosmetic implications are similar to the MOOKP. Additionally, the device is not currently available for use.

7.6.5 LVP Keratoprosthesis

To avoid the multiple surgeries needed in MOOKP, an attempt was made to use a Boston type 1 KPro under an MMG. With the LVP KPro, the mucosa is tucked directly under the front plate along with the corneal graft as compared to the Lux, where the mucosa is tucked in the ledge above the front plate, which then acts as a barrier [19].

7.6.6 Pintucci KPro

The Pintucci KPro is similar to OOKP except that the skirt around the PMMA cylinder comprises a bio-integratable, filamentous Dacron mesh, simplifying the implantation procedure; however, it is no longer readily available [20].

7.6.7 Titanium Skirt KPro

Titanium skirt KPros are used widely in Ukraine, Russia, and China. All the devices require a two-staged procedure and are inserted in the host corneal lamellae; thus, having a host cornea with adequate strength and thickness is an essential prerequisite. Though anecdotal reports have claimed usage of these in wet and dry eyes, long-term, multicenter studies are required to assess outcomes [22–24]. The various devices in use are described below:

(a) ***Filatov Institute, Ukraine***

The latest and the most widely used model available now is known as the "Iakymenko-Golubenko model." It consists of a threaded PMMA cylinder with a ring titanium skirt having three ring-shaped flanges.

(b) ***Moscow Eye Microsurgery Complex in Russia (MICOF) KPro***

The MICOF KPro is similar to the Filatov KPro, except that it has two ear-shaped solid flanges.

(c) ***Fyodorov-Zuev Kpr.***

In the Fyodorov-Zuev design, the flanges are ear shaped and contain large holes. The device is first placed into a donor allograft lamella and then sutured to the host cornea like a penetrating keratoplasty.

7.7 Surgical Technique

7.7.1 Preoperative Evaluation

Detailed preoperative evaluation forms an important aspect of surgical decision-making in determining the suitability of a KPro for the patient and the type of KPro that would be best-suited for the individual.

A detailed ocular, systemic, and psychological evaluation, in addition to a thorough history, must be undertaken. Though the type of KPro implanted will guide more specific discussion with the patient and family, the general recommendations governing KPro surgery are elucidated in Table 7.2. Counseling the patient and the family is of utmost importance as the surgical procedure is the beginning of a long journey with extensive follow-ups and the high possibility of complications and subsequent supplementary procedures. It is important to communicate realistic expectations to the patient and family regarding the visual and cosmetic outcome of the procedure. Strict compliance with long-term postoperative care, restrictions, and follow-ups must also be discussed preoperatively. Any patient not willing to comply with these stipulations should not be considered a candidate for KPro implantation [9, 28].

Table 7.2 General recommendations governing KPro surgery

General preoperative considerations	**Type 1 specific**
Detailed history to establish etiology and age of onset of blindness for prognosis (considered poor if the age of onset is before five years of age) Previous surgery Perception of light present Detailed slit-lamp evaluation Anterior segment optical coherence tomography, ultrasound biomicroscopy Ultrasound B scan with axial length measurement Digital tonometry Realistic patient expectation Psychological counseling Willingness to comply with postoperative follow-up and care Preoperative checklist	Blink adequacy Schirmer's I (>5 mm) Ability to wear and retain a contact lens Absence of immune conditions **Type 2 specific** Detailed tooth and oral mucosal evaluation Dental X-ray/spiral CT scan to determine width and girth of a canine tooth Fitness for general anesthesia
General recommendations KPro should be performed only in bilaterally blind patients KPro should be performed in only one eye The fellow eye is a spare, for KPro to be performed later, if required Selection of the type of KPro is as crucial as the selection of a patient for KPro	

7.8 Ordering the KPro

Depending upon the patient's age (pediatric or adult), the axial length of the eyeball, and lens status (pseudophakic or aphakic), a specific KPro is ordered for the patient. Two KPros are always ordered for a patient in the event of intraoperative damage to the device, especially during assembly.

7.9 Surgical Steps

7.9.1 Type 1 KPro

The surgical technique for type 1 KPro is very similar to that of penetrating keratoplasty after the assembly of the KPro device [29, 30]. Type 1 KPro can be performed under local anesthesia.

7.9.2 KPro Assembly

The KPro is assembled such that the donor corneal graft is sandwiched between the optic and backplate. The donor graft is preferably sized 0.25 mm more than the size of the backplate (typically 8.5 mm) but is dependent on the host corneal status and the degree of host trephination needed. A KPro with a 7 mm backplate can be used in eyes with smaller corneas. The central 3 mm of the donor corneal graft is trephined to accommodate the optic cylinder stem of the front plate. The KPro is then assembled in a sandwich fashion and locked together with the assembly tool that accompanies the KPro kit. The host cornea is trephined and excised, and the carrier graft of the assembled KPro is then sutured to the host cornea with 16 interrupted 9–0 nylon sutures. At the end of the procedure, a large diameter bandage contact lens (BCL) is placed on the eye. It can be customized based on the individual patient. Available customization for the Kontur Precision Sphere BCL (Kontur Kontact Lens Co., Hercules, CA) includes various base curves (6.8 mm to 9.8 mm), diameters (12.00 mm to 24.00 mm), spherical powers (+12.00D to −20.00D), and cylindrical powers (−0.75 to −5.00D). Other less-expensive BCLs with more limited parameters include AirOptix Night&Day Aqua (Alcon, Fort Worth, TX), PureVision2 (Bausch & Lomb, Rochester, NY), and Acuvue Oasys (Vistakon, Jacksonville, FL).

7.9.3 Type 2 KPro

7.9.3.1 Boston Type 2 KPro

The Boston type 2 KPro is a single-stage surgery that is preferably performed under general anesthesia. However, in cases unfit for general anesthesia, the procedure can be performed under local anesthesia with sedation. In addition to the steps of the type 1 KPro, an iris sphincterotomy, pars plana vitrectomy, and Ahmed glaucoma valve implantation is performed in all cases. The ocular surface epithelium is removed from eyelid margin to eyelid margin to facilitate adhesion to the surface. At the end of the procedure, the lid margins are extirpated to ensure the complete removal of hair follicles and lashes. The eyelid skin is closed in two layers around the protruding nub of the optic, and a notch is cut out on the upper lid around the optic [33].

7.9.3.2 MOOKP

MOOKP is performed under general anesthesia only, as a three-stage procedure per the Rome-Vienna protocol, with slight modifications practiced by different groups [38, 39]. The first stage is subcategorized into two or three parts based on the group's preference. First, the operative eye is prepared by removing the iris, lens, and anterior vitreous through a near 180-degree superior limbal incision. An intracapsular cataract extraction technique with cryotherapy is used to remove the lens. A tectonic penetrating keratoplasty can be considered if the host cornea is thin. A conjunctival hooding or flap to cover the cornea, with or without a tarsorrhaphy, is performed and concludes stage 1A of the procedure. A month later, stage 1B + C is performed. Stage 1B involves harvesting 3 cm of buccal mucosa and securing it over the ocular surface by suturing it to the recti muscles. Stage 1C consists of harvesting the selected canine tooth from the patient for fashioning the osteo-odonto alveolar lamina and incorporating the PMMA cylinder in it. The whole assembly is then placed in a subcutaneous pocket of the contralateral cheek in the patient's mouth to promote fibrovascular coverage. Three months later, stage 2 is performed, where the lamina with the cylinder is removed from the subcutaneous pocket and placed in the eye after reflecting the buccal mucosa with an inferior hinge. The host cornea is trephined to accommodate the PMMA cylinder, and the lamina is sutured. After reflecting the mucosa, a central hole is created to allow the cylinder to protrude out.

The surgical technique and steps for the other varieties of type 2 KPros mentioned above are not described in detail here. The osteo-KPro is performed like the MOOKP but involves harvesting the tibial bone instead of the canine tooth. The LUX, LVP, Ukraine, MICOF, and Fyodrov KPros are two-stage procedures where primarily the oral mucosa is anchored to the eye, and then subsequently, three months later, the assembled KPro is sutured to the host cornea after reflecting the mucosa. A central opening is created in the mucosa for the optic to protrude through after suturing the mucosa back in place.

7.10 Postoperative Regimen, Care, and Follow-Up

Postoperative care and follow-up are more stringent in type 1 than type 2.

Patients with type 1 KPros are on a topical fourth-generation fluoroquinolone four times a day, topical vancomycin once a day, and topical steroids four times a day postoperatively. The fluoroquinolone is reduced to twice-daily indefinitely around the 2-week mark, and the steroids are tapered over 6 months. Topical lubricants are also used as needed. The BCL placed at the end of the surgery needs to be replaced once every three months, mandating regular three-month follow-ups [28, 29].

In type 2 KPro, since either the lids are apposed or there is oral mucosa covering the ocular surface, the need for long-term topical antibiotics and steroids is minimal, with most patients requiring just an antibiotic ointment once a day along with lubricants, indefinitely, once the topical and systemic steroids are tapered and stopped in the immediate postoperative period. In general, patients with the Boston type 2 KPro require regular three-month follow-ups, while those with the MOOKP require six-month follow-ups [33, 38, 39].

A detailed slit-lamp evaluation, a slit-lamp/external photograph, visual acuity, intraocular pressure by finger tension, and optic nerve head and posterior pole status are documented at each follow-up visit. For a type 1 KPro, the surface is examined for defects in the epithelium and microleaks with fluorescein staining after BCL removal. Ultrasound B scan is performed once a year and visual fields once every six months.

7.11 Outcomes and Complications

Outcomes and complications have been extensively reported with each type of commonly used KPro and vary with the indication and cohort of patients and the follow-up period. Most studies report favorable short-term outcomes (less than two years of follow-up); however, studies with longer follow-ups are needed to appropriately characterize long-term visual and anatomical outcomes.

7.12 Type 1 KPro

7.12.1 Visual Outcome

Most studies report an improvement in visual acuity after type 1 KPro, with a postoperative vision of ≥20/200 present in 72–87% of eyes at two years and 56–65% of eyes at six to eight years of follow-up [40, 41, 42]. The largest prospective study of type 1 KPro involving 300 eyes of 300 patients demonstrated the maintenance of ≥20/200 vision or better for an average of 47.8 months in the Boston type 1 KPro [41]. The underlying etiology of corneal disease was found to have the most significant impact on visual outcomes. Best-corrected visual acuity (BCVA) improved to ≥20/200 in 64–67% of eyes and ≥ 20/60 in 55% of eyes implanted with Boston KPro for chemical injury [25, 42, 43]. Similar outcomes were reported for silicon oil–filled eyes, failed grafts, and limbal stem cell deficiency [44–46]. However, in patients with autoimmune disorders like SJS, OCP, and herpes zoster, less than 50% of eyes maintained visual acuity of ≥20/200 [47–49].

Similar outcomes have been demonstrated with the Auro KPro [15, 32, 50]. Short-term and long-term results of the Lucia KPro remain to be elucidated [14].

7.12.2 Anatomical Retention

Various intermediate and long-term studies have demonstrated an 80–95% anatomical retention rate for Boston type 1 KPro [44, 51]. As with visual acuity, the anatomical retention rate is less (below 55%) in a patient with an autoimmune cicatrizing disorder [47, 48]. This emphasizes the importance of selecting the most appropriate KPro for the patient; generally, type 1 KPro is not routinely recommended in cases of immunological conditions of the eye.

7.13 Type 2 KPro

7.13.1 Visual Outcome

SJS and OCP are the most common indications for type 2 KPro. Chemical injuries form another important indication. Mid-term outcomes with Boston type 2 KPro have reported BCVAs of ≥20/200 in 70% of eyes at a mean follow-up of 2.75 years; however, Lee et al. reported that at a mean follow-up of 5.9 years, 37.5% of patients had a BCVA of ≥20/200 with 33.3% having ≥20/100 [34, 35]. Pujari et al. noted that visual acuity of ≥20/200 was maintained in 57.1% of patients who had at least one year of follow-up and in 46.2% with five or more years of follow-up [33].

For MOOKP and OKP, functional success defined as BCVA ≥20/400 at ten years was reported to occur in 49% and 25% of eyes, respectively [52]. The functional outcome was similar between the two procedures when performed in comparable clinical scenarios of chemical injury. At 5 years, functional success was reported in 86% of eyes with MOOKP, 84% with OKP, and 71% with Boston type 1 KPro. In contrast, functional success in autoimmune disorders was 44% and 15% in eyes with osteo-KPro and Boston type 1 KPro, respectively, highlighting the type 1 KPro as a poor choice in autoimmune disease [53]. Of 181 patients who underwent MOOKP, Falcinelli et al. reported that the cumulative probability of retaining post-operative BCVA at nine years was 70% and more than 50% at 18 years after the surgery [54].

Short-term outcomes in nine patients who underwent Lux KPro demonstrated maintenance of BCVA ≥20/200 at the last follow-up (mean 18.7 months) [18]. LVP KPro implantation has shown maintenance of ≥20/400 vision in 61.5% of patients at one year postoperatively [19].

7.13.2 Anatomical Retention

Among type 2 KPros, the resistance of dentine in teeth to resorption makes MOOKP a durable device, and long-term studies, with almost two decades of follow-up, have reported device retention rates ranging from 80 to 98% [54, 55]. In another study, the anatomical survival of OKP is reported to range from 47 to 54%, not differing significantly from the 67–85% in OOKP [52, 53]. Primary indication for surgery has been found to influence the anatomical outcome, with OOKP demonstrating better results in SJS and the OKP in OCP. In the elderly, the anatomical success of OKP may be lower due to hormonal changes leading to osteoporosis; however, conclusive evidence is not available [52]. The retention rate of Boston type 2 is 90% at 2.7 years and 50% at five years [33–35]. In one study of nine patients who received the Lux KPro, anatomical success and device retention were achieved in all nine eyes. Retention was found to be 76.6% at 3–5 years in eyes that underwent LVP KPro implantation [18, 19].

The outcomes for the other type 2 KPros have shown favorable and comparable results; however, due to their limited usage, conclusive comparisons with other devices cannot be made.

7.14 Complications

The complications are categorized as ocular and device (KPro) related (Fig. 7.3).

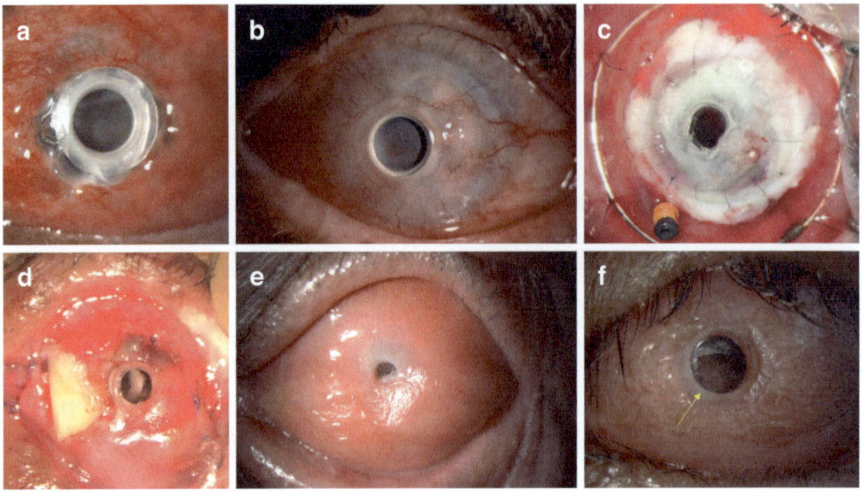

Fig. 7.3 Ocular and KPro-related complications associated with distinct types of KPros (**a**) Diffuse periprosthetic sterile melt around the optic in a type 1 KPro, requiring a KPro exchange. (**b**) Visually disabling RPM in a type 1 KPro, requiring surgical membranectomy. (**c**) Endophthalmitis with graft infiltrate following type 1 KPro, requiring KPro removal with pars plana vitrectomy along with a therapeutic penetrating keratoplasty. Six months later, the patient underwent a repeat type 1 KPro with improvement in visual acuity to 20/400. (**d**) Peripheral mucosal ulceration in MOOKP causing lamina exposure 15 years post procedure. Patient underwent a KPro swap with removal of the MOOKP lamina and replacement with a type 2 Boston KPro through the mucosa. (**e**) Mucosal overgrowth over the optic in MOOKP, addressed by surgical excision of the mucosa. (**f**) Aqueous leak (yellow arrow) 12 years post-MOOKP, due to laminar resorption. The osteo-odonto lamina was removed, and the patient underwent a type 2 Boston kpro through the mucosa with maintenance of a best-corrected visual acuity of 20/80

7.15 Ocular

7.15.1 Glaucoma

Glaucoma is one of the leading causes of visual loss in anatomically successful KPro implantations. It can either occur as new onset after KPro implantation (de novo) or as progression of existing disease. The incidence of preexisting glaucoma is 36%–76%, 44% -72%, and 20%–40% in type 1 Boston KPro, type 2 Boston KPro, and MOOKP, respectively. The incidence of de novo glaucoma is 13%–28%, 8%, and 10%–15% in type 1 Boston KPro, type 2 Boston KPro, and MOOKP, respectively [33, 34, 54, 56–59]. In addition to primary disease, distorted angles, peripheral anterior synechia, retroprosthetic membrane (RPM), and progressive angle closure are the causative mechanisms for glaucoma development and progression in KPro patients.

Managing glaucoma in the setting of KPro is far more challenging than in an eye without a KPro. Progression of glaucoma can be rapid and needs immediate attention. Measurement of IOP is unreliable with traditional instruments, and digital tonometry, though inaccurate, is the method most commonly used. In a type 1 Boston KPro, a tonopen may be used at the limbus but provides inaccurate readings. Furthermore, the optical cylinder limits visual field monitoring. However, optic disc photography, nerve fiber layer optical coherence tomography, and Heidelberg retinal tomography are helpful tools in diagnosing and monitoring glaucoma onset and progression and treatment response. The treatment options available include topical medications, drainage devices (required in the majority), and cyclophotocoagulation. Topical medications have a limited role in MOOKP due to a thick MMG, thus necessitating oral acetazolamide or surgical intervention. Surgical treatment consists of simultaneous or sequential drainage device implantation and ciliary body ablation. Li et al. found that 37.7% of type 1 Boston KPro patients required tube insertion, of which 59% had tube erosions [60]. Ciliary body ablation (endoscopic/transscleral) is performed in patients unresponsive to drainage tube devices. Tube/valve insertion is performed at the time of a type 2 Boston KPro [28]. Iyer et al. have described the technique, timing, and outcomes of Ahmed glaucoma valve in eyes undergoing MOOKP and recommend placing the tube before mucosal graft placement, when the ocular surface anatomy is least altered, though it can be performed at any stage as is warranted [61].

1. Vitreoretinal Complications

The commonly encountered vitreoretinal complications in a KPro patient are retinal detachment (RD), sterile vitritis, choroidal detachment (CD), choroidal/suprachoroidal hemorrhage, vitreous hemorrhage, cystoid macular edema (CME), choroidal effusion, and epiretinal membrane. These complications are more common during the first five years postimplantation. Retinal detachment is one of the most common complications of Boston KPro implantation ranging in incidence from 3.5% to 18.6% with type 1 and 18% with type 2.[34,44,62.] In MOOKP, an incidence of 3%–26% for retinal detachment, with a 20% success rate following surgical intervention has been reported [39, 63, 64]. Retinal detachment can be rhegmatogenous or tractional and can occur months or years following KPro surgery. Diagnosis is primarily made by ultrasound sonography unless it can be clinically visualized. Managing RDs in KPro eyes brings forth unique challenges, particularly with limited visualization through the optic [62–65].

Vitritis in a type 1 Boston KPro is always presumed infectious unless proven otherwise. Vitritis in an MOOKP has largely been reported to be sterile and responds to medical management with systemic steroids and antibiotics. This sterile vitritis is thought to be secondary to an inflammatory spillover associated with laminar resorption [39, 66].

7.15.2 Endophthalmitis

The incidence of endophthalmitis in Boston KPros is found to be 0–12.5%, while in MOOKP, it is reported to be 2–8% [34, 39, 54, 63, 67, 68]. Lack of complete bio-integration, chronic steroid use, multiple procedures, continuous contact lens wear, altered ocular flora secondary to continued antibiotic use, multiple surgeries, the underlying pathology, presence of glaucoma drainage devices, and periprosthetic melts or sterile keratolysis make eyes with a type 1 KPro more susceptible to infections. In MOOKP or OKP, preoperative dental/bone health is the most important predictor for subsequent endophthalmitis. Both bacteria and fungi are equally implicated as the causative organism [67, 68]. However, with the introduction of topical vancomycin as prophylaxis in type 1 KPro, a noticeable decline in the incidence of bacterial endophthalmitis was noted, but was accompanied by an increase in fungal infections [65].

Prophylactic use of broad-spectrum antibiotics, intermittent courses of topical antifungals, and weekly use of povidone-iodine along with a regular change of BCL has helped reduce the incidence of endophthalmitis in type 1 KPro.

The management of endophthalmitis in eyes with type 1 KPro is similar to the management in that of a non-KPro eye [65, 67, 68]. In the case of worsening despite medical management, intravitreal injections, and vitrectomy, it is advisable to remove the KPro and replace it with a donor corneal graft. Rarely, evisceration may be needed in nonresponsive eyes. The possibility of infection or carrier graft melt beneath the mucosa still exists. The diagnosis and management of endophthalmitis in eyes with type 2 KPro is more complex. In eyes with MOOKP, vitreous inflammation is usually sterile and responds to a systemic steroid-antibiotic combination. However, in cases of suspected infective etiology, any surgical intervention would involve reflection of the mucosa and/or lamina removal to proceed with measures for diagnosis and management [63, 64, 67]. Similarly, in eyes with Boston type 2 KPro, surgical intervention may proceed after reflecting the skin [34, 35].

7.16 Device/KPro Related

7.16.1 Retroprosthetic Membrane (RPM)

RPM is the most common complication of KPro, with the incidence ranging from 25% to 65% for Boston type 1 and 2 KPros, and 1%–7% for MOOKP [33, 34, 39, 44, 54, 69]. It occurs due to a fibrovascular growth on the inner surface of the optic from stromal downgrowth, metaplastic lens epithelium, or native iris stroma [70]. There are various risk factors for the development of an RPM, especially in type 1 Boston KPro, including anterior segment inflammation, previous keratitis, and simultaneous other surgery [71]. It primarily causes a drop in vision but can secondarily lead to graft melts and retinal detachment.

Removal of the native iris and lens, and anterior vitrectomy at the time of KPro surgery, reduces the chances of RPM formation. This is considered a critical factor contributing to the significantly reduced incidence of RPM in MOOKP as compared to Boston KPro. However, other factors might also come into play in such cases.

Modifying the design of the Boston type 1 KPro to use a titanium backplate has improved biocompatibility over PMMA, but studies comparing outcomes of devices with different backplate materials have found no significant difference in the incidence of RPM [72].

Visually insignificant RPMs can be observed while RPMs affecting vision may be treated with either YAG laser or surgical membranectomy [70, 71].

7.16.2 Sterile Melts

Incidence rates of 35–50% have been reported for sterile melts in type 1 KPro in eyes with chemical injury; it is higher in eyes with underlying autoimmune etiology [25, 73]. Dellen, RPM, or infectious keratitis further act as a risk factor, thus necessitating a detailed, careful slit-lamp evaluation at each visit [73]. The management of a sterile melt is mainly dependent on the presence or absence of an associated aqueous leak. Small epithelial defects and early melts involving less than 2 clock hours can be managed by applying cyanoacrylate glue. In contrast, the larger ones will require a crescentic annular/lamellar graft. In very severe cases or those with recurrent melts, explantation of the existing device and replacement with a new one is recommended. Medical treatment to reduce the lysis can be given simultaneously at various stages. Topical medroxyprogesterone, systemic tetracyclines, and copious lubricants can also be used [74].

7.16.3 Lamina Resorption

Similar to sterile melts, the periprosthetic tissue loss in MOOKP/OKP is called lamina resorption, in which the thickness of the lamina decreases, resulting in an aqueous leak in severe cases [75]. It is considered the most common cause of anatomical failure in MOOKP/OKP, with an incidence of 2%–28% [39, 54]. Central resorption can lead to a loose cylinder, aqueous leak, altered refraction, lamina tilt, and endophthalmitis [75].Apart from the natural course of the bone lamina, the risk factors associated with lamina resorption are allograft, young age, tibial lamina, persistent inflammation, RPM, smoking, and steroid used [38, 54, 66].

Lamina resorption is challenging to diagnose as it is a slow process and not visible on slit-lamp due to the MMG cover; however, early subtle clinical signs like a cylinder tilt and a boggy feel on palpation due to the dead space under the mucosa or an increased protrusion of the cylinder can aid in diagnosis along with serial CT scans, showing the linear dimensions and volumetric data [76]. To reduce the chances of lamina resorption, the lamina can be fashioned under a pool of fluid to eliminate thermal and desiccation-induced damage [77]. Canine tooth bone augmentation with mandibular bone graft and bone morphogenic protein has shown promise in delaying resorption and enhancing anatomic survival, respectively [75, 78].

7.17 Mucous Membrane/Skin Related

7.17.1 Ulceration

The mucosa in MOOKP can ulcerate due to inadequate vascularization immediately following stage 1B, though dryness and infection can also be responsible. It varies in incidence from 8% to 48% [38, 39, 54]. The trophic changes can cause lamina exposure either centrally near the optic or peripherally in the case of a bulky lamina. In mild cases, adequate lubricants will suffice; however, moderate to severe cases can be treated surgically with a bucket-handle flap, tarsal pedicle flap, new mucosal patch graft, or rarely, a through-the-lid KPro [79]. Similarly, retraction of the skin around the optic of the Boston type 2 KPro needs to be addressed surgically by resuturing the skin edges so that they are flush with the optic edge.

7.17.2 Overgrowth

Mucosal overgrowth in the MOOKP and skin overgrowth in the Boston type 2 occur in 2%–33% and > 50% of cases, respectively [34, 39, 54, 58]. Surgical excision is usually required. In recurrent mucous membrane overgrowth, trimming with off-label application of mitomycin C at the margins has been performed [80].

7.18 Future Directions

The ideal KPro is still far from reality, and current research aims to improve anatomical outcomes by enhancing bio-integration of the KPro with the host tissue, either with better materials or surface coating, or by using synthetic biomimetic substitutes for tooth or bone [75, 78]. Methods to facilitate early diagnosis and management of possible complications are being actively investigated.

Constant efforts have been underway to overcome the unreliability of IOP measurement in post-KPro eyes. This has led to the development of a device that can be fixed in the sulcus intraocularly during KPro surgery to allow telemetric assessment of IOP and has shown satisfactory results in Boston type 1 KPro implantation [81]. Another device, a micro-optomechanical pressure sensor, which can be incorporated into KPro assembly is currently under development [30]. Additionally, new glaucoma shunt devices specially designed for KPro patients and contact lens drug delivery of antiglaucoma medications have shown promising results in animal trials [82, 83].

Slow-releasing antibiotic contact lenses are being tested in Boston type 1 KPro to reduce the chances of endophthalmitis. To minimize the chances of a melt and its associated complications, cross-linked tissue as a carrier is being studied for high risk patients [84]. To address the global shortage of corneal donor tissue, the use of gamma-irradiated donor grafts, glycerin-preserved grafts, and xenografts are being evaluated for use as a carrier for Boston KPro [30].

Apart from technical modifications, biological agents such as antitumor necrosis factor-α are being studied in patients with chemical burns to reduce the chances of chronic inflammation and its associated complications post-KPro [85].

7.19 Conclusion

Boston type 1 KPro and MOOKP are the most popular choices of KPro currently available. While there is ample evidence of success in restoring vision, there is a high risk of sight-threatening complications. Judicious selection of patients and devices is of utmost importance. Despite the long-term successes that have been reported for various KPros, associated complications indicate the need for further research. Decision-making and counseling are the most crucial aspects of KPro surgery and cannot be overemphasized.

Declarations of Interest None.

Conflict of Interest None.

References

1. Khan B, Dudenhoefer EJ, Dohlman CH. Keratoprosthesis: an update. Curr Opin Ophthalmol. 2001;12(4):282–7. https://doi.org/10.1097/00055735-200108000-00007.
2. Sangwan VS, Tseng SC. New perspectives in ocular surface disorders. An integrated approach for diagnosis and management. Indian J Ophthalmol. 2001;49(3):153–68.
3. Dogru M, Tsubota K. Current concepts in ocular surface reconstruction. Semin Ophthalmol. 2005;20(2):75–93. https://doi.org/10.1080/08820530590931142.
4. Iyer G, Srinivasan B, Agarwal S. Ocular sequelae of Stevens-Johnson syndrome: a comprehensive approach. Cornea. 2020;39(Suppl 1):S3–6. https://doi.org/10.1097/ICO.0000000000002532.
5. Chirila TV, Hicks CR. The origins of the artificial cornea: Pellier de Quengsy and his contribution to the modern concept of keratoprosthesis. Gesnerus. 1999;56(1–2):96–106.
6. Barber JC. Keratoprosthesis: past and present. Int Ophthalmol Clin. 1988;28(2):103–9. https://doi.org/10.1097/00004397-198802820-00002.
7. Cardona H. Mushroom Transcorneal Keratoprosthesis: bolt and nut. Am J Ophthalmol. 1969;68(4):604–12. https://doi.org/10.1016/0002-9394(69)91239-2.
8. Dohlman CH, Schneider HA, Doane MG. Prosthokeratoplasty. Am J Ophthalmol. 1974;77(5):694–700. https://doi.org/10.1016/0002-9394(74)90534-0.
9. Liu C, Hille K, Tan D, Hicks C, Herold J. Keratoprosthesis surgery. Surg Dry Eye. 2008;41:171–86. https://doi.org/10.1159/000131088.
10. Dohlman CH, Doane MG. Some factors influencing outcome after keratoprosthesis surgery. Cornea. 1994;13(3):214–8. https://doi.org/10.1097/00003226-199405000-00004.
11. Dohlman CH, Harissi-Dagher M. The Boston Keratoprosthesis: a new Threadless design. Digital J Ophthalmol. 2007;13(3)
12. Harissi-Dagher M, Khan BF, Schaumberg DA, Dohlman CH. Importance of nutrition to corneal grafts when used as a carrier of the Boston Keratoprosthesis. Cornea. 2007;26(5):564–8. https://doi.org/10.1097/ICO.0b013e318041f0a6.

13. Avadhanam VS, Smith HE, Liu C. Keratoprostheses for corneal blindness: a review of contemporary devices. Clin Ophthalmol Auckl NZ. 2015;9:697–720. https://doi.org/10.2147/OPTH.S27083.
14. Bakshi SK, Paschalis EI, Graney J, Chodosh J. Lucia and beyond: development of an affordable Keratoprosthesis. Cornea. 2019;38(4):492–7. https://doi.org/10.1097/ICO.0000000000001880.
15. Venugopal A, Rathi H, Rengappa R, Ravindran M, Raman R. Outcomes after Auro Keratoprosthesis implantation: a low-cost design based on the Boston Keratoprosthesis. Cornea. 2016;35(10):1285–8. https://doi.org/10.1097/ICO.0000000000000936.
16. Strampelli B. Keratoprosthesis with osteodontal tissue. Am J Ophthalmol. 1963;89:1029–39.
17. Temprano J. Keratoprosthesis with tibial autograft. Refract Corneal Surg. 1993;9:192–3.
18. Bakshi SK, Graney J, Paschalis EI, et al. Design and outcomes of a novel Keratoprosthesis: addressing unmet needs in end-stage Cicatricial corneal blindness. Cornea. 2020;39(4):484–90. https://doi.org/10.1097/ICO.0000000000002207.
19. Basu S, Nagpal R, Serna-Ojeda JC, Bhalekar S, Bagga B, Sangwan V. LVP keratoprosthesis: anatomical and functional outcomes in bilateral end-stage corneal blindness. Br J Ophthalmol. 2018. Published online June 11, 2018 bjophthalmol-2017-311649; https://doi.org/10.1136/bjophthalmol-2017-311649.
20. Pintucci S, Pintucci F, Cecconi M, Caiazza S. New Dacron tissue colonisable keratoprosthesis: clinical experience. Br J Ophthalmol. 1995;79(9):825–9. https://doi.org/10.1136/bjo.79.9.825.
21. Kim MK, Lee SM, Lee JL, et al. Long-term outcome in ocular intractable surface disease with Seoul-type keratoprosthesis. Cornea. 2007;26(5):546–51. https://doi.org/10.1097/ICO.0b013e3180415d35.
22. Iakymenko S. Forty-five years of keratoprosthesis study and application at the Filatov institute: a retrospective analysis of 1 060 cases. Int J Ophthalmol. 2013;6(3):375–80. https://doi.org/10.3980/j.issn.2222-3959.2013.03.22.
23. Huang Y, Yu J, Liu L, Du G, Song J, Guo H. Moscow eye microsurgery complex in Russia keratoprosthesis in Beijing. Ophthalmology. 2011;118(1):41–6. https://doi.org/10.1016/j.ophtha.2010.05.019.
24. Ghaffariyeh A, Honarpisheh N, Karkhaneh A, et al. Fyodorov-Zuev keratoprosthesis implantation: long-term results in patients with multiple failed corneal grafts. Graefes Arch Clin Exp Ophthalmol Albrecht Von Graefes Arch Klin Exp Ophthalmol. 2011;249(1):93–101. https://doi.org/10.1007/s00417-010-1493-8.
25. Iyer G, Srinivasan B, Gupta N, Padmanabhan P. Outcome of Boston Keratoprosthesis in a developing country-importance of patient selection, education, and perioperative care: the Indian experience. Asia-Pac J Ophthalmol Phila Pa. 2012;1(4):202–7. https://doi.org/10.1097/APO.0b013e3182607e5d.
26. Traish AS, Chodosh J. Expanding application of the Boston type I keratoprosthesis due to advances in design and improved post-operative therapeutic strategies. Semin Ophthalmol. 2010;25(5–6):239–43. https://doi.org/10.3109/08820538.2010.518895.
27. Aldave AJ, Kamal KM, Vo RC, Yu F. The Boston type I keratoprosthesis: improving outcomes and expanding indications. Ophthalmology. 2009;116(4):640–51. https://doi.org/10.1016/j.ophtha.2008.12.058.
28. Iyer G, Srinivasan B, Agarwal S, et al. Keratoprosthesis: current global scenario and a broad Indian perspective. Indian J Ophthalmol. 2018;66(5):620–9. https://doi.org/10.4103/ijo.IJO_22_18.
29. Saeed HN, Shanbhag S, Chodosh J. The Boston keratoprosthesis. Curr Opin Ophthalmol. 2017;28(4):390–6. https://doi.org/10.1097/ICU.0000000000000373.
30. Nonpassopon M, Niparugs M, Cortina MS. Boston type 1 Keratoprosthesis: updated perspectives. Clin Ophthalmol Auckl NZ. 2020;14:1189–200. https://doi.org/10.2147/OPTH.S219270.
31. Sayegh RR, Diaz LA, Vargas-Martín F, Webb RH, Dohlman CH, Peli E. Optical functional properties of the Boston Keratoprosthesis. Invest Ophthalmol Vis Sci. 2010;51(2):857–63. https://doi.org/10.1167/iovs.09-3372.

32. Sharma N, Falera R, Arora T, Agarwal T, Bandivadekar P, Vajpayee RB. Evaluation of a low-cost design keratoprosthesis in end-stage corneal disease: a preliminary study. Br J Ophthalmol. 2016;100(3):323–7. https://doi.org/10.1136/bjophthalmol-2015-306982.
33. Pujari S, Siddique SS, Dohlman CH, Chodosh J. The Boston keratoprosthesis type II: the Massachusetts eye and ear infirmary experience. Cornea. 2011;30(12):1298–303. https://doi.org/10.1097/ICO.0b013e318215207c.
34. Lee R, Khoueir Z, Tsikata E, Chodosh J, Dohlman CH, Chen TC. Long-term visual outcomes and complications of Boston Keratoprosthesis type II implantation. Ophthalmology. 2017;124(1):27–35. https://doi.org/10.1016/j.ophtha.2016.07.011.
35. Iyer G, Srinivasan B, Agarwal S, et al. Boston type 2 keratoprosthesis- mid term outcomes from a tertiary eye care Centre in India. Ocul Surf. 2019;17(1):50–4. https://doi.org/10.1016/j.jtos.2018.08.003.
36. Falcinelli G. Personal changes and innovations in Strampelli's osteo-odonto-keratoprosthesis. Inst BarraquerBarc. 1998;28:47–8.
37. Lee RMH, Ong GL, Lam FC, et al. Optical functional performance of the osteo-odonto-keratoprosthesis. Cornea. 2014;33(10):1038–45. https://doi.org/10.1097/ICO.0000000000000235.
38. Hille K, Grabner G, Liu C, et al. Standards for modified osteoodontokeratoprosthesis (OOKP) surgery according to Strampelli and Falcinelli: the Rome-Vienna protocol. Cornea. 2005;24(8):895–908. https://doi.org/10.1097/01.ico.0000157401.81408.62.
39. Iyer G, Pillai VS, Srinivasan B, et al. Modified osteo-odonto keratoprosthesis–the Indian experience–results of the first 50 cases. Cornea 2010;29(7):771–776. doi:https://doi.org/10.1097/ICO.0b013e3181ca31fc.
40. Kang KB, Karas FI, Rai R, et al. Five year outcomes of Boston type I keratoprosthesis as primary versus secondary penetrating corneal procedure in a matched case control study. PLoS One. 2018;13(2):e0192381. https://doi.org/10.1371/journal.pone.0192381.
41. Rudnisky CJ, Belin MW, Guo R, Ciolino JB. Boston type 1 Keratoprosthesis study group. Visual acuity outcomes of the Boston Keratoprosthesis type 1: multicenter study results. Am J Ophthalmol. 2016;162:89–98.e1. https://doi.org/10.1016/j.ajo.2015.10.023.
42. Phillips DL, Hager JL, Goins KM, et al. Boston type 1 keratoprosthesis for chemical and thermal injury. Cornea. 2014;33(9):905–9. https://doi.org/10.1097/ICO.0000000000000204.
43. Shanbhag SS, Saeed HN, Paschalis EI, Chodosh J. Boston keratoprosthesis type 1 for limbal stem cell deficiency after severe chemical corneal injury: a systematic review. Ocul Surf. 2018;16(3):272–81. https://doi.org/10.1016/j.jtos.2018.03.007.
44. Zerbe BL, Belin MW, Ciolino JB. Boston type 1 Keratoprosthesis study group. Results from the multicenter Boston type 1 Keratoprosthesis study. Ophthalmology. 2006;113(10):1779.e1–7. https://doi.org/10.1016/j.ophtha.2006.05.015.
45. Iyer G, Srinivasan B, Gupta J, et al. Boston Keratoprosthesis for keratopathy in eyes with retained silicone oil: a new indication. Cornea. 2011;30(10):1083–7. https://doi.org/10.1097/ICO.0b013e318213a8b5.
46. Aravena C, Yu F, Aldave AJ. Long-term visual outcomes, complications, and retention of the Boston type I Keratoprosthesis. Cornea. 2018;37(1):3–10. https://doi.org/10.1097/ICO.0000000000001405.
47. Sayegh RR, Ang LPK, Foster CS, Dohlman CH. The Boston keratoprosthesis in Stevens-Johnson syndrome. Am J Ophthalmol. 2008;145(3):438–44. https://doi.org/10.1016/j.ajo.2007.11.002.
48. Palioura S, Kim B, Dohlman CH, Chodosh J. The Boston keratoprosthesis type I in mucous membrane pemphigoid. Cornea. 2013;32(7):956–61. https://doi.org/10.1097/ICO.0b013e318286fd73.
49. Brown CR, Wagoner MD, Welder JD, et al. Boston keratoprosthesis type 1 for herpes simplex and herpes zoster keratopathy. Cornea. 2014;33(8):801–5. https://doi.org/10.1097/ICO.0000000000000164.
50. Basu S, Serna-Ojeda JC, Senthil S, Pappuru RR, Bagga B, Sangwan V. The Aurolab Keratoprosthesis (KPro) versus the Boston type I KPro: 5-year clinical outcomes in 134 cases of bilateral corneal blindness. Am J Ophthalmol. 2019;205:175–83. https://doi.org/10.1016/j.ajo.2019.03.016.

51. Greiner MA, Li JY, Mannis MJ. Longer-term vision outcomes and complications with the Boston type 1 keratoprosthesis at the University of California, Davis. Ophthalmology. 2011;118(8):1543–50. https://doi.org/10.1016/j.ophtha.2010.12.032.
52. Charoenrook V, Michael R, de la Paz MF, Temprano J, Barraquer RI. Comparison of long-term results between osteo-odonto-keratoprosthesis and tibial bone keratoprosthesis. Ocul Surf. 2018;16(2):259–64. https://doi.org/10.1016/j.jtos.2018.02.003.
53. de la Paz MF, Salvador-Culla B, Charoenrook V, et al. Osteo-odonto-, Tibial bone and Boston keratoprosthesis in clinically comparable cases of chemical injury and autoimmune disease. Ocul Surf. 2019;17(3):476–83. https://doi.org/10.1016/j.jtos.2019.04.006.
54. Falcinelli G, Falsini B, Taloni M, Colliardo P, Falcinelli G. Modified osteo-odonto-keratoprosthesis for treatment of corneal blindness: long-term anatomical and functional outcomes in 181 cases. Arch Ophthalmol Chic Ill 1960. 2005;123(10):1319–1329. doi:https://doi.org/10.1001/archopht.123.10.1319.
55. Marchi V, Ricci R, Pecorella I, Ciardi A, Di Tondo U. Osteo-odonto-keratoprosthesis. Description of surgical technique with results in 85 patients. Cornea. 1994;13(2):125–30.
56. Talajic JC, Agoumi Y, Gagné S, Moussally K, Harissi-Dagher M. Prevalence, progression, and impact of glaucoma on vision after Boston type 1 keratoprosthesis surgery. Am J Ophthalmol. 2012;153(2):267–274.e1. https://doi.org/10.1016/j.ajo.2011.07.022.
57. Netland PA, Terada H, Dohlman CH. Glaucoma associated with keratoprosthesis. Ophthalmology. 1998;105(4):751–7. https://doi.org/10.1016/S0161-6420(98)94034-9.
58. Tan A, Tan DT, Tan X-W, Mehta JS. Osteo-odonto keratoprosthesis: systematic review of surgical outcomes and complication rates. Ocul Surf. 2012;10(1):15–25. https://doi.org/10.1016/j.jtos.2012.01.003.
59. Zarei-Ghanavati M, Avadhanam V, Vasquez Perez A, Liu C. The osteo-odonto-keratoprosthesis. Curr Opin Ophthalmol. 2017;28(4):397–402. https://doi.org/10.1097/ICU.0000000000000388.
60. Li JY, Greiner MA, Brandt JD, Lim MC, Mannis MJ. Long-term complications associated with glaucoma drainage devices and Boston keratoprosthesis. Am J Ophthalmol. 2011;152(2):209–18. https://doi.org/10.1016/j.ajo.2011.01.034.
61. Iyer G, Srinivasan B, Agarwal S, et al. Glaucoma in modified osteo-odonto-keratoprosthesis eyes: role of additional stage 1A and Ahmed glaucoma drainage device-technique and timing. Am J Ophthalmol. 2015;159(3):482–489.e2. https://doi.org/10.1016/j.ajo.2014.11.030.
62. Khair D, Salimi A, Harissi-Dagher M. Vitreoretinal complications in Boston Keratoprosthesis type 1. Am J Ophthalmol. 2021;231:101–8. https://doi.org/10.1016/j.ajo.2021.06.002.
63. Rishi P, Rishi E, Agarwal V, et al. Vitreoretinal complications and outcomes in 92 eyes undergoing surgery for modified Osteo-Odonto-Keratoprosthesis: a 10-year review. Ophthalmology. 2018;125(6):832–41. https://doi.org/10.1016/j.ophtha.2017.12.003.
64. Lim LS, Ang CL, Wong E, Wong DWK, Tan DTH. Vitreoretinal complications and vitreoretinal surgery in Osteo-Odonto-Keratoprosthesis surgery. Am J Ophthalmol. 2014;157(2):349–54. https://doi.org/10.1016/j.ajo.2013.08.033.
65. Modjtahedi BS, Eliott D. Vitreoretinal complications of the Boston Keratoprosthesis. Semin Ophthalmol. 2014;29(5–6):338–48. https://doi.org/10.3109/08820538.2014.959204.
66. Avadhanam V, Liu C. Managing laminar resorption in osteo-odonto-keratoprosthesis. Am J Ophthalmol. 2014;158(2):213–214.e2. https://doi.org/10.1016/j.ajo.2014.04.011.
67. Rishi P, Rishi E, Manchegowda P, Iyer G, Srinivasan B, Agarwal S. Endophthalmitis in eyes with Osteo-odonto Keratoprosthesis. Ocul Immunol Inflamm. Published online October 7, 2020:1–5. https://doi.org/10.1080/09273948.2020.1770807.
68. Robert M-C, Moussally K, Harissi-Dagher M. Review of endophthalmitis following Boston keratoprosthesis type 1. Br J Ophthalmol. 2012;96(6):776–80. https://doi.org/10.1136/bjophthalmol-2011-301263.
69. De La Paz MF, De Toledo JÁ, Charoenrook V, et al. Impact of clinical factors on the long-term functional and anatomic outcomes of osteo-odonto-keratoprosthesis and tibial bone keratoprosthesis. Am J Ophthalmol. 2011;151(5):829–839.e1. https://doi.org/10.1016/j.ajo.2010.11.011.

70. Stacy RC, Jakobiec FA, Michaud NA, Dohlman CH, Colby KA. Characterization of retrokeratoprosthetic membranes in the Boston type 1 keratoprosthesis. Arch Ophthalmol Chic Ill 1960. 2011;129(3):310–316. doi:https://doi.org/10.1001/archophthalmol.2011.26.
71. Rudnisky CJ, Belin MW, Todani A, et al. Risk factors for the development of retroprosthetic membranes with Boston keratoprosthesis type 1: multicenter study results. Ophthalmology. 2012;119(5):951–5. https://doi.org/10.1016/j.ophtha.2011.11.030.
72. Talati RK, Hallak JA, Karas FI, de la Cruz J, Cortina MS. Retroprosthetic membrane formation in Boston Keratoprosthesis: a case-control-matched comparison of titanium versus PMMA Backplate. Cornea. 2018;37(2):145–50. https://doi.org/10.1097/ICO.0000000000001462.
73. Bouhout S, Robert M-C, Deli S, Harissi-Dagher M. Corneal melt after Boston Keratoprosthesis: clinical presentation, management, outcomes and risk factor analysis. Ocul Immunol Inflamm. 2018;26(5):693–9. https://doi.org/10.1080/09273948.2016.1269930.
74. Hicks CR, Crawford GJ. Melting after keratoprosthesis implantation: the effects of medroxyprogesterone. Cornea. 2003;22(6):497–500. https://doi.org/10.1097/00003226-200308000-00001.
75. Iyer G, Srinivasan B, Agarwal S, Shanmugasundaram S, Rajan G. Structural & functional rehabilitation in eyes with lamina resorption following MOOKP--can the lamina be salvaged? Graefes Arch Clin Exp Ophthalmol Albrecht Von Graefes Arch Klin Exp Ophthalmol. 2014;252(5):781–790. doi:https://doi.org/10.1007/s00417-014-2598-2.
76. Stoiber J, Forstner R, Csáky D, Ruckhofer J, Grabner G. Evaluation of bone reduction in osteo-odontokeratoprosthesis (OOKP) by three-dimensional computed tomography. Cornea. 2003;22(2):126–30. https://doi.org/10.1097/00003226-200303000-00009.
77. Aguilar M, Sawatari Y, Gonzalez A, et al. Improvements in the modified osteo-odonto Keratoprosthesis (MOOKP) surgery technique. Invest Ophthalmol Vis Sci. 2013;54(15):3481.
78. Iyer G, Srinivasan B, Agarwal S, et al. Bone augmentation of the osteo-odonto alveolar lamina in MOOKP--will it delay laminar resorption? Graefes Arch Clin Exp Ophthalmol Albrecht Von Graefes Arch Klin Exp Ophthalmol 2015;253(7):1137–1141. doi:https://doi.org/10.1007/s00417-015-3055-6.
79. Avadhanam VS, Vasquez-Perez A, Chervenkoff JV, El-Zahab S, Liu C. Mucosal complications in osteo-odonto keratoprosthesis (OOKP) surgery. J EuCornea. 2020;6:13–23. https://doi.org/10.1016/j.xjec.2020.01.001.
80. Avadhanam VS, Herold J, Thorp S, Liu CSC. Mitomycin-C for mucous membrane overgrowth in OOKP eyes. Cornea. 2014;33(9):981–4. https://doi.org/10.1097/ICO.0000000000000183.
81. Enders P, Hall J, Bornhauser M, Mansouri K, Altay L, Schrader S, Dietlein TS, Bachmann BO, Neuhann T, Cursiefen C. Telemetric intraocular pressure monitoring after Boston Keratoprosthesis surgery using the Eyemate-IO sensor: dynamics in the first year. Am J Ophthalmol. 2019;206:256–63.
82. Paschalis EI, Chodosh J, Sperling RA, Salvador-Culla B, Dohlman C. A novel implantable glaucoma valve using ferrofluid. PLoS One. 2013;8(6):e67404. https://doi.org/10.1371/journal.pone.0067404.
83. Ciolino JB, Stefanescu CF, Ross AE, et al. In vivo performance of a drug-eluting contact lens to treat glaucoma for a month. Biomaterials. 2014;35(1):432–9. https://doi.org/10.1016/j.biomaterials.2013.09.032.
84. Robert M-C, Arafat SN, Ciolino JB. Collagen cross-linking of the Boston keratoprosthesis donor carrier to prevent corneal melting in high-risk patients. Eye Contact Lens. 2014;40(6):376–81. https://doi.org/10.1097/ICL.0000000000000081.
85. Cade F, Paschalis EI, Regatieri CV, Vavvas DG, Dana R, Dohlman CH. Alkali burn to the eye: protection using TNF-α inhibition. Cornea. 2014;33(4):382–9. https://doi.org/10.1097/ICO.0000000000000071.

Corneal Endothelial Diseases

8

Xueyang Wang, Hajirah N. Saeed, and Ula V. Jurkunas

Summary

- Fuchs endothelial dystrophy, postinfectious endotheliitis, bullous keratopathy, iridocorneal endothelial syndrome, posterior polymorphous dystrophy, and congenital hereditary endothelial dystrophy are all diseases of the endothelium that can result in irreversible corneal edema and opacity.
- Pachymetry, specular microscopy, confocal microscopy, and anterior segment optical coherence tomography are all modalities that aid in the diagnosis and characterization of endothelial disease by assessing corneal thickness and endothelial cell morphology, allowing the visualization of all layers of the cornea.
- While corneal transplantation is currently the mainstay of treatment, novel therapies, including corneal endothelial cell expansion and pharmacological agents targeting endothelial cell degeneration, are on the horizon. Other investigational therapies include human embryonic stem cells, induced pluripotent stem cells, and endothelial stem cell regeneration.

X. Wang · U. V. Jurkunas (✉)
Department of Ophthalmology, Massachusetts Eye and Ear, Harvard Medical School, Boston, MA, USA
e-mail: ula_jurkunas@meei.harvard.edu

H. N. Saeed
Department of Ophthalmology and Visual Sciences, Illinois Eye and Ear Infirmary, University of Illinois Chicago, Chicago, IL, USA

Department of Ophthalmology, Massachusetts Eye and Ear Infirmary, Harvard Medical School, Boston, MA, USA

Department of Ophthalmology, Loyola University Medical Center, Maywood, IL, USA

H. N. Saeed, R. B. Singh (eds.), *Corneal Disorders*, Current Practices in Ophthalmology, https://doi.org/10.1007/978-981-96-5294-5_8

8.1 Introduction

The endothelial cell layer of the cornea lines the inner surface of the cornea and regulates corneal stromal hydration. This single, approximately 5-μm thick layer of polygonal cells serves as a passive barrier to imbibing fluid from the aqueous humor and actively pumping fluid out of the cornea. Endothelial dysfunction or damage results in corneal edema, reducing corneal transparency. This can lead to painful blistering of the corneal epithelium, called bullae. This chapter provides an overview of the diagnosis and management of endothelial diseases.

8.2 Fuchs Endothelial Corneal Dystrophy

8.2.1 Epidemiology and Etiology

Fuchs endothelial corneal dystrophy (FECD) is the most common primary corneal endothelial dystrophy and the leading indication for corneal transplantation in the world [1]. It is typically a late-onset disease characterized by slow, progressive degeneration of the endothelium, leading to corneal edema and vision loss. The onset of FECD is typically in the fifth or sixth decades of life, with a greater incidence in women, at a ratio of 3–4:1 [2–5]. A higher frequency of more advanced FECD has also been reported in women than men [6]. The disease prevalence ranges from 3.7% to 9.2%, affecting approximately 3.9–6.62% of the population in the United States over the age of 40 [7–13].

FECD is characterized by the buildup of extracellular matrix excrescences, called guttae, on the posterior Descemet membrane. There is an increased rate of thickening and disorganization of the extracellular matrix, and the endothelial cell density declines faster. The pathogenesis of FECD involves a combination of multiple genes and environmental factors. It is a heterogeneous genetic disease with variable expressivity and incomplete penetrance, meaning individuals within a given family do not conform to a specific clinical presentation [14, 15]. One exception is early-onset FECD associated with *COL8A2* mutations, which can occur in the third decade of life [16]. Mutation in the transcription factor 4 (*TCF4*) gene is a causal variant in the majority of FECD patients [17]. Other risk factors for FECD include family history, ultraviolet ray exposure, smoking, and diabetes [12, 18–20].

8.2.2 Symptoms

Patients are usually asymptomatic in early disease. As FECD progresses, patients experience glare at night and reduced vision in the morning, secondary to increased corneal edema after eye closure overnight. Patients with advanced FECD develop decreased vision, photophobia, epiphora, and pain throughout the day. Increased stromal and epithelial edema can lead to ruptured epithelial bullae, resulting in a persistent epithelial defect or a corneal ulcer [18].

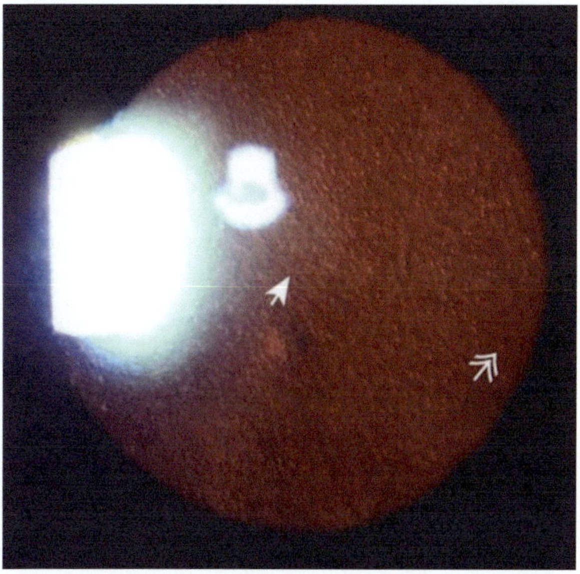

Fig. 8.1 Slit-lamp photograph of a cornea with Fuchs endothelial corneal dystrophy. Retroillumination shows confluent (solid arrowhead) and individual (double arrowhead) guttae. (Reprinted with permission from Taylor and Francis. doi: 10.1080/08820538.2019.1632355)

8.2.3 Examination Findings and Clinical Grading

Slit-beam illumination with a thin beam can reveal epithelial bullae, corneal edema, and guttae. Guttae are excrescences of abnormal collagen deposited by the corneal endothelium, and their presence is the first clinical sign of FECD (Fig. 8.1). Retroillumination of the cornea after pupillary dilation is an important technique in assessing the distribution and number of guttae [21–23]. Guttae typically originate in the central cornea and radiate toward the periphery (Figs. 8.2, 8.3 and 8.4).

Four clinical stages of FECD were described by Adamis et al. in 1993 [24]. Patients in stage 1 usually have normal vision with central corneal guttae, pigment on the posterior cornea, and a gray, thickened Descemet membrane. Patients with stage 2 FECD have a painless decrease in vision and presence of significant glare, typically worse upon waking. On examination, guttae are confluent and extend toward the peripheral cornea, and mild corneal edema can be seen. Stage 3 is defined by worsening vision and recurrent episodes of pain due to rupture of epithelial bullae. Stage 4 is characterized by chronic severe edema resulting in subepithelial scarring, which decreases bullae formation but severely limits vision. Other grading scales of FECD include the Krachmer and modified Krachmer grading scale, which assess the confluence of guttae and the presence of stromal or epithelial corneal edema [3, 4].

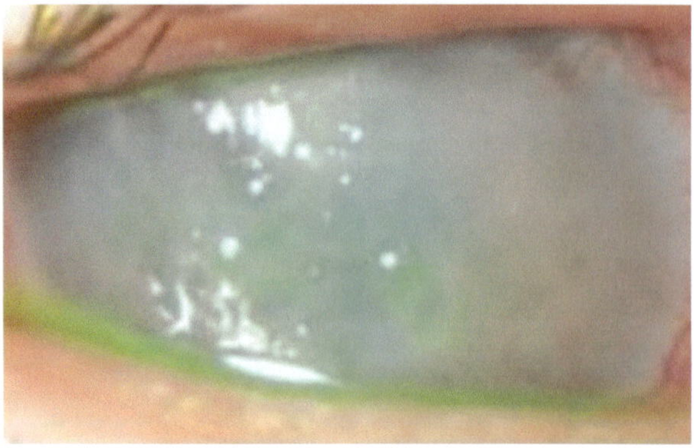

Fig. 8.2 Slit-lamp photograph of a cornea with bullous keratopathy. Corneal edema and bullae can be seen along with diffuse haze. (Reprinted with permission from Elsevier. doi: 10.1016/j.ajoc.2022.101287)

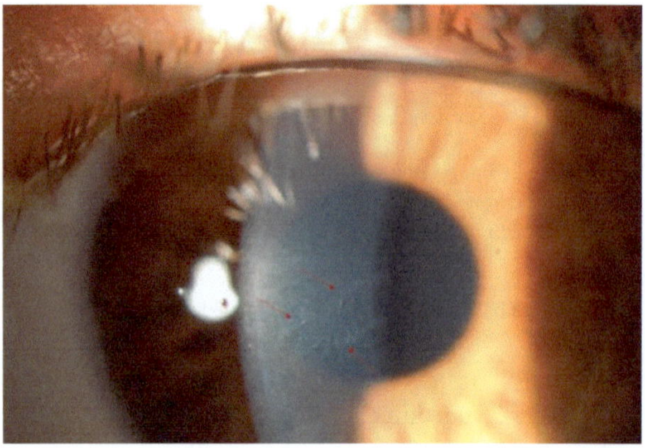

Fig. 8.3 Slit-lamp photograph showing scalloped band lesions, also known as "snail tracks"(red arrows) at Descemet membrane, characteristic of PPCD. (Reprinted with permission from Wolters Kluwer Health, Inc. doi: 10.1097/ICO.0000000000002847)

Fig. 8.4 Noncontact specular microscopy and in vivo confocal microscopy (IVCM) in healthy and Fuchs endothelial corneal dystrophy (FECD) subjects. (**a**) Noncontact specular microscopy in a healthy subject. (**b**) IVCM in a healthy subject. (**c**) Noncontact specular microscopy in a FECD subject with stage 3 guttae (solid arrowhead). (**d**) IVCM in a FECD subject with stage 1 guttae (arrow). (**e**) Noncontact specular microscopy in a FECD subject with stage 2 guttae (solid arrowhead) and stage 3 guttae (double arrowhead). (**f**) IVCM in a FECD subject with stage 1 guttae (arrow) and stage 2 guttae (solid arrowhead). (Reprinted with permission from Taylor and Francis. doi: 10.1080/08820538.2019.1632355)

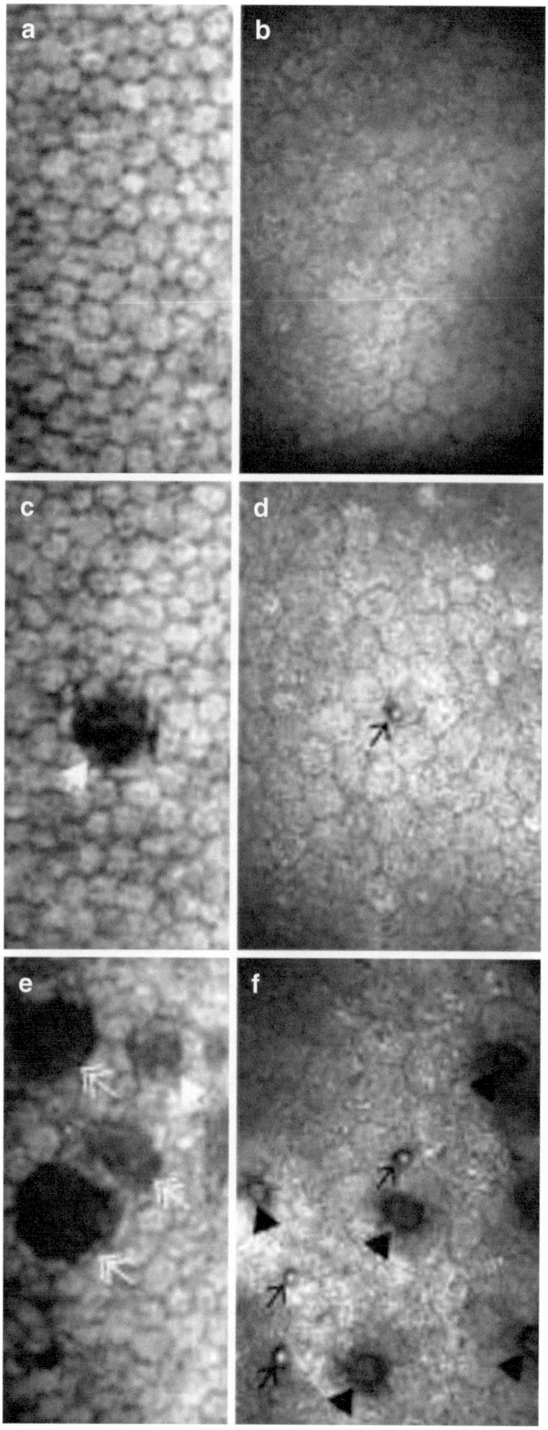
a
b
c
d
e
f

8.3 Endothelial Disease from Surgical or Laser Trauma

Bullous keratopathy is a condition in which corneal edema, and resultant epithelial bullae, occurs from injury to the corneal endothelium, often due to intraocular surgery. Corneal edema following cataract surgery is called pseudophakic bullous keratopathy (PBK), which can occur from endothelial cell loss during or after cataract surgery and is affected by surgeon experience, nuclear density, intraocular lens position (especially in the anterior chamber), and postsurgical inflammation. Patient factors including advanced age, previous intraocular surgery, previous trauma, shallow anterior chamber, glaucoma, and diabetes can also increase the risk of PBK. In the United States, about 4500 keratoplasty procedures are performed annually to treat PBK, representing 9% of the annual keratoplasty procedures. Glaucoma surgery and laser peripheral iridotomy have also been associated with increased risk of corneal decompensation [25].

8.4 Postinfectious Endotheliitis

Corneal endotheliitis can result from infectious anterior uveitis, resulting in corneal decompensation. Herpes simplex virus (HSV), varicella-zoster virus (VZV), and cytomegalovirus (CMV) have all been reported to cause this condition. Patients commonly present with eye pain, photophobia, and vision changes. Examination reveals corneal edema, keratic precipitates, and anterior chamber inflammation. While there are no established guidelines for the dosage of treatment for viral endotheliitis, patients with HSV/VZV endotheliitis are treated with oral acyclovir or valacyclovir, and those with CMV endotheliitis are treated with oral valganciclovir. Patients are also placed on topical corticosteroids to reduce inflammation [26].

8.5 Iridocorneal Endothelial Syndrome

Iridocorneal endothelial syndrome (ICE) is a group of three ocular conditions (Chandler syndrome, progressive iris atrophy, and Cogan-Reese syndrome) associated with corneal edema and secondary glaucoma. It is caused by the proliferation of endothelial cells toward the iridocorneal angle and iris surface. It is most common in young women and is usually unilateral. Chandler syndrome presents with a cobblestone or hammered silver appearance of the endothelium with corectopia. There is often less iris involvement in Chandler syndrome than in the other variants. Progressive iris atrophy often presents with corectopia, ectropion uveae, iris atrophy, and polycoria and iris holes. In Cogan-Reese syndrome, patients have pigmented nodules on the iris, loss of iris crypts and collarettes, hypochromia, ectropion uveae, and corectopia. Pathogenesis is thought to be of viral etiology, including HSV and Epstein-Barr virus (EBV) [27].

8.6 Other Corneal Dystrophies

Posterior polymorphous corneal dystrophy (PPMD) is an autosomal dominant bilateral disease of early childhood onset that can often be asymptomatic. Endothelial plaque-like lesions are seen on examination with railroad track alterations. The endothelium is replaced with flat epithelial-like cells that can form blisters. Patients can develop corneal steepening and edema, requiring corneal transplantation in approximately 20–25% of patients. About 25% of the patients can also develop peripheral iridocorneal adhesions with elevated intraocular pressure occurring in about 15% of patients with adhesions [28].

Congenital hereditary endothelial dystrophy (CHED) is an autosomal recessive bilateral disease characterized by corneal clouding and thickening. Patients are born with corneal clouding and blurred vision, often with the development of nystagmus. The course is relatively nonprogressive. Patients can be treated with corneal transplantation [28].

8.7 Diagnostic Testing in Corneal Endothelial Disease

Pachymetry measures corneal thickness, which can be used to monitor endothelial disease progression. Patients with FECD and a preoperative corneal thickness of 640 μm or less have a 95% chance of not requiring a corneal transplant within the first year of cataract surgery [29]. The central-to-peripheral corneal thickness ratio has also been described to correlate with the clinical grade of FECD. The thickness ratio is measured at 4 mm from the center [30].

Specular microscopy uses specular reflection for in vivo visualization of the corneal endothelium. This noninvasive technology can determine endothelial cell density (ECD), polymegethism (variation in size), pleomorphism (percentage of hexagonal cells), and central corneal thickness and can visualize guttae. Patients with ECD <1000 cells/mm^2, polymegethism >0.40, and/or pleomorphism $<50\%$ may not tolerate intraocular surgery [18, 31].

Confocal microscopy is a contact-based imaging modality that visualizes all corneal layers in vivo. Guttae, thickened Descemet membrane, epithelial bullae, and cystic lesions can be seen. In patients with advanced FECD where central ECD is unreliable, confocal microscopy is superior to specular microscopy since it can image through corneal edema and capture both the central and peripheral cornea [32–35].

Anterior segment optical coherence tomography (AS-OCT) uses light reflection to produce high-resolution cross-sectional images of the corneal layers. In FECD, the Descemet membrane appears hyper-reflective, thickened, irregular, and multilayered. Epithelial bullae, thickening of the epithelium, and subepithelial fibrosis can also be seen in advanced FECD and other endothelial diseases [36–38]. It is also a useful modality in postoperative follow-up of endothelial keratoplasty to assess for endothelial graft detachment and evaluate the graft-host interface [39].

8.8 Treatment of Corneal Endothelial Disease

8.8.1 Penetrating Keratoplasty

Since 1905, penetrating keratoplasty (PK), or full-thickness corneal transplantation, has been used to treat corneal endothelial disease. In PK, the central 7–9 mm of the host cornea is removed, and a comparably sized cadaver cornea is sutured into its place. The sutures typically remain in place for months to years, and transplant recipients receive chronic corticosteroid eye drops to prevent immunologic graft rejection. PK has been reported to restore best corrected visual acuity (BCVA) of 20/40 or better in 47–65% of patients treated for FECD and 20–40% of patients treated for PBK. High astigmatism (4-5D or greater) can prevent functional success in 10–20% of treated eyes [40–44].

The two most common causes of PK failure are endothelial decompensation due to immunologic rejection and late endothelial decompensation in the absence of clinically diagnosed rejection [45]. The PK grafts used to treat FECD patients have a reported 10-year survival rate of 67% to 90%, and those used to treat PBK have a survival rate of 36% to 80% [43, 45, 46]. PK is also a relatively risky procedure as the eye is completely open during the procedure and can be lost if a suprachoroidal hemorrhage occurs. Patients also have a 5% lifetime risk of wound dehiscence with minor trauma, leading to permanent vision loss from expulsion of the intraocular contents [47]. Given the more favorable risk-to-benefit ratio and visual outcomes, endothelial keratoplasty has now replaced PK as the current standard of treatment for corneal endothelial disease.

8.8.2 Descemet Stripping Endothelial Keratoplasty

Descemet stripping endothelial keratoplasty (DSEK) is a procedure that was first described in 2004, in which the dysfunctional host endothelium and Descemet membrane are stripped off and replaced with a partial thickness graft including donor stroma, Descemet membrane, and endothelium. It is performed through a small (2–5 mm) incision and is a closed-eye procedure, virtually eliminating risks of intraoperative suprachoroidal hemorrhage or postoperative wound dehiscence [48, 49]. As the microkeratome began to be used to create a smoother dissection plane of donor tissue to offset the challenges of manual dissection, a variation of DSEK called Descemet stripping automated endothelial keratoplasty (DSAEK) was introduced. DSEK refers to both of these techniques, and the former is rarely performed when a microkeratome is available [50].

During DSEK, the patient's cornea is marked for an appropriate stripping diameter with a trephination mark. Small incisions are made at the limbus, followed by scoring of the Descemet membrane on the trephination mark 360 degrees. The Descemet membrane is then stripped and removed from the anterior chamber. Using one of a variety of insertion techniques, the donor tissue is inserted into the anterior chamber via an enlarged corneal wound between 4 and 5 mm in size. The corneal wound is then sutured closed, and the graft is unfolded. Injection of an air bubble or balanced salt solution into the anterior chamber then ensures apposition between the donor and host corneal stroma. Peripheral iridotomy done preoperatively or peripheral iridectomy performed intraoperatively is needed to reduce the risk of pupillary block. Alternatively, pupillary dilation can be performed perioperatively to minimize the risk of pupillary block.

DSEK provides rapid visual recovery, better visual acuity, and less astigmatism than PK. DSEK is associated with a hyperopic shift in the spherical equivalent refraction of about 1.0–1.5D, which should be considered when calculating the appropriate intraocular lens power for combined cataract surgery [49]. Thinner DSAEK tissue is associated with better visual acuity [51, 52]. DSEK has a similar rate of endothelial cell loss compared to PK at 3 and 10 years [53, 54]. Patients with FECD tend to have a slower chronic endothelial cell loss rate than those with pseudophakic or aphakic corneal edema [54, 55]. Glaucoma surgery, including implantation of an aqueous shunt, can lead to accelerated cell loss. Nonetheless, at 5 years, the overall DSEK graft survival rate has been reported to be 96% in eyes without glaucoma, 90% in eyes with medically managed glaucoma, and 48% in eyes with previous glaucoma filtration surgery [56–58].

8.8.3 Descemet Membrane Endothelial Keratoplasty

Descemet membrane endothelial keratoplasty (DMEK) is a procedure that was first described in 2006 that involves replacing the dysfunctional Descemet membrane and endothelium from the host with Descemet membrane and endothelium alone. This uses a thinner donor tissue compared to DSEK as it does not include the posterior donor stroma [59]. Preparation of DMEK tissue requires more refined peeling techniques and selective donor selection than that for DSEK. It is also more challenging to discern tissue orientation, often requiring intraoperative OCT or an orientation stamp that is added on the donor graft during tissue preparation. Many eye banks now provide prestamped, pre-stripped, pre-stained, and preloaded DMEK tissues [60–62]. Insertion techniques include using glass tubes, intraocular lens inserters, or glides. After injection of donor tissue, it is partially uncurled using tapping maneuvers on the outer surface of the recipient cornea. A small air bubble can be injected beneath the donor tissue to help keep it uncurled and pressed against the recipient's cornea. At the end of the surgery, the anterior chamber is injected with a larger air or gas bubble to help with graft attachment [63, 64].

Visual acuity after DMEK is significantly better compared to that after DSEK [65, 66]. The median best corrected distance vision 3 months after DMEK has been demonstrated to be 20/25 compared to 20/30 6 months after DSEK [63]. At 1 year, best corrected distance vision of ≥20/20 occurred in 49% of treated eyes after DMEK, which improved to 64% of eyes at 10 years. At 10 years, 98% of eyes had ≥20/40 vision [67]. Similar to DSEK, DMEK is associated with a hyperopic shift in refraction, although to a lesser extent, ranging from 0.25 to 0.5D [63].

DMEK and DSEK experience similar rates of endothelial cell loss, and the 5-year survival rate of DMEK and DSEK is identical to the 5-year survival of PK for FECD [68]. At 1 year, secondary graft failure was significantly lower with DMEK than DSEK [69]. At 5 years, the survival rates of DMEK, DSEK, and PK for the treatment of FECD have been reported to be 97%, 95%, and 73%, respectively [70]. Two-year rejection rates with PK, DSEK, and DMEK have been reported to be 20%, 12%, and 1%, respectively [58]. Five-year rejection rates with PK, DSEK, and DMEK have been reported to be 14%, 5.0%, and 1.7%, respectively [70]. While DMEK provides better visual acuity and a lower risk of rejection, it is a more challenging surgery to perform.

The most common complication in the early postoperative period of EK is graft detachment. In DSEK, the donor stromal tissue is more adherent than the bare Descemet membrane in DMEK. Therefore, partial DSEK detachments often reseal spontaneously over time, while partial DMEK detachments are more common and less likely to resolve on their own. The DSEK detachment rate has been reported to be 8%, while the rate of complete DMEK detachment is about 30% [71, 72]. Partial DMEK detachment rates have been reported to be between 34.6% to 63% [73]. To reattach an EK graft, air needs to be reinjected into the anterior chamber.

Both DMEK and DSEK patients receive topical antibiotics for 1 week and topical corticosteroids for months to years. DMEK patients can resume normal activities within a few weeks, while DSEK patients can resume activity within a few months. Complications of EK include graft detachment, immunologic rejection, intraocular pressure elevation, and ocular infection.

8.8.4 Descemet Stripping Only

Descemet stripping only (DSO) or Descemet stripping without endothelial keratoplasty (DWEK) is a procedure in which the central Descemet membrane is removed without the transplantation of donor tissue. Surgeons began to adopt this procedure after reports in 2012 of FECD patients experiencing a corneal clearing and visual recovery despite having their DSEK grafts removed without replacement or having their DMEK grafts detach completely [74, 75]. The surgery comprises stripping off the central 4–5 mm in diameter of Descemet membrane and endothelium, then awaiting the migration of peripheral endothelial cells over the denuded area. Care is taken to avoid roughening the underlying stroma during removal, as endothelial cells do not adhere well to rough areas [76, 77].

Rho-associated coiled-coil-containing protein kinase (ROCK) inhibitor eye drops have been anecdotally reported to accelerate endothelial cell migration and corneal clearing. ROCK inhibitors are serine/threonine kinases that act on small Rho GTPases, and they have been shown to promote cell adhesion, inhibit apoptosis, and increase proliferation in vitro [78–80]. In 2013, topical ROCK inhibitor Y-27632 cleared corneal edema in an FECD patient following trans-corneal freezing [81]. Ripasudil, another ROCK inhibitor, has been used as a salvage agent in cases of DSO where the corneas fail to clear [82]. It has also been used to enhance clearing and visual improvement following DSO [83]. Clinical trials are ongoing to study ROCK inhibitors after DSO in FECD patients.

8.9 Future Directions

Corneal endothelial cell expansion is being studied using cultured human corneal endothelial cells. Various delivery modalities are currently being developed, including cell injection, tissue graft, ultrathin carrier, and magnetic particles [25]. A group in Japan injected 11 eyes with bullous keratopathy with cultured human corneal endothelial cells and a ROCK inhibitor. At 5 years, 10 of 11 eyes had normal corneal endothelial function with a mean endothelial cell density of 1257 cells/mm^2 [84, 85]. Furthermore, human embryonic stem cells, induced pluripotent stem cells, and endothelial stem cell regeneration are also being investigated as possible strategies for human corneal endothelial-like cells [25].

Pharmacological agents targeting endothelial cell degeneration are also under investigation. Compounds that may protect cells against oxidative stress and upregulation of unfolded protein response can be potentially therapeutic for corneal endothelial cell disease. An in vitro study with bovine corneal endothelial cells showed that oxotremorine, a muscarinic receptor agonist, and mefenamic acid, a nonsteroidal anti-inflammatory drug, could protect against oxidative stress [86]. N-acetylcysteine (NAC) is an antioxidant and free radical scavenger that has been shown to decrease endoplasmic reticulum stress in a mouse model of early-onset FECD [87]. Systemic administration of NAC in mice has also been reported to reduce UVA-induced corneal endothelial cell loss and corneal edema [88]. Clinical trials are underway to investigate the administration of small molecules in FECD patients.

A depiction of current, frontier, and developing therapies in endothelial disease can be seen in Fig. 8.5.

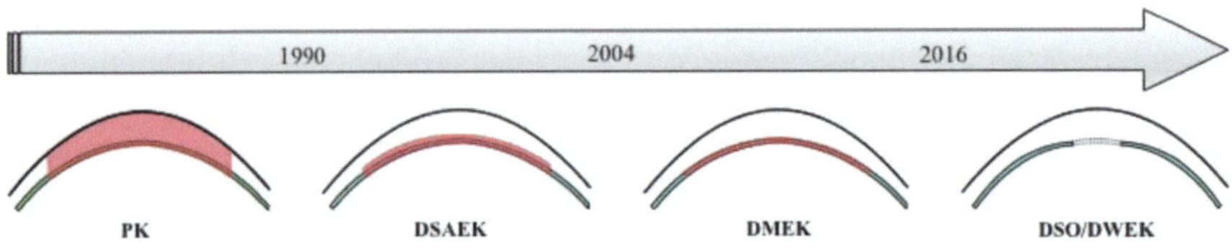

Treatment						
Current			Frontier	Developing Therapies		
Endothelial Keratoplasty	DMEK	Standard DMEK	DSO/DWEK	Cell Therapy	Cell injection	
		Hemi-DMEK			Tissue Engineered Endothelial Keratoplasty	
		Quarter-DMEK		Descemet Membrane Transplantation	ROCKi (-)	ROCKi (+)
	DSAEK	Standard DSAEK				
		UT-DSAEK				
		NT-DSAEK				

Fig. 8.5 Current, frontier and developing therapies for endothelial disease. PK depicts full-thickness corneal transplantation; DSAEK depicts partial-thickness corneal transplantation with host Descemet membrane replaced by donor Descemet membrane and adjacent stroma; DMEK depicts partial-thickness corneal transplantation with host Descemet membrane replaced by donor Descemet membrane. DSO/DWEK depicts central host endothelium being stripped. *PK* penetrating keratoplasty, *DSAEK* Descemet stripping automated endothelial keratoplasty, *DMEK* Descemet membrane endothelial keratoplasty, *DWEK* Descemetorhexis without endothelial keratoplasty, *DSO* Descemet stripping only, *UT-DSAEK* ultrathin-DSAEK, *NT-DSAEK* nanothin-DSAEK; *ROCKi* Rho kinase inhibitor. (Reprinted with permission from Elsevier. doi: 10.1080/08820538.2019.1632355)

References

1. Gain P, Jullienne R, He Z, et al. Global survey of corneal transplantation and eye banking. JAMA Ophthalmol. 2016;134(2):167–73. https://doi.org/10.1001/jamaophthalmol.2015.4776.
2. Afshari NA, Pittard AB, Siddiqui A, Klintworth GK. Clinical study of Fuchs corneal endothelial dystrophy leading to penetrating keratoplasty: a 30-year experience. Arch Ophthalmol. 2006;124(6):777–80. https://doi.org/10.1001/archopht.124.6.777.
3. Krachmer JH, Purcell JJ Jr, Young CW, Bucher KD. Corneal endothelial dystrophy: a study of 64 families. Arch Ophthalmol. 1978;96(11):2036–9. https://doi.org/10.1001/archopht.1978.03910060424004.
4. Louttit MD, Kopplin LJ, Igo RP, et al. A multi-center study to map genes for Fuchs' endothelial corneal dystrophy: baseline characteristics and heritability. Cornea. 2012;31(1):26–35. https://doi.org/10.1097/ICO.0b013e31821c9b8f.
5. Minear MA, Li Y-J, Rimmler J, et al. Genetic screen of African Americans with Fuchs endothelial corneal dystrophy. Mol Vis. 2013;19:2508–16.
6. Hogan MJ, Wood I, Fine M. Fuchs' endothelial dystrophy of the cornea: 29th Sanford Gifford memorial lecture. Am J Ophthalmol. 1974;78(3):363–83. https://doi.org/10.1016/0002-9394(74)90224-4.
7. Eghrari AO, McGlumphy EJ, Iliff BW, et al. Prevalence and severity of Fuchs corneal dystrophy in Tangier Island. Am J Ophthalmol. 2012;153(6):1067–72. https://doi.org/10.1016/j.ajo.2011.11.033.
8. Higa A, Sakai H, Sawaguchi S, et al. Prevalence of and risk factors for cornea Guttata in a population-based study in a Southwestern Island of Japan: the Kumejima study. Arch Ophthalmol. 2011;129(3):332–6. https://doi.org/10.1001/archophthalmol.2010.372.

9. Kitagawa K, Kojima M, Sasaki H, et al. Prevalence of primary cornea Guttata and morphology of corneal endothelium in aging Japanese and Singaporean subjects. Ophthalmic Res. 2002;34(3):135–8. https://doi.org/10.1159/000063656.
10. Lorenzetti DWC, Uotila MH, Parikh N, Kaufman HE. Central cornea Guttata: incidence in the general population. Am J Ophthalmol. 1967;64(6):1155–8. https://doi.org/10.1016/0002-9394(67)93073-5.
11. Nagaki Y, Hayasaka S, Kitagawa K, Yamamoto S. Primary cornea Guttata in Japanese patients with cataract: specular microscopic observations. Jpn J Ophthalmol. 1996;40(4):520–5.
12. Zoega GM, Fujisawa A, Sasaki H, et al. Prevalence and risk factors for cornea Guttata in the Reykjavik eye study. Ophthalmology. 2006;113(4):565–9. https://doi.org/10.1016/j.ophtha.2005.12.014.
13. Goar EL. Dystrophy of the corneal endothelium (cornea Guttata), with report of a histologic examination. Trans Am Ophthalmol Soc. 1933;31:48–59.
14. Jurkunas UV. Fuchs endothelial corneal dystrophy through the prism of oxidative stress. Cornea. 2018;37:S50. https://doi.org/10.1097/ICO.0000000000001775.
15. Schmedt T, Silva MM, Ziaei A, Jurkunas U. Molecular bases of corneal endothelial dystrophies. Exp Eye Res. 2012;95(1):24–34. https://doi.org/10.1016/j.exer.2011.08.002.
16. Biswas S, Munier FL, Yardley J, et al. Missense mutations in COL8A2, the gene encoding the alpha2 chain of type VIII collagen, cause two forms of corneal endothelial dystrophy. Hum Mol Genet. 2001;10(21):2415–23. https://doi.org/10.1093/hmg/10.21.2415.
17. Fautsch MP, Wieben ED, Baratz KH, et al. TCF4-mediated Fuchs endothelial corneal dystrophy: insights into a common trinucleotide repeat-associated disease. Prog Retin Eye Res. 2021;81:100883. https://doi.org/10.1016/j.preteyeres.2020.100883.
18. Ong Tone S, Kocaba V, Böhm M, Wylegala A, White TL, Jurkunas UV. Fuchs endothelial corneal dystrophy: the vicious cycle of Fuchs pathogenesis. Prog Retin Eye Res. 2021;80:100863. https://doi.org/10.1016/j.preteyeres.2020.100863.
19. Zhang X, Igo RP, Fondran J, et al. Association of smoking and other risk factors with Fuchs' endothelial corneal dystrophy severity and corneal thickness. Invest Ophthalmol Vis Sci. 2013;54(8):5829–35. https://doi.org/10.1167/iovs.13-11918.
20. Liu C, Miyajima T, Melangath G, et al. Ultraviolet a light induces DNA damage and estrogen-DNA adducts in Fuchs endothelial corneal dystrophy causing females to be more affected. Proc Natl Acad Sci. 2020;117(1):573–83. https://doi.org/10.1073/pnas.1912546116.
21. Eghrari AO, Mumtaz AA, Garrett B, et al. Automated retroillumination photography analysis for objective assessment of Fuchs corneal dystrophy severity. Cornea. 2017;36(1):44–7. https://doi.org/10.1097/ICO.0000000000001056.
22. Gottsch JD, Sundin OH, Rencs EV, et al. Analysis and documentation of progression of Fuchs corneal dystrophy with retroillumination photography. Cornea. 2006;25(4):485–9. https://doi.org/10.1097/01.ico.0000178726.11693.14.
23. Graves B. Report to the lang clinical research committee, Royal London Ophthalmic Hospital: a bilateral chronic affection of the endothelial face of the cornea of elderly persons with an account of the technical and clinical principles of its slit-lamp observation. Br J Ophthalmol. 1924;8(11):502–44. https://doi.org/10.1136/bjo.8.11.502.
24. Adamis AP, Filatov V, Tripathi BJ, Tripathi RA, mesh C. Fuchs' endothelial dystrophy of the cornea. Surv Ophthalmol. 1993;38(2):149–68. https://doi.org/10.1016/0039-6257(93)90099-S.
25. Price MO, Mehta JS, Jurkunas UV, Price FW. Corneal endothelial dysfunction: evolving understanding and treatment options. Prog Retin Eye Res. 2021;82:100904. https://doi.org/10.1016/j.preteyeres.2020.100904.
26. Moshirfar M, Murri MS, Shah TJ, et al. A review of corneal endotheliitis and endotheliopathy: differential diagnosis, evaluation, and treatment. Ophthalmol Ther. 2019;8(2):195–213. https://doi.org/10.1007/s40123-019-0169-7.
27. Silva L, Najafi A, Suwan Y, Teekhasaenee C, Ritch R. The iridocorneal endothelial syndrome. Surv Ophthalmol. 2018;63(5):665–76. https://doi.org/10.1016/j.survophthal.2018.01.001.
28. Weiss JS, Møller HU, Aldave AJ, et al. IC3D classification of corneal dystrophies--edition 2. Cornea. 2015;34(2):117–59. https://doi.org/10.1097/ICO.0000000000000307.

29. Seitzman GD, Gottsch JD, Stark WJ. Cataract surgery in patients with Fuchs' corneal dystrophy: expanding recommendations for cataract surgery without simultaneous keratoplasty. Ophthalmology. 2005;112(3):441–6. https://doi.org/10.1016/j.ophtha.2004.10.044.
30. Repp DJ, Hodge DO, Baratz KH, McLaren JW, Patel SV. Fuchs' endothelial corneal dystrophy: subjective grading versus objective grading based on the central-to-peripheral thickness ratio. Ophthalmology. 2013;120(4):687–94. https://doi.org/10.1016/j.ophtha.2012.09.022.
31. McCarey BE, Edelhauser HF, Lynn MJ. Review of corneal endothelial specular microscopy for FDA clinical trials of refractive procedures, surgical devices, and new intraocular drugs and solutions. Cornea. 2008;27(1):1–16. https://doi.org/10.1097/ICO.0b013e31815892da.
32. Cavanagh HD, Jester JV, Essepian J, Shields W, Lemp MA. Confocal microscopy of the living eye. CLAO J Off Publ Contact Lens Assoc Ophthalmol Inc. 1990;16(1):65–73.
33. Fujimoto H, Maeda N, Soma T, et al. Quantitative regional differences in corneal endothelial abnormalities in the central and peripheral zones in Fuchs' endothelial corneal dystrophy. Invest Ophthalmol Vis Sci. 2014;55(8):5090–8. https://doi.org/10.1167/iovs.14-14249.
34. Syed ZA, Tran JA, Jurkunas UV. Peripheral endothelial cell count is a predictor of disease severity in advanced Fuchs endothelial corneal dystrophy. Cornea. 2017;36(10):1166–71. https://doi.org/10.1097/ICO.0000000000001292.
35. Ong Tone S, Bruha MJ, Böhm M, Prescott C, Jurkunas U. Regional variability in corneal endothelial cell density between guttae and non-guttae areas in Fuchs endothelial corneal dystrophy. Can J Ophthalmol. 2019;54(5):570–6. https://doi.org/10.1016/j.jcjo.2018.12.009.
36. Kaluzny BJ, Szkulmowska A, Szkulmowski M, Bajraszewski T, Kowalczyk A, Wojtkowski M. Fuchs' endothelial dystrophy in 830-nm spectral domain optical coherence tomography. Ophthalmic Surg Lasers Imaging Off J Int Soc Imaging Eye. 2009;40(2):198–200. https://doi.org/10.3928/15428877-20090301-11.
37. Shousha MA, Perez VL, Wang J, et al. Use of ultra-high-resolution optical coherence tomography to detect in vivo characteristics of Descemet's membrane in Fuchs' dystrophy. Ophthalmology. 2010;117(6):1220–7. https://doi.org/10.1016/j.ophtha.2009.10.027.
38. Iovino C, Fossarello M, Giannaccare G, et al. Corneal endothelium features in Fuchs' endothelial corneal dystrophy: a preliminary 3D anterior segment optical coherence tomography study. PLoS One. 2018;13(11):e0207891. https://doi.org/10.1371/journal.pone.0207891.
39. Satue M, Idoipe M, Sanchez-Perez A, et al. Evaluation of early graft detachment after Descemet membrane endothelial keratoplasty using new swept-source optical coherence tomography. Cornea. 2016;35(10):1279–84. https://doi.org/10.1097/ICO.0000000000000925.
40. Price FW, Whitson WE, Marks RG. Progression of visual acuity after penetrating keratoplasty. Ophthalmology. 1991;98(8):1177–85. https://doi.org/10.1016/S0161-6420(91)32136-5.
41. Claesson M, Armitage WJ, Fagerholm P, Stenevi U. Visual outcome in corneal grafts: a preliminary analysis of the Swedish corneal transplant register. Br J Ophthalmol. 2002;86(2):174–80.
42. Pineros O, Cohen EJ, Rapuano CJ, Laibson PR. Long-term results after penetrating keratoplasty for Fuchs' endothelial dystrophy. Arch Ophthalmol. 1996;114(1):15–8. https://doi.org/10.1001/archopht.1996.01100130013002.
43. Williams KA, Keane MC, Coffey NE, Jones VJ, Mills RA, Coster DJ. The Australian corneal graft registry 2018 report. South Australian Health and Medical Research Institute; 2018. Accessed 23 Aug 2021. https://dspace.flinders.edu.au/xmlui/handle/2328/37917.
44. Riddle HKJ, Parker DAS, Price FWJ. Management of postkeratoplasty astigmatism. Curr Opin Ophthalmol. 1998;9(4):15–28.
45. Thompson RW, Price MO, Bowers PJ, Price FW. Long-term graft survival after penetrating keratoplasty. Ophthalmology. 2003;110(7):1396–402. https://doi.org/10.1016/S0161-6420(03)00463-9.
46. Writing Committee for the Cornea Donor Study Research Group. Factors associated with corneal graft survival in the cornea donor study. JAMA Ophthalmol. 2015;133(3):246–54. https://doi.org/10.1001/jamaophthalmol.2014.3923.
47. Elder MJ, Stack RR. Globe rupture following penetrating keratoplasty: how often, why, and what can we do to prevent it? Cornea. 2004;23(8):776–80. https://doi.org/10.1097/01.ico.0000133996.99520.c4.

48. Melles GRJ, Wijdh RHJ, Nieuwendaal CP. A technique to excise the Descemet membrane from a recipient cornea (descemetorhexis). Cornea. 2004;23(3):286–8. https://doi.org/10.1097/00003226-200404000-00011.
49. Price FW, Price MO. Descemet's stripping with endothelial keratoplasty in 50 eyes: a refractive neutral corneal transplant. J Refract Surg Thorofare NJ 1995. 2005;21(4):339–45.
50. Gorovoy MS. Descemet-stripping automated endothelial keratoplasty. Cornea. 2006;25(8):886–9. https://doi.org/10.1097/01.ico.0000214224.90743.01.
51. Neff KD, Biber JM, Holland EJ. Comparison of central corneal graft thickness to visual acuity outcomes in endothelial keratoplasty. Cornea. 2011;30(4):388–91. https://doi.org/10.1097/ICO.0b013e3181f236c6.
52. Dickman MM, Kruit PJ, Remeijer L, et al. A randomized multicenter clinical trial of ultrathin Descemet stripping automated endothelial keratoplasty (DSAEK) versus DSAEK. Ophthalmology. 2016;123(11):2276–84. https://doi.org/10.1016/j.ophtha.2016.07.036.
53. Price MO, Gorovoy M, Price FW, Benetz BA, Menegay HJ, Lass JH. Descemet's stripping automated endothelial keratoplasty: three-year graft and endothelial cell survival compared with penetrating keratoplasty. Ophthalmology. 2013;120(2):246–51. https://doi.org/10.1016/j.ophtha.2012.08.007.
54. Price MO, Calhoun P, Kollman C, Price FW, Lass JH. Descemet stripping endothelial keratoplasty: ten-year endothelial cell loss compared with penetrating keratoplasty. Ophthalmology. 2016;123(7):1421–7. https://doi.org/10.1016/j.ophtha.2016.03.011.
55. Terry MA, Aldave AJ, Szczotka-Flynn LB, et al. Donor, recipient, and operative factors associated with graft success in the cornea preservation time study. Ophthalmology. 2018;125(11):1700–9. https://doi.org/10.1016/j.ophtha.2018.08.002.
56. Aldave AJ, Chen JL, Zaman AS, Deng SX, Yu F. Outcomes after DSEK in 101 eyes with previous trabeculectomy and tube shunt implantation. Cornea. 2014;33(3):223–9. https://doi.org/10.1097/ICO.0000000000000028.
57. Nahum Y, Mimouni M, Busin M. Risk factors predicting the need for graft exchange after Descemet stripping automated endothelial keratoplasty. Cornea. 2015;34(8):876–9. https://doi.org/10.1097/ICO.0000000000000455.
58. Anshu A, Price MO, Price FW. Descemet's stripping endothelial keratoplasty: long-term graft survival and risk factors for failure in eyes with preexisting glaucoma. Ophthalmology. 2012;119(10):1982–7. https://doi.org/10.1016/j.ophtha.2012.04.031.
59. Melles GRJ, Ong TS, Ververs B, van der Wees J. Descemet membrane endothelial keratoplasty (DMEK). Cornea. 2006;25(8):987–90. https://doi.org/10.1097/01.ico.0000248385.16896.34.
60. Veldman PB, Dye PK, Holiman JD, et al. The S-stamp in Descemet membrane endothelial keratoplasty safely eliminates upside-down graft implantation. Ophthalmology. 2016;123(1):161–4. https://doi.org/10.1016/j.ophtha.2015.08.044.
61. Tenkman LR, Price FW, Price MO. Descemet membrane endothelial keratoplasty donor preparation: navigating challenges and improving efficiency. Cornea. 2014;33(3):319–25. https://doi.org/10.1097/ICO.0000000000000045.
62. LMM V, Stoeger CG, Galloway JD, et al. Risk factors for eye bank preparation failure of Descemet membrane endothelial keratoplasty tissue. Am J Ophthalmol. 2015;159(5):829–34.e2. https://doi.org/10.1016/j.ajo.2015.01.030.
63. Price MO, Giebel AW, Fairchild KM, Price FW. Descemet's membrane endothelial keratoplasty: prospective multicenter study of visual and refractive outcomes and endothelial survival. Ophthalmology. 2009;116(12):2361–8. https://doi.org/10.1016/j.ophtha.2009.07.010.
64. Tan T-E, Devarajan K, Seah X-Y, et al. Descemet membrane endothelial keratoplasty with a pull-through insertion device: surgical technique, endothelial cell loss, and early clinical results. Cornea. 2020;39(5):558–65. https://doi.org/10.1097/ICO.0000000000002268.
65. Dunker SL, Dickman MM, Wisse RPL, et al. Descemet membrane endothelial keratoplasty versus ultrathin Descemet stripping automated endothelial keratoplasty: a multicenter randomized controlled clinical trial. Ophthalmology. 2020;127(9):1152–9. https://doi.org/10.1016/j.ophtha.2020.02.029.

66. Chamberlain W, Lin CC, Austin A, et al. Descemet endothelial thickness comparison trial: a randomized trial comparing ultrathin Descemet stripping automated endothelial keratoplasty with Descemet membrane endothelial keratoplasty. Ophthalmology. 2019;126(1):19–26. https://doi.org/10.1016/j.ophtha.2018.05.019.
67. Vasiliauskaitė I, Oellerich S, Ham L, et al. Descemet membrane endothelial keratoplasty: ten-year graft survival and clinical outcomes. Am J Ophthalmol. 2020;217:114–20. https://doi.org/10.1016/j.ajo.2020.04.005.
68. Price DA, Kelley M, Price FW, Price MO. Five-year graft survival of Descemet membrane endothelial keratoplasty (EK) versus Descemet stripping EK and the effect of donor sex matching. Ophthalmology. 2018;125(10):1508–14. https://doi.org/10.1016/j.ophtha.2018.03.050.
69. Lin SR, Prapaipanich P, Yu F, et al. Comparison of endothelial keratoplasty techniques in patients with prior glaucoma surgery: a case-matched study. Am J Ophthalmol. 2019;206:94–101. https://doi.org/10.1016/j.ajo.2019.03.020.
70. Woo J-H, Ang M, Htoon HM, Tan D. Descemet membrane endothelial keratoplasty versus Descemet stripping automated endothelial keratoplasty and penetrating keratoplasty. Am J Ophthalmol. 2019;207:288–303. https://doi.org/10.1016/j.ajo.2019.06.012.
71. Aldave AJ, Terry MA, Szczotka-Flynn LB, et al. Effect of graft attachment status and intraocular pressure on Descemet stripping automated endothelial keratoplasty outcomes in the cornea preservation time study. Am J Ophthalmol. 2019;203:78–88. https://doi.org/10.1016/j.ajo.2019.02.029.
72. Melles GRJ, Ong TS, Ververs B, van der Wees J. Preliminary clinical results of Descemet membrane endothelial keratoplasty. Am J Ophthalmol. 2008;145(2):222–7. https://doi.org/10.1016/j.ajo.2007.09.021.
73. Parekh M, Leon P, Ruzza A, et al. Graft detachment and rebubbling rate in Descemet membrane endothelial keratoplasty. Surv Ophthalmol. 2018;63(2):245–50. https://doi.org/10.1016/j.survophthal.2017.07.003.
74. Dirisamer M, Yeh R-Y, van Dijk K, Ham L, Dapena I, Melles GRJ. Recipient endothelium may relate to corneal clearance in Descemet membrane endothelial transfer. Am J Ophthalmol. 2012;154(2):290–296.e1. https://doi.org/10.1016/j.ajo.2012.02.032.
75. Shah RD, Randleman JB, Grossniklaus HE. Spontaneous corneal clearing after Descemet's stripping without endothelial replacement. Ophthalmology. 2012;119(2):256–60. https://doi.org/10.1016/j.ophtha.2011.07.032.
76. Arbelaez JG, Price MO, Price FW. Long-term follow-up and complications of stripping Descemet membrane without placement of graft in eyes with Fuchs endothelial dystrophy. Cornea. 2014;33(12):1295–9. https://doi.org/10.1097/ICO.0000000000000270.
77. Borkar DS, Veldman P, Colby KA. Treatment of Fuchs endothelial dystrophy by Descemet stripping without endothelial keratoplasty. Cornea. 2016;35(10):1267–73. https://doi.org/10.1097/ICO.0000000000000915.
78. Okumura N, Ueno M, Koizumi N, et al. Enhancement on primate corneal endothelial cell survival in vitro by a ROCK inhibitor. Invest Ophthalmol Vis Sci. 2009;50(8):3680–7. https://doi.org/10.1167/iovs.08-2634.
79. Okumura N, Fujii K, Kagami T, et al. Activation of the rho/rho kinase signaling pathway is involved in cell death of corneal endothelium. Invest Ophthalmol Vis Sci. 2016;57(15):6843–51. https://doi.org/10.1167/iovs.16-20123.
80. Pipparelli A, Arsenijevic Y, Thuret G, Gain P, Nicolas M, Majo F. ROCK inhibitor enhances adhesion and wound healing of human corneal endothelial cells. PLoS One. 2013;8(4):e62095. https://doi.org/10.1371/journal.pone.0062095.
81. Koizumi N, Okumura N, Ueno M, Nakagawa H, Hamuro J, Kinoshita S. Rho-associated kinase inhibitor eye drop treatment as a possible medical treatment for Fuchs corneal dystrophy. Cornea. 2013;32(8):1167–70. https://doi.org/10.1097/ICO.0b013e318285475d.
82. Moloney G, Petsoglou C, Ball M, et al. Descemetorhexis without grafting for Fuchs endothelial dystrophy-supplementation with topical Ripasudil. Cornea. 2017;36(6):642–8. https://doi.org/10.1097/ICO.0000000000001209.

83. Huang MJ, Kane S, Dhaliwal DK. Descemetorhexis without endothelial keratoplasty versus DMEK for treatment of Fuchs endothelial corneal dystrophy. Cornea. 2018;37(12):1479–83. https://doi.org/10.1097/ICO.0000000000001742.
84. Kinoshita S, Koizumi N, Ueno M, et al. Injection of cultured cells with a ROCK inhibitor for bullous keratopathy. N Engl J Med. 2018;378(11):995–1003. https://doi.org/10.1056/NEJMoa1712770.
85. Numa K, Imai K, Ueno M, et al. Five-year follow-up of first 11 patients undergoing injection of cultured corneal endothelial cells for corneal endothelial failure. Ophthalmology. 2021;128(4):504–14. https://doi.org/10.1016/j.ophtha.2020.09.002.
86. Kim EC, Toyono T, Berlinicke CA, et al. Screening and characterization of drugs that protect corneal endothelial cells against unfolded protein response and oxidative stress. Invest Ophthalmol Vis Sci. 2017;58(2):892–900. https://doi.org/10.1167/iovs.16-20147.
87. Kim EC, Meng H, Jun AS. N-Acetylcysteine increases corneal endothelial cell survival in a mouse model of Fuchs endothelial corneal dystrophy. Exp Eye Res. 2014;127:20–5. https://doi.org/10.1016/j.exer.2014.06.002.
88. Liu C, Miyajima T, Vasanth S, Miyai T, Farinelli B, Jurkunas UV. N-acetylcysteine alleviates progression of Fuchs endothelial corneal dystrophy in a UVA irradiation-induced mouse model. Invest Ophthalmol Vis Sci. 2018;59(9):1356.

Anterior Segment Disease and Pediatric Keratoplasty

9

Ken K. Nischal

Key Points

- Deep phenotype of pediatric corneal disease must include appropriate imaging including high frequency ultrasound (or linear ultrasound) and high-definition OCT (optical coherence tomography).
- Management includes control of ocular comorbidities (e.g., glaucoma) and systemic comorbidities (e.g., renal or cardiac disease).
- Choice of intervention depends on the deep phenotype classification but includes no intervention, optical iridectomy, selective endothelial removal, deep anterior lamellar keratoplasty (DALK), endothelial keratoplasty (EK), and penetrating keratoplasty (PKP).
- Severe visual impairment has a profound effect on global development in an infant and toddler. Therefore, even if keratoplasty fails after 12–18 months, the gain in global development should justify the intervention.
- Visual function (e.g., contrast sensitivity functions, visual field, temporal-spatial coordination) is more important than central visual acuity.

Pediatric anterior segment disease is a broad subject, but, in this chapter, we will focus largely on the latest developments affecting congenital disease, techniques of pediatric keratoplasty as they pertain to specific corneal diseases, and select, common acquired diseases for which newer therapies have become available. A classification [1] to help differentiate corneal opacities in children is useful in categorizing and managing disease and is used in this chapter to order the below diseases.

K. K. Nischal (✉)
UPMC Children's Hospital of Pittsburgh, Pittsburgh, PA, USA
e-mail: nischalkk@upmc.edu

H. N. Saeed, R. B. Singh (eds.), *Corneal Disorders*, Current Practices in Ophthalmology, https://doi.org/10.1007/978-981-96-5294-5_9

9.1 Primary Congenital Corneal Opacity

9.1.1 Corneal Dystrophies

There are only three corneal dystrophies that can present with corneal clouding at birth: congenital hereditary endothelial dystrophy (CHED), posterior polymorphous corneal dystrophy (PPCD), and X-linked endothelial corneal dystrophy [2].

9.1.1.1 Congenital Hereditary Endothelial Dystrophy

There is only one type of CHED, and this is caused by biallelic mutations in the *SLC4A11* gene [3]. Mutations in this gene can also cause Harboyan syndrome-CHED with progressive sensorineural hearing loss. There is bilateral, usually asymmetric, corneal clouding which can have a diffuse haziness or a milky ground-glass appearance. The cornea is often thickened with significant reduction in endothelial cell count.

Management involves appropriate evaluation for amblyopia and refractive correction. Hypertonic saline is usually not effective, and if the vision is significantly affected, then endothelial keratoplasty is the procedure of choice. Surgical techniques are discussed later in this chapter.

9.1.1.2 Posterior Polymorphous Corneal Dystrophy

There are four types of posterior polymorphous dystrophy (PPCD), each type caused by a mono-allelic mutation in a different gene. PPCD 1 is caused by a mutation in the *OVOL2* gene, PPCD 2 in *COL8A2* gene, PPCD3 in the *ZEB1* gene, and PPCD 4 in the *GRHL2* gene [4]. This condition is often asymmetric, and presentation varies between asymptomatic or severe clouding of the corneas, which usually exhibits itself around the second to third decade of life but can present at birth. Clinically, you can see vesicles, polymorphous opacities at the level of Descemet membrane and the corneal endothelium, and track-like changes that resemble a "snail track." There can be involvement of the iris into the angle causing glaucoma. The endothelial cells in this condition develop epithelial characteristics, staining with cytokeratin and often producing abnormal basement membrane.

Management depends on the severity of presentation, but hypertonic saline can be helpful. When this condition presents at birth, treatment is either endothelial keratoplasty or penetrating keratoplasty depending on how shallow the anterior chamber of the infant is. Glaucoma management is extremely important, and glaucoma must be assessed for in these patients.

9.1.1.3 X-Linked Endothelial Corneal Dystrophy

This is an X-linked dominant condition which maps to a locus on Xp25 [5]. The condition can present at birth as a ground glass-appearing cornea. Otherwise, female carriers and affected males may show moon-crater-like changes at the level of the endothelium and Descemet membrane.

Clearing of this can be facilitated by hypertonic saline and by managing any associated raised intraocular pressure. However, most cases, when presenting at birth, end up needing surgical intervention either through endothelial keratoplasty or penetrating keratoplasty depending on how shallow the anterior chamber of the infant is.

9.1.2 Corneal Dermoids

There are three distinct types of corneal dermoid (see Fig. 9.1):

9.1.2.1 Limbal Dermoid

These may be isolated to the limbus and usually tend to be in the inferior half of the eye but can be found superiorly as well. They can be associated with a lipodermoid extending around the bulbar conjunctiva. Indications for surgery are an extremely elevated dermoid causing inability to close the lids, hair growing from the dermoid and causing punctate epitheliopathy, an elevated dermoid that is causing a dellen adjacent to it on the cornea, and improved cosmesis, especially in teenagers. The amount of astigmatism present is not an indication for removal, as removing the dermoid usually results in an unchanged or worse astigmatism. One exception to this is in the setting of high astigmatism where removal of the dermoid will allow for refractive correction with hybrid contact lenses to correct the amblyopia that is likely present because of the high astigmatism.

Limbal dermoids usually are not complex in that they do not invade the anterior chamber; if invasion is found, evaluation for another underlying cause in terms of systemic disease other than Goldenhar syndrome [6] should be undertaken. It is important to recognize localized ectasia at the limbus and differentiate this from a simple dermoid. In the former, there is a a dark blue discoloration indicating thinning of the overlying sclera and tissue. This is not seen in true, simple limbal dermoids (see Fig. 9.1).

Management consists of either simple excision or excision with lamellar keratoplasty. There is no sound evidence that either technique is better than the other, and it really depends on the preference of the surgeon. Lubrication at night should be undertaken to prevent epitheliopathy. The hairs that might grow from a limbal dermoid should not be epilated as they will grow back thicker and more problematic than before.

9.1.2.2 Diffuse Corneal Dermoid with Lipodermoids Component

Postzygotic *KRAS*, *HRAS*, *NRAS*, and *FGFR1* mutations (genes involved in the RAS/MAPK signaling pathway) result in a group of mosaic RASopathies characterized by related developmental anomalies in the eye, skin, heart, and brain [7]. These oculocutaneous disorders include oculoectodermal syndrome (OES), encephalo-cranio-cutaneous lipomatosis (ECCL), and Schimmelpenning-Feuerstein-Mims syndrome (SFMS) (also known as linear sebaceous nevus syndrome). These conditions exhibit a variety of anomalies that include scalp lesions (nevus psiloliparus or waxy alopecia), epilepsy, epibulbar and corneal dermoids, eyelid coloboma, coarctation of the aorta, and skin pigmentation abnormalities. In ECCL and SFMS, cortical atrophy can be seen resulting in seizure disorder and developmental delay.

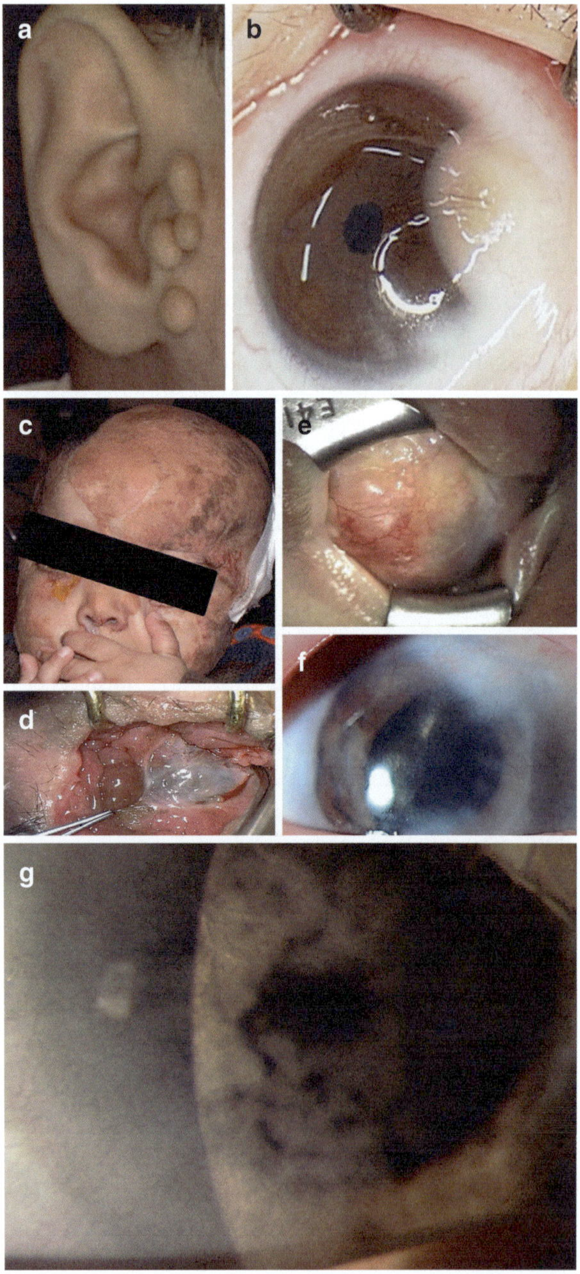

Fig. 9.1 Composite figure showing 4 patients, all with different types of dermoids. (**a**) shows the preauricular skin tags in a patient with Goldenhar syndrome. (**b**) shows the same patient's left eye with a limbal corneal dermoid which has hair growing out of the surface. (**c**) shows a patient with linear sebaceous nevus syndrome with typical skin changes. (**d**) shows the right eye of the same patient with an extensive dermoid affecting the cornea with contiguous lipodermoids. (**e** and **f**) are the pre and post pictures of a child with oculoectodermal syndrome; 1e shows an extensive vascularized dermoid with a lipodermoid component. (**f**) shows a successful corneal transplant 7 years post graft of the same eye as in (**e**). (**g**) is a reticular dermoid seen in a patient with Trisomy 8 mosaicism

In all three conditions, diffuse flat dermoids which have contiguous and adjacent vessels in the cornea are often seen with a dermolipoma component extending into the orbit [8]. The corneal dermoids are often full thickness or close to full thickness and can be extensive.

Management involves oculoplastic intervention for lid colobomas, topical lubrication, and mild steroids to help with the corneal neovascularization. However, in the presence of extensive corneal opacity due to dermoid, penetrating keratoplasty (PKP) needs to be considered (see Fig. 9.1).

9.1.2.3 Reticular Dermoid

This type of dermoid is extremely rare but is seen in trisomy 8 mosaicism [9]. The lesion is reticular in morphology and superficial (see Fig. 9.1). If occluding the visual axis, pupil dilation should be attempted with patching of the better eye. The lesions can be bilateral but often are unilateral. If conservative therapy is unsuccessful, superficial keratectomy can be performed.

9.1.3 CYP1B1 Cytopathy

This condition has been reported only recently. The *CYP1B1* gene when affected by biallelic mutations is most commonly known for causing primary congenital glaucoma [10]. However, there are now cases reported of associated corneal opacity which presents as a ground-glass appearance. The cornea is not enlarged horizontally, and the opacity remains even when the glaucoma is adequately controlled. Histologically, there is absence of Bowman's layer, endothelium, and Descemet's membrane centrally with fibrotic changes of the stroma centrally. The glaucoma in this condition can be relentless and must always be controlled. Management entails control of the glaucoma followed by PKP [10]. The published cases suggest that the corneal grafts do well, but that the glaucoma can be very difficult to control.

9.2 Secondary Congenital Corneal Opacity

9.2.1 Kerato-Irido-Lenticular Dysgenesis KILD

Much has been written about the genetic causes of developmental anomalies of the anterior segment that lead to corneal opacification [11]. However, Mataftsi et al. [12] showed very clearly that terminology such as sclerocornea without adequate anterior segment imaging was often inaccurate. Studies have confirmed that a clinical diagnosis often is changed after anterior segment imaging is done in cases of congenital corneal opacity. It is this difficulty in the phenotyping of congenital corneal opacities that has led to confusion in molecular etiology of disease. There are a plethora of genes that have been implicated in causing conditions termed "Peters anomaly." The problem is that Peters anomaly is a very heterogeneous term for a clinical sign. It is not a diagnosis, and therefore it is not a surprise that the causes in terms of molecular diagnosis are extremely varied [13].

9.2.1.1 Iridocorneal Adhesions Only

This entity is also known as Peters anomaly type 1. The phenotype can vary between a central, eccentric, or extensive opacity of the cornea with or without microcornea. The adhesions of the iris can often stop the pupil from being dilated. Management depends on the degree of extension of the corneal opacity. If the opacity is involving the whole cornea, then often penetrating keratoplasty is the only option. Studies have shown that the prognosis for PKP in these cases is reasonably good [14]. If, however, the opacity is eccentric, then optical iridectomy can be considered to try and improve the vision. More recently, a procedure called selective endothelial removal (see later) has been described when the opacity is more central.

9.2.1.2 Lens Fails to Separate from Cornea

This entity is also known as Peters anomaly type 2 [1, 12]. Often, keratolenticular adhesion occurs with iridocorneal adhesions [15]. The phenotype varies from a central opacity to a diffuse opacity. Often, when the lens is attached to the cornea because it failed to separate, there are blood vessels in the opacity with vascularization often coming from the limbus. If the opacity is more central and there is clear cornea in the periphery, an optical iridectomy is often preferred because PKP under these circumstances necessitates a lensectomy at the same time as the corneal transplant. When this is done, survival of the corneal transplant is much worse due to the formation of retro corneal membranes.

9.2.1.3 Lens Fails to Form (Primary Congenital Aphakia)

There is a consistent phenotype in this condition, and it is one of a silvery-grey appearing cornea, which is usually thin [16, 17]. Most cases of this condition are due to biallelic mutations in *FOXE3*, which is expressed in the lens epithelial cell [18]. There is variation in the presence of microphthalmos or extreme microphthalmos with these being most commonly seen in cases of homozygous mutations. Management consists of control of the intraocular pressure either by transscleral cyclodiode laser or by a drainage tube. The glaucoma occurs because the lens is needed to induce the tertiary vitreous, which is in turn needed to induce normal development of the trabecular meshwork. PKP often fails because the eye becomes phthisical due to the formation of tenacious vitreous membranes; the speculation is that the vitreous is abnormal due to the primary absence of the lens, leading to the formation of such membranes and causing either cyclitic membranes and/or retinal detachment.

9.2.1.4 Lens Separates But Fails to Form Thereafter (Secondary Congenital Aphakia)

In this scenario, the cornea is often completely opaque and may display a silver-gray appearance. This has been termed sclerocornea, and unfortunately this does not necessarily define the phenotype accurately enough. Invariably, the only treatment is penetrating keratoplasty in at least one eye in bilateral cases. The prognosis in such cases, however, is guarded because of graft failure and the formation of retro-corneal membranes and/or tenacious vitreous membranes causing phthisis, depending on the stage at which the lens failed to develop after separating from the cornea.

9.2.2 Persistent Fetal Vasculature

In all cases of diffuse corneal opacity without vascularization, the possibility of the lens being pushed forward up against the cornea by a lens plaque due to persistent fetal vasculature (PFV) must be considered, particularly in unilateral cases [19, 20]. The clue in the diagnosis is the loss of the anterior chamber and an uninterrupted endothelium/Descemet membrane on anterior segment imaging of the cornea (see Fig. 9.2). The treatment here is control of the intraocular pressure and a lensectomy either endoscopically or with endoillumination. While a residual corneal opacity often remains, the prognosis for visual rehabilitation is often better than what the cornea would indicate; a corneal graft would necessitate removal of the lens, with an increased risk of graft failure, usually due to the formation of retro-corneal membranes.

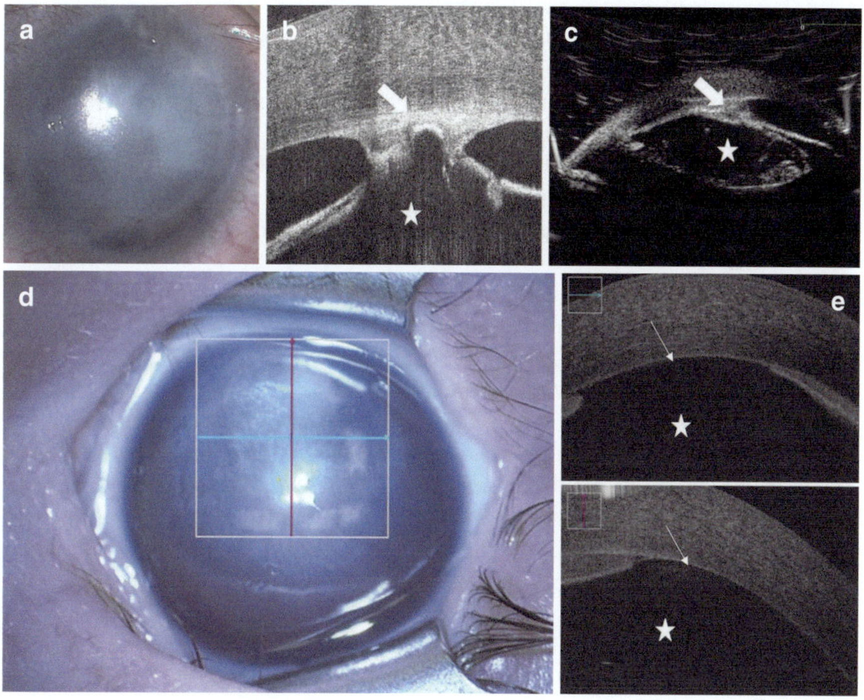

Fig. 9.2 Composite figure showing a case of keratolenticular adhesion where the lens (white star) failed to separate from the cornea (**a**, **b**, and **c**), and a case of persistent fetal vasculature causing a central corneal opacity due to the lens mechanically touching the cornea (**d** and **e**). Note the keratolenticular adhesion on OCT (**b**) and high frequency ultrasound (**c**) disrupting the endothelial/Descemet membrane complex (thick white arrow). In (**e** and **f**), the endothelial/Descemet membrane complex remains intact suggesting this is a mechanical and not an embryological failure

9.2.3 Irido-trabecular Dysgenesis

This group of conditions entails developmental anomalies of the iris including iris hypoplasia, complete absence of the iris, and infantile or congenital glaucoma.

9.2.3.1 Infantile Glaucoma

Infantile glaucoma is most commonly due to biallelic mutations in *CYP1B1* but has also been reported to be due to biallelic mutations in *LTBP2* and least commonly as monoallelic mutations of the *TEK* gene [21]. The cardinal clinical signs are buphthalmos, cloudy corneas, Haab striae, and intense lacrimation due to photophobia. Control of the glaucoma results in clearing of the corneal opacity. In some cases where this control is delayed, there is stromal fibrosis and opacification of the cornea necessitating PKP. In cases where the glaucoma is controlled but there are Haab striae across the visual axis, reports of endothelial keratoplasty, especially in the setting of secondary corneal decompensation, have been reported [22–24].

9.2.3.2 Axenfeld-Rieger Syndrome

Axenfeld-Rieger syndrome is caused by monoallelic mutations in *PITX2* or *FOXC1*. Posterior embryotoxon (though not seen in every case) is often present, along with iris hypoplasia with or without corectopia, aniridia, pseudopolycoria, and often glaucoma [25, 26]. Iridocorneal adhesions can be seen to cause congenital corneal opacities (CCO) consistent with Peters anomaly type 1. Glaucoma can be treated with filtering surgery or with drainage tube placement. In cases with CCO, a PKP is often needed, but glaucoma control is essential for graft survival.

9.2.3.3 Aniridia

Aniridia is an absent or partially absent iris that is present from birth. It may be due to mutations in *PAX6*, *FOXC1*, *PITX2*, *CYP1B1*, *FOXD3*, and *TRIM44* genes [27]. Classic aniridia is due to monoallelic mutations in *PAX6* and is a panocular disorder affecting the cornea (pannus and limbal stem cell dysfunction), lens (anterior and posterior subcapsular lens opacities), fovea (hypoplasia), and optic disc (hypoplasia), with the latter two leading to nystagmus. Rarely, keratolenticular adhesions (Peters anomaly type 2) can be seen in anridia due to monoallelic mutations in *PAX6* [28]. In these cases, it is better to consider doing a lensectomy with or without an intraocular implant, since there is usually enough clear cornea around the central opacity [29].

9.2.4 Corneal Dystrophies

There are extensive publications that discuss the different types of corneal dystrophies that we are aware of, most notably the IC3D classification system [2]. It is worth noting that in children up until the third decade of life, corneal dystrophies often present in an unusual manner. Surgical intervention is usually not indicated except in the aforementioned primary congenital opacities where corneal clouding is present at birth. The exceptions to these are the anterior stromal corneal dystrophies due to monolithic mutations in the *TGFBI* gene, namely granular, granular lattice, and lattice dystrophies. Results after phototherapeutic keratectomy have been shown to vary depending on the exact mutation found in the *TGFBI* gene [30–32]. Genotyping of these conditions is therefore very important before any surgical intervention is done [33].

Other non-TGFB1-related dystrophies such as macular dystrophy can cause visual deterioration in the second decade of life and necessitates PKP. Meesmann dystrophy is a superficial dystrophy that can cause intense photophobia in the first decade of life; patients benefit from alcohol delamination, which can be repeated.

9.3 Acquired Corneal Opacity

It is not possible to cover all the acquired corneal opacities that may benefit from pediatric keratoplasty. However, there are some that merit special mention. These include metabolic disorders, exposure and neurotrophic keratopathy, infectious keratitis, and keratoconus. Metabolic disorders, namely mucopolysaccharidoses, necessitate either DALK or PKP. It is also worth noting that both exposure keratopathy and neurotrophic keratopathy can lead to the formation of descemetoceles or corneal melts, which necessitate a tectonic corneal transplant. In cases of corneal anesthesia, the advent of corneal neurotization has improved ocular and visual outcomes. Similarly, cases of corneal scarring or severe infectious disease burden after infectious keratitis sometimes benefit from either DALK or PKP. Keratoconus is worth mentioning mainly because collagen cross-linking (CXL) has become a much more accepted treatment modality for use in the pediatric population [34]. Techniques have evolved to include accelerated CXL, largely outside of the United States, but the advantage of other modifications such as epithelium on vs epithelium off is still not clear. Even with the advent of CXL, many patients still do not receive timely care, meaning that DALK and PKP are still options that are needed in the treatment of KCN.

9.4 Pediatric Keratoplasty Techniques

Techniques for pediatric keratoplasty have evolved in the last 20 years. While PKP has been the mainstay of corneal transplant surgery in children and especially in infants, increasingly, lamellar keratoplasty is being utilized. There are alternatives to pediatric keratoplasty and, when available, should be considered in appropriate cases. These include optical iridectomy and selective endothelial removal.

9.4.1 Assessment

The assessment of the child is extremely important. It should include systemic evaluation by a pediatrician, and evaluation of visual potential using visual electrophysiology namely visual evoked potential and electroretinogram. Anterior segment imaging is essential and for practitioners who do not have access to high frequency ultrasound, ultrasound with a linear ultrasound probe is often available in a children's hospital. Even if the practitioner is in stand-alone eye institute, the anesthesiology department often has a linear ultrasound which is used to detect veins in difficult cannulations and this type of ultrasound can be used to give adequate images of the anterior chamber. Verification that the probe is safe for use on the eye can be done with a phone call to the manufacturer or to sales representative. Ultrasound can then be used to assess whether there are keratolenticular and/or iridocorneal adhesions, or if the anterior chamber is otherwise completely healthy. These findings affect the surgical approach.

9.4.2 Anesthesia

In order to minimize the risk of expulsive hemorrhage, the child undergoes systemic muscle paralysis, is hyperventilated to keep the end-tidal CO_2 around 30 mmHg if possible, and is given IV mannitol [35, 36].

9.5 Penetrating Keratoplasty

The technique for penetrating keratoplasty varies for children when compared to adults, and this variation is greater the younger the child. Children's eyes over the age of 4 years behave more like those of an adult but still display a greater degree of scleral elasticity. In infants, the eye is very elastic. Non-spring lid specula increase the intraocular pressure less than spring ones [37]. In infants under 6 months of age, a lateral canthotomy may be necessary to reduce pressure of the lids on the globe. The elasticity of the sclera necessitates the use of a Flieringa ring secured to the episcleral with four interrupted 8–0 nylon sutures, with one end of each suture secured to the brow or cheek. This reduces th0065 risk of an expulsive hemorrhage [38]. Vacuum trephines can be used in almost all cases except for developmental or congenital cases in infants. In the latter, a manual partial trephination is done, with penetration performed using a super blade to avoid hitting the lens. Prior to trephination, a small paracentesis is made and the anterior chamber is hyperinflated with heavy viscoelastic. This provides counter tension and also avoids inadvertent lens damage. Corneal scissors are used to excise the recipient tissue (see Fig. 9.3). In cases of extreme ectasia or where the preoperative intraocular pressure was high, a "sandwich technique" can be used to safeguard against the possibility of an expulsive hemorrhage [39] (see Fig. 9.4).

In developmental or congenital opacities, the anterior chamber is always shallow. It is, therefore, advisable to oversize the donor by 1 mm relative to the host trephination. This is not the case for acquired cases of corneal opacification. The graft is secured with at least sixteen 10–0 nylon sutures.

Early suture removal is essential in infants for both DALK and PKP to avoid epithelial graft rejection.

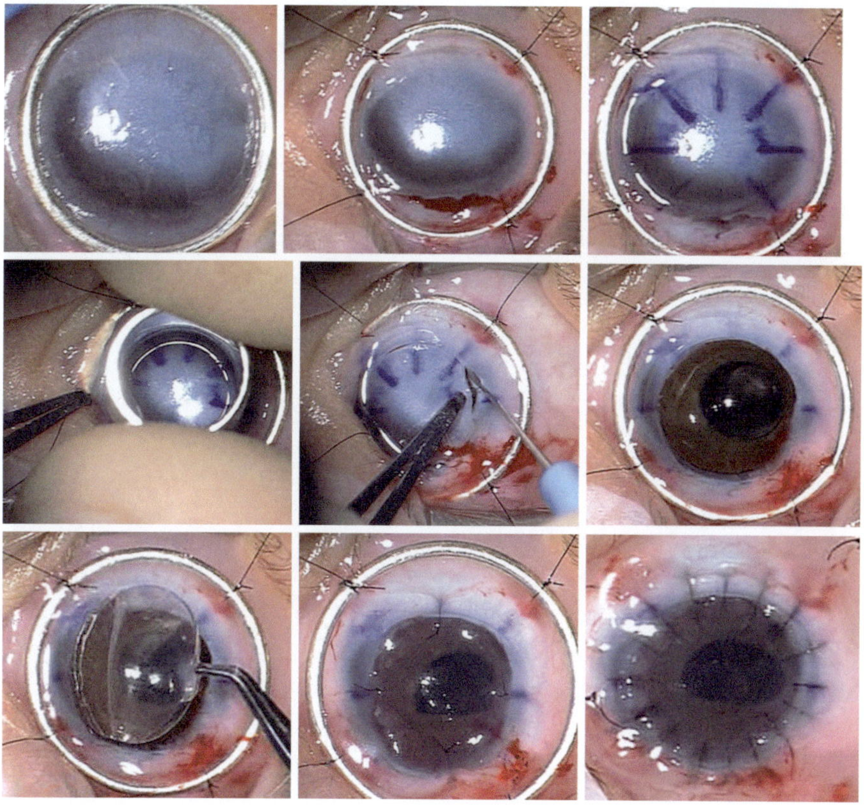

Fig. 9.3 Composite figure showing steps of a penetrating keratoplasty in an infant. See text for details

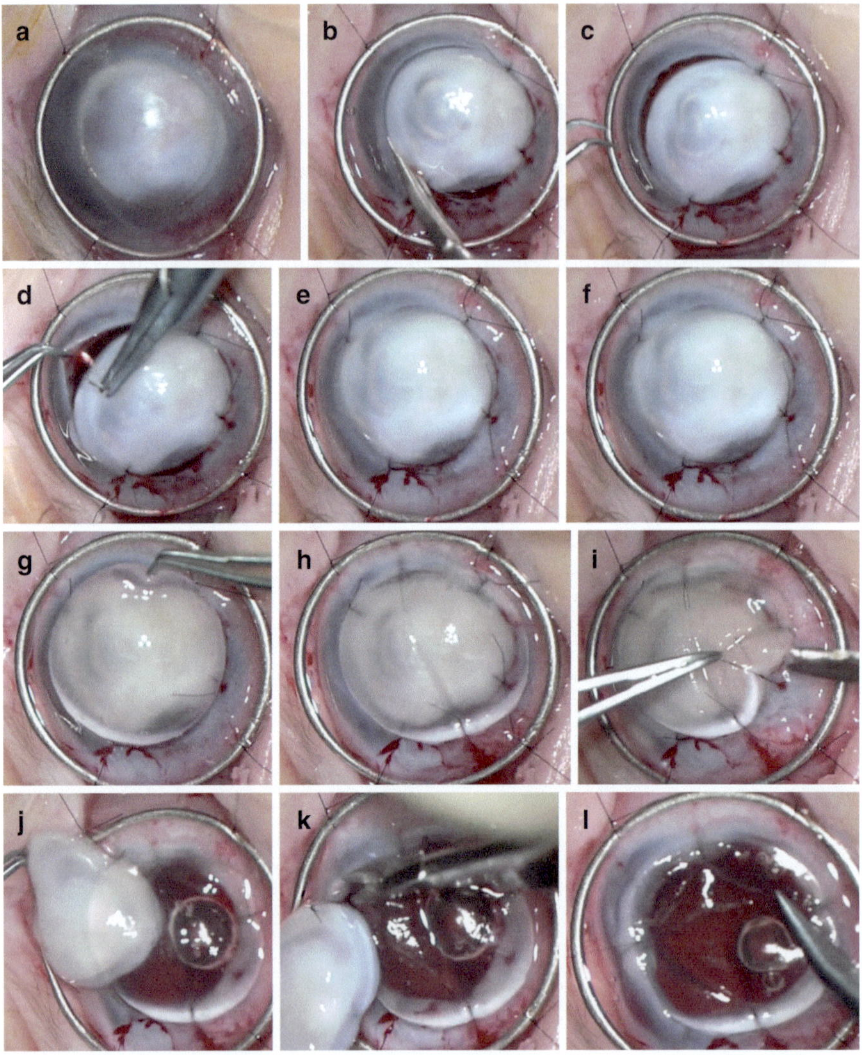

Fig. 9.4 Composite figure showing the 'sandwich technique' in a case of corneal opacity. After penetration of a quadrant, an 8–0 nylon suture is placed to appose the recently cut edges of host tissue (**b**, **c**, and **d**). In this way, the host tissue is held in place by four interrupted 10–0 nylon sutures (**e**). The graft is placed over the host button with copious viscoelastic sandwiched between the two (**g** and **h**). The donor is secured at the 12 and 6 o'clock positions with interrupted 10–0 nylon sutures (**i**). Once this is done, the four nylon sutures holding the host button in place are cut and the host button is slid out from underneath the donor button (**j**, **k**, and **l**). In this way, the child's eye is never totally in the "open-sky" state

9.6 Deep Anterior Lamellar Keratoplasty

All the precautions described for penetrating keratoplasty are necessary for DALK in case of conversion to PKP. The technique of DALK depends in large part on the surgeon's comfort level with the various techniques used in adults [40, 41]. The younger the child, the more difficult the big-bubble technique [42]. The use of femtosecond laser-assisted big-bubble technique has been recently described for DALK in children [43].

Viscodissection [44] appears to be a reliable method even in children and infants. In cases of severe corneal clouding, a manual technique is utilized, but (ultrasound biomicrosocpy) UBM is used to define the trephine-cut depth in order to get as close to posterior stroma as possible prior to starting manual trephination [40]. A graduated vacuum trephine is necessary for such cases. The Hessburg-Barron (Barron Precision Instruments, Grand Blanc, MI) trephine is one such trephine whereby each quarter turn of the handle is equal to a 60 micron depth.

The viscodissection technique requires an air bubble in the anterior chamber to allow visualization of the air-Descemet interface. Using Healon (Johnson & Johnson, Santa Ana, CA) on a 27G needle, the needle is advanced in the periphery until a triple reflex of the needle point is seen. At this point, with the bevel face-down, the Healon is injected and a visco-bubble forms. Once formed, manual trephination is performed and the viscoelastic is thoroughly washed away with jets of Balanced salt solution (BSS) on a cannula. In such cases, the donor is either the same, 0.25 mm, or 0.5 mm larger than the host trephine. In cases of marked keratoconus, the same size or 0.25 mm larger may be used (see Fig. 9.5).

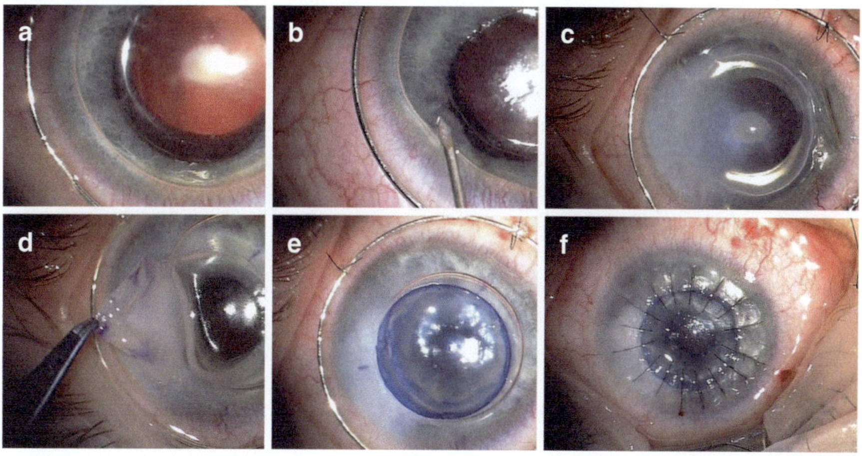

Fig. 9.5 Composite figure showing the viscodissection technique for deep anterior lamellar keratoplasty. Air is placed in the anterior chamber (**a**). A 27G or 30G needle is introduced into the corneal stroma in the periphery until a triple reflection is seen of the needle tip at the air-DM interface (**b**). Viscoelastic is injected through this needle creating a wave of viscoelastic separating posterior stroma from the Descemet membrane (**c** and **d**). Once the host tissue is excised, the donor tissue is secured with 16 10-0 nylon interrupted sutures (**e** and **f**)

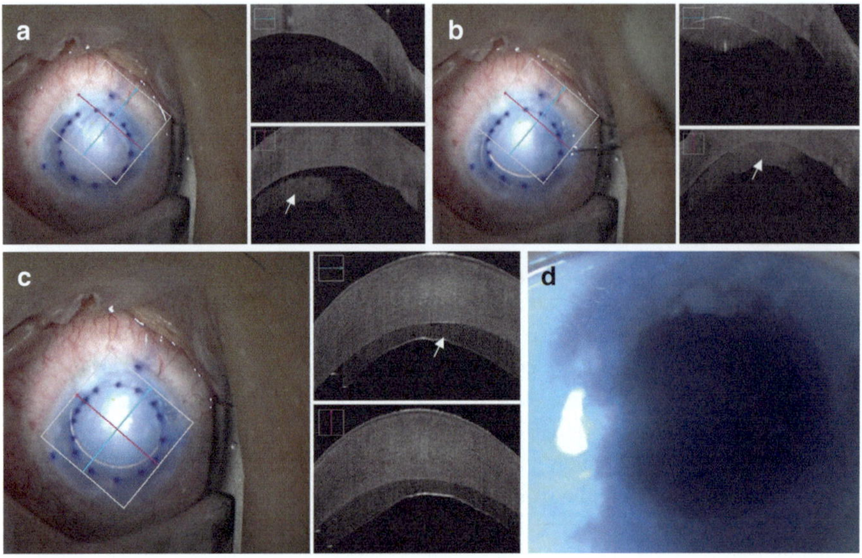

Fig. 9.6 Composite figure of a child undergoing endothelial keratoplasty. Integrated intraoperative OCT allows visualization of the donor graft (white arrow; **a**, **b**, and **c**). Good apposition of the graft can be seen in (**c**). Clearing of the cornea can be seen 8 weeks post-surgery (**d**)

9.6.1 Endothelial Keratoplasty

The technique for endothelial keratoplasty used in children in the past 5 years is Descemet stripping automated endothelial keratoplasty (DSAEK) [45–49]. The younger the child, the shallower the anterior chamber and the more likely the anterior chamber is to collapse, making unfolding the donor material more difficult. Although it can be harder to remove the Descemet membrane in children, it is important to strip it to ensure a successful endothelial keratoplasty. There are various methods of introducing the precut donor tissue into the eye, ranging from the use of an endo-inserter to suture to a Busin glide *(Moria, Doylestown, PA)*. Puncturing the stroma with a 30G needle to gently impale the donor in order to position it or get rid of any small folds may be needed. The advent of intraoperative OCT has meant that the endothelial graft can be visualized very easily, flattening the learning curve for this procedure in children (see Fig. 9.6).

The anesthesiologist should be aware that after the procedure is complete, the child may need to be brought back to the operating room (OR) in 1–2 hours to reduce the air bubble, check the intraoular pressure (IOP), or manipulate any dislocated graft.

9.6.2 Selective Endothelial Removal

In this procedure, endothelial cells are removed using a low vacuum aspiration cannula in the area of the opacity, encouraging adjacent endothelial cells to migrate into the area of opacity and encouraging clearing of the cornea [50].

9.6.3 Optical Iridectomy

In cases of eccentric corneal opacities, an optical iridectomy can be a low-risk, high-gain procedure [51]. It is best to do a limbal peritomy and create a short scleral tunnel to perform a broad peripheral iridectomy. Corneal incisions can result in an opacity of the clear cornea, thereby reducing the effect of the iridectomy. Doing an optical iridectomy under the upper lid is probably not useful.

9.6.4 The Future

Measuring success beyond the clarity of the cornea includes assessment of gains in global development. Standardizing and evaluating these gains with developmental pediatricians will become standard practice in assessing success.

The development of tissue-engineered cornea is a reality now with decellularized human corneal transplantation already in phase I trials for humans in cases of marked tissue loss and keratoconus [52].

Stem cell research also shows promising results for the clearing of acquired corneal scars with mesenchymal stem cells [53, 54]. If this can be safely developed, it may have a role in clearing congenital corneal opacities, thereby avoiding pediatric keratoplasty altogether.

References

1. Nischal KK. Genetics of congenital corneal opacification--impact on diagnosis and treatment. Cornea. 2015;34(Suppl 10):S24–34.
2. Weiss JS, Møller HU, Aldave AJ, Seitz B, Bredrup C, Kivelä T, Munier FL, Rapuano CJ, Nischal KK, Kim EK, Sutphin J, Busin M, Labbé A, Kenyon KR, Kinoshita S, Lisch W. IC3D classification of corneal dystrophies--edition 2. Cornea. 2015 Feb;34(2):117–59.
3. Liu M, Xia JL, Yang H, Yu L. Compound heterozygous mutations in the *SLC4A11* gene associated with congenital hereditary endothelial dystrophy in a Chinese family. Ophthalmic Genet. 2022;16:1–5.
4. Davidson AE, Hafford-Tear NJ, Dudakova L, Sadan AN, Pontikos N, Hardcastle AJ, Tuft SJ, Liskova P. CUGC for posterior polymorphous corneal dystrophy (PPCD). Eur J Hum Genet. 2020;28(1):126–31.
5. Schmid E, Lisch W, Philipp W, Lechner S, Göttinger W, Schlötzer-Schrehardt U, Müller T, Utermann G, Janecke AR. A new, X-linked endothelial corneal dystrophy. Am J Ophthalmol. 2006;141(3):478–87.
6. Singh M, Kaur M, Grewal AM, Yangzes S, Yadav D, Zadeng Z, Gupta P. Ophthalmic features and management outcomes of 30 children having Goldenhar syndrome. Int Ophthalmol. 2020;40(3):667–75.
7. Chacon-Camacho OF, Lopez-Moreno D, Morales-Sanchez MA, Hofmann E, Pacheco-Quito M, Wieland I, Cortes-Gonzalez V, Villanueva-Mendoza C, Zenker M, Zenteno JC. Expansion of the phenotypic spectrum and description of molecular findings in a cohort of patients with oculocutaneous mosaic RASopathies. Mol Genet Genomic Med. 2019;7(5):e625.
8. Kapoor S, Scanga HL, Reyes-Múgica M, Nischal KK. Somatic KRAS mutation affecting codon 146 in linear sebaceous nevus syndrome. Am J Med Genet A. 2021;185(12):3825–30.
9. Stark DJ, Gilmore DW, Vance JC, Pearn JH. A corneal abnormality associated with trisomy 8 mosaicism syndrome. Br J Ophthalmol. 1987;71(1):29–31.

10. Kelberman D, Islam L, Jacques TS, Russell-Eggitt I, Bitner-Glindzicz M, Khaw PT, Nischal KK, Sowden JC. CYP1B1-related anterior segment developmental anomalies novel mutations for infantile glaucoma and von Hippel's ulcer revisited. Ophthalmology. 2011;118(9):1865–73.
11. Weh E, Reis LM, Happ HC, Levin AV, Wheeler PG, David KL, Carney E, Angle B, Hauser N, Semina EV. Whole exome sequence analysis of Peters anomaly. Hum Genet. 2014;133(12):1497–511.
12. Mataftsi A, Islam L, Kelberman D, Sowden JC, Nischal KK. Chromosome abnormalities and the genetics of congenital corneal opacification. Mol Vis. 2011;17:1624–40.
13. Nischal KK. A new approach to the classification of neonatal corneal opacities. Curr Opin Ophthalmol. 2012;23(5):344–54.
14. Zaidman GW, Flanagan JK, Furey CC. Long-term visual prognosis in children after corneal transplant surgery for Peters anomaly type I. Am J Ophthalmol. 2007;144(1):104–8.
15. Shah PR, Chauhan B, Chu CT, Kofler J, Nischal KK. Ocular Phenotype of Peters-Plus Syndrome. Cornea. 2022;41(2):219–23.
16. Ernst J, Medsinge A, Scanga HL, Hiasat J, Moore W, Ali A, Levin AV, Stahl ED, Nischal KK. Congenital primary aphakia. J AAPOS. 2022;26(1):4.e1–5.
17. Zinn KM. Changes in corneal ultrastructure resulting from early lens removal in the developing chick embryo. Investig Ophthalmol. 1970;9(3):165–82.
18. Islam L, Kelberman D, Williamson L, Lewis N, Glindzicz MB, Nischal KK, Sowden JC. Functional analysis of FOXE3 mutations causing dominant and recessive ocular anterior segment disease. Hum Mutat. 2015;36(3):296–300.
19. Muslubas IS, Hocaoglu M, Arf S, Karacorlu M. A case of morning glory syndrome associated with persistent hyperplastic primary vitreous and Peters' anomaly. GMS Ophthalmol Cases. 2017;7:Doc02.
20. Singh N, Agrawal S, Mishra P. Bilateral primary hyperplastic persistent vitreous: report of two cases. GMS Ophthalmol Cases. 2020;10:Doc42.
21. Mocan MC, Mehta AA, Aref AA. Update in genetics and surgical management of primary congenital glaucoma. Turk J Ophthalmol. 2019;49(6):347–55.
22. Beltz J, Madi S, Santorum P, Scorcia V, Busin M. Descemet stripping automated endothelial keratoplasty for endothelial decompensation in buphthalmos. Am J Ophthalmol. 2013;156(3):608–15.
23. Hirano K, Kachi S, Matsuura M, Kawase K. Non-descemet stripping automated endothelial keratoplasty for bullous keratopathy in buphthalmic eye. Case Rep Ophthalmol. 2016;7(2):279–84.
24. Quilendrino R, Yeh RY, Dapena I, Ham L, Dirisamer M, van Niekerk J, Melles GR. Large diameter Descemet membrane endothelial keratoplasty in buphthalmic eyes. Cornea. 2013;32(5):e74–8.
25. Zepeda EM, Branham K, Moroi SE, Bohnsack BL. Surgical outcomes of Glaucoma associated with Axenfeld-Rieger syndrome. BMC Ophthalmol. 2020;20(1):172.
26. Seifi M, Walter MA. Axenfeld-Rieger syndrome. Clin Genet. 2018 Jun;93(6):1123–30.
27. Samant M, Chauhan BK, Lathrop KL, Nischal KK. Congenital aniridia: etiology, manifestations and management. Expert Rev Ophthalmol. 2016;11(2):135–44.
28. Sawada M, Sato M, Hikoya A, Wang C, Minoshima S, Azuma N, Hotta Y. A case of aniridia with unilateral Peters anomaly. J AAPOS. 2011;15(1):104–6.
29. Medsinge A, Nischal KK. Cataract surgery in children with congenital keratolenticular adhesion (Peters anomaly type 2). J AAPOS. 2015;19(1):24–8.
30. Han KE, Choi SI, Kim TI, Maeng YS, Stulting RD, Ji YW, Kim EK. Pathogenesis and treatments of TGFBI corneal dystrophies. Prog Retin Eye Res. 2016;50:67–88.
31. Jun RM, Tchah H, Kim TI, Stulting RD, Jung SE, Seo KY, Lee DH, Kim EK. Avellino corneal dystrophy after LASIK. Ophthalmology. 2004;111(3):463–8.
32. Zeng L, Zhao J, Chen Y, Shang J, Aruma A, Zhou X. Multiple phototherapeutic keratectomy treatments in a Chinese pedigree with corneal dystrophy and an R124L mutation: a 20-year observational study. BMC Ophthalmol. 2019;19(1):191.

33. Gruenauer-Kloevekorn C, Braeutigam S, Froster UG, Duncker GI. Surgical outcome after phototherapeutic keratectomy in patients with TGFBI-linked corneal dystrophies in relation to molecular genetic findings. Graefes Arch Clin Exp Ophthalmol. 2009;247(1):93–9.
34. Lalgudi VG, Nischal KK. Pediatric corneal collagen cross-linking for keratoconus: not an experimental procedure. J AAPOS. 2019;23(2):63–5.
35. Pillar A, Jeng BH, Munir WM. Positive End-Expiratory Pressure as a Risk Factor for Severe Positive Vitreous Pressure During Combined Penetrating Keratoplasty and Cataract Extraction. Cornea. 2016;35(11):1491–4.
36. Chronopoulos A, Thumann G, Schutz J. Positive vitreous pressure: pathophysiology, complications, prevention, and management. Surv Ophthalmol. 2017;62(2):127–33.
37. Epley KD, Tychsen L, Lueder GT. The effect of an eyelid speculum on intraocular pressure measurement in children. Am J Ophthalmol. 2002;134(6):926–7.
38. Soong H. Corneal transplantation. In: Spaeth GL, editor. Ophthalmic surgery. Philadelphia: Elsevier; 2003. p. 139–59.
39. Arslan OS, Unal M, Arici C, et al. Novel method to avoid the open-sky condition in penetrating keratoplasty: covered cornea technique. Cornea. 2014;33(9):994–8.
40. Harding SA, Nischal KK, Upponi-Patil A, et al. Indications and outcomes of deep anterior lamellar keratoplasty in children. Ophthalmology. 2010;117(11):2191–5.
41. Sharma N, Agarwal R, Jhanji V, Bhaskar S, Kamalakkannan P, Nischal KK. Lamellar keratoplasty in children. Surv Ophthalmol. 2020;65(6):675–90.
42. Ashar JN, Pahuja S, Ramappa M, et al. Deep anterior lamellar keratoplasty in children. Am J Ophthalmol. 2013;155(3):570–4.
43. Buzzonetti L, Petrocelli G, Valente P. Big-bubble deep anterior lamellar keratoplasty assisted by femtosecond laser in children. Cornea. 2012;31(9):1083–6.
44. Melles GR, Remeijer L, Geerards AJ, et al. A quick surgical technique for deep, anterior lamellar keratoplasty using visco-dissection. Cornea. 2000;19(4):427–32.
45. Patil M, Soh YQ, Yu HC, Nischal KK, Mehta JS. Recent advances in pediatric endothelial keratoplasty. Int Ophthalmol Clin. 2021;61(1):57–75.
46. Panahi-Bazaz M, Sharifipour F, Malekahmadi M. Modified Descemet's stripping automated endothelial keratoplasty for congenital hereditary endothelial dystrophy. J Ophthalmic Vis Res. 2014;9(4):522–5.
47. Gonnermann J, Klamann MK, Maier AK, et al. Descemet membrane endothelial keratoplasty in a child with corneal endothelial dysfunction in Kearns-Sayre syndrome. Cornea. 2014;33(11):1232–4.
48. Anwar HM, El-Danasoury A. Endothelial keratoplasty in children. Curr Opin Ophthalmol. 2014;25(4):340–6.
49. Mittal V, Mittal R. Challenges in pediatric endothelial keratoplasty. Indian J Ophthalmol. 2014;62(2):251–4.
50. Soh YQ, Mehta JS. Selective endothelial removal for peters anomaly. Cornea. 2018;37(3):382–5.
51. Donoso Rojas R, López Garin JP, Jara UG. Long-term experience and visual acuity outcomes in Peters anomaly cases. Arch Soc Esp Oftalmol (Engl Ed). 2022;97(1):3–8.
52. Porzionato A, Stocco E, Barbon S, Grandi F, Macchi V, De Caro R. Tissue-engineered grafts from human decellularized extracellular matrices: a systematic review and future perspectives. Int J Mol Sci. 2018;19(12):4117. https://doi.org/10.3390/ijms19124117. PMID: 30567407; PMCID: PMC6321114
53. Basu S, Hertsenberg AJ, Funderburgh ML, Burrow MK, Mann MM, Du Y, Lathrop KL, Syed-Picard FN, Adams SM, Birk DE, Funderburgh JL. Human limbal biopsy-derived stromal stem cells prevent corneal scarring. Sci Transl Med. 2014;6(266):266ra172.
54. Sangwan VS, Jain R, Basu S, Bagadi AB, Sureka S, Mariappan I, Macneil S. Transforming ocular surface stem cell research into successful clinical practice. Indian J Ophthalmol. 2014 Jan;62(1):29–40.

Ocular Chemical Burns and Stevens-Johnson Syndrome

10

Tanvi Mudgil, Anahita Kate, and Swapna S. Shanbhag

Key Points

1. Both ocular chemical burn (OCB) and Stevens-Johnson syndrome/toxic epidermal necrolysis (SJS/TEN) can cause chronic cicatricial disease of the ocular surface. Chronic disease can be prevented by rigorous acute care.
2. While both OCB and SJS/TEN can cause limbal stem cell deficiency, disease is usually unilateral in OCB and bilateral in SJS/TEN. Available interventions are more limited in cases of bilateral LSCD.
3. In the acute phase of disease, removal/discontinuation of the offending agent and suppression of inflammation are critical components of management.
4. In the chronic phase of disease in OCB and SJS/TEN, a multimodal approach is necessary where the main goals are minimizing ocular discomfort and maximizing visual potential. Because the underlying pathogenesis of disease is inflammatory in OCB and immunological in SJS/TEN, chronic management options and outcomes vary between the two.

T. Mudgil
Shantilal Shanghvi Cornea Institute, L. V. Prasad Eye Institute, Vishakhapatnam, Andhra Pradesh, India
e-mail: tanvimudgil@lvpei.org

A. Kate
Shantilal Shanghvi Cornea Institute, L. V. Prasad Eye Institute, Vijayawada, Andhra Pradesh, India
e-mail: dranahitakate@lvpei.org

S. S. Shanbhag (✉)
Shantilal Shanghvi Cornea Institute, L. V. Prasad Eye Institute, Hyderabad, Telangana, India
e-mail: swapnashanbhag@lvpei.org

H. N. Saeed, R. B. Singh (eds.), *Corneal Disorders*, Current Practices in Ophthalmology, https://doi.org/10.1007/978-981-96-5294-5_10

10.1 Introduction

Ocular chemical injuries are true ophthalmic emergencies that require immediate and intensive intervention to minimize severe complications and profound visual loss [1, 2]. Improvements in the understanding of the pathophysiology of chemical injuries, as well as advancements in ocular surface reconstruction, have provided hope for patients who would otherwise have had a dismal visual prognosis. The major sight-threatening complications in the acute stage include corneal persistent epithelial defects (PED), stromal scarring, and corneal perforation. Chronic sequelae include limbal stem cell deficiency (LSCD), symblepharon formation, and glaucomatous changes. Various management strategies exist to mitigate the severity of acute and chronic disease. This chapter details those strategies and discusses novel therapies in ocular chemical injuries.

10.2 Epidemiology

Ocular chemical burns (OCBs) are a major cause of corneal blindness, particularly in economically developing countries. The incidence of OCBs varies widely between different regions of the world. In the United States, which has a significantly lower incidence of ocular burns than much of the world, the incidence may be 51.1 new cases per million persons per year [3]. OCBs most commonly occur in the workplace (industrial, agriculture, construction sites), in domestic circumstances, or as a criminal assault [4]. Young men in the 20–40 year age group are at greatest risk of OCBs in their work environments [5]. As such, OCBs can have dramatic social and economic effects [6].

10.3 Etiological Agents and Their Pathophysiology

The severity of chemical injury is determined by several factors, such as the chemical and physical characteristics of the offending agent (particularly the pH), its specific reactivity with tissues, concentration, volume, temperature, and impact force. Alkalis (ammonia, lime, sodium hydroxide, potassium hydroxide, calcium hydroxide) are present in commonly used cleaning agents and are the most common culprit agents of OCBs. Alkalis (pH of >11.5) are highly lipophilic and penetrate the eye more readily than other substances, including acids, and therefore threaten both ocular surface tissues and intraocular structures such as the trabecular meshwork, ciliary body, and lens [1, 7]. In contrast, acidic substances cause protein coagulation in the epithelium, limiting further penetration into the eye. The most common cause of acid ocular injury is sulfuric acid, which is much less likely to result in severe ocular injury than alkalis unless associated with thermal or high-velocity injury such as that of a battery explosion. Unlike other acids, however, hydrofluoric acid in particular has a powerful dissolving action on cell membranes and has a similar ability to penetrate the anterior chamber as alkalis [1, 8].

Damage to the corneal and conjunctival epithelium from OCBs may also damage the pluripotent limbal epithelial stem cells (LESC), causing partial or total LSCD [9]. Cicatricial entropion or ectropion can cause further damage to the cornea secondary to lagophthalmos and exposure [1]. An acute rise in intraocular pressure (IOP) due to shrinkage and contraction of the cornea and sclera may occur. Long-term IOP elevation can occur from the accumulation of inflammatory debris within the trabecular meshwork and direct damage to the trabecular meshwork. Damage to the conjunctiva can cause extensive scarring, perilimbal ischemia, and forniceal shortening and loss of goblet cells, and conjunctival inflammation can lead to dry eyes.

10.4 Classification System for Ocular Injuries

It is crucial to classify OCBs at every visit to titrate the treatment. The two main classification systems used commonly in clinical practice are the Roper Hall classification and Dua classification [10, 11].

The Roper Hall classification divides OCBs into four grades based on corneal clarity and degree of limbal ischemia [10]. Although easier to use in an emergency setting, this classification system does not include the degree of conjunctival injury, and all injuries with >50% limbal ischemia are classified as grade IV and designated as "poor prognosis." The Dua classification was developed to allow for a more accurate stratification of prognosis, particularly for severe injuries, by incorporating the clock hours of limbal and bulbar conjunctival involvement as determined by fluorescein staining [11]. Although limbal involvement is considered in this classification, the extent of limbal de-epithelialization may not correlate with the extent of ischemia [12]. A more objective means of assessing limbal ischemia is required.

10.5 Clinical Course

McCulley categorized the pathophysiology and course of the disease process into four distinct clinical phases: immediate, acute (0–7 days), early repair (7–21 days), and late repair (after 21 days) [13].

The immediate phase begins as soon as the chemical agent encounters the ocular surface. At this stage, the main prognostic factors are the extent of corneal and conjunctival epithelial defects, the clock hours of limbal blanching, the area and density of corneal opacification, degree of IOP elevation, and loss of lens clarity. During the acute phase, the ocular tissue may attempt to recover by removing the noxious substance and reestablishing the superficial protective layer of corneal epithelium. In the early repair phase, the acute inflammation may decrease, and the ocular surface may progress to a stage of chronic inflammation, stromal repair, and scarring. Three weeks after the acute OCB, chronic sequelae such as dry eyes, corneal scarring, symblepharon, ankyloblepharon, glaucoma, uveitis, cataract, LSCD, and adnexal abnormalities such as lagophthalmos, entropion, ectropion, and trichiasis can occur.

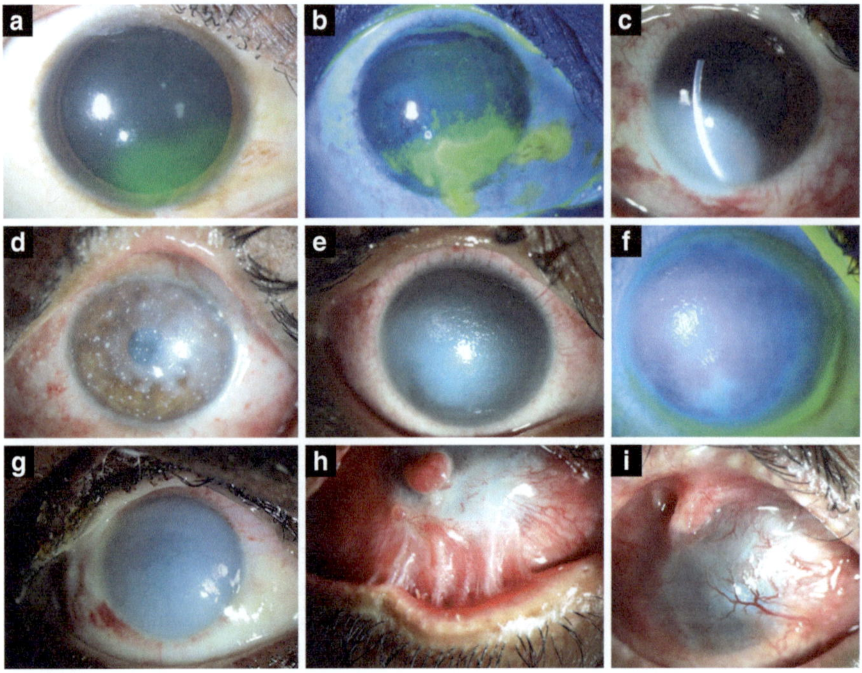

Fig. 10.1 Images depicting the spectrum of clinical features in ocular chemical burns. (**a**, **b**) Image of the cornea showing an epithelial defect inferiorly. Fluorescein staining reveals an adjacent conjunctival defect. (**c**) Inferonasal area of dense stromal haze and edema. The perilimbal conjunctival shows blanching in all quadrants. (**d**) Multiple corneal foreign bodies dispersed within the stroma. (**e**, **f**) A total cornea epithelial defect with the margins delineated on fluorescein staining. The stroma shows diffuse edema. (**g**) Total corneal epithelial defect with stromal edema, limbal ischemia and conjunctival blanching. (**h**) Inferior conjunctival cicatrization with symblepharon formation and total limbal stem cell deficiency (LSCD). (**i**) Superior symblepharon with total LSCD, conjunctivalization, and corneal neovascularization

Figure 10.1 is a representative collage of the spectrum of clinical manifestations in OCB.

10.6 Management

1. **Immediate phase:** The first step is to eradicate the chemical agent with thorough irrigation of the ocular surface [1]. Readily available tap water can be used immediately. In hospital settings, lactated Ringers or a balanced salt solution is preferred [14].
2. **Acute phase:** The main objective in this phase is to suppress inflammation, enhance re-epithelization, reduce corneal exposure, and prevent stromal breakdown [15]. Figure 10.2 depicts the different treatment modalities in cases of acute ocular chemical burns.

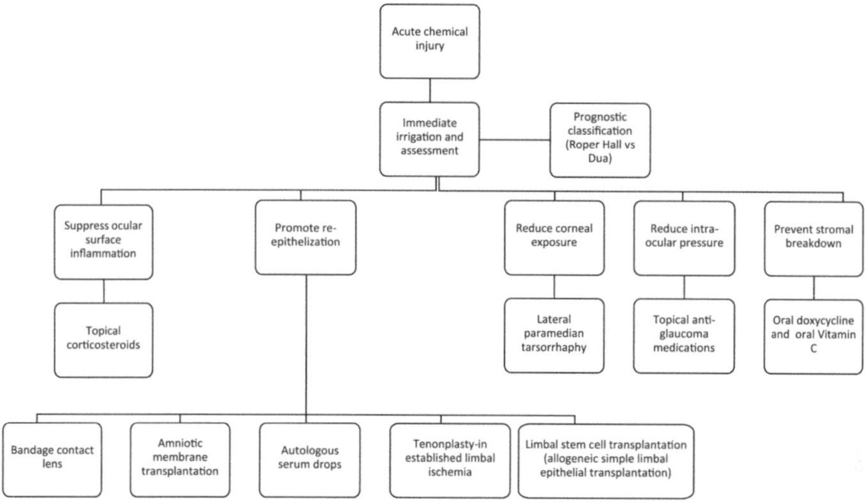

Fig. 10.2 Different modalities for management of acute chemical ocular burn

10.6.1 Anti-inflammatory Therapy

Topical corticosteroids are critical in the acute phase as they suppress inflammation by inhibiting neutrophilic infiltration, stabilizing lysosomal membranes, and subsequent release of matrix-degrading enzymes [16]. Topical steroids help to reduce ocular surface inflammation and increase the resolution rate of corneal epithelial defects.

Agents such as prednisolone acetate 1% can be used at a high frequency in the first few days (i.e., every hour).

10.6.2 Prevention of Stromal Breakdown

Corneal thinning and stromal melting may be precipitated by collagenases and matrix metalloproteinases (MMP) released by the reactive inflammatory cells [17]. Collagenase inhibitors [e.g., tetracyclines, citrate, cysteine, acetylcysteine, sodium ethylenediamine tetra acetic acid (EDTA), penicillamine] and proteinase inhibitors (e.g., aprotinin) have been found to prevent corneal thinning after chemical injuries [18]. Additionally, supplementation with ascorbic acid can directly enhance collagen synthesis and promote wound healing [19].

10.6.3 Promotion of Re-epithelization of the Ocular Surface

10.6.3.1 Bandage Contact Lens (BCL)

BCLs may aid in faster re-epithelization of the cornea by preventing the direct exposure of MMPs to the denuded corneal stroma and by protecting the ocular surface from the windshield wiper effect of the eyelids. It also increases patient comfort [1, 20].

10.6.3.2 Amniotic Membrane Transplantation (AMT)

AMT is an adjunct to medical therapy in severe chemical burns [21]. Amniotic membrane (AM) works like a biological BCL by protecting the denuded cornea. The AM also traps inflammatory cells and mediators, thus exerting anti-inflammatory effects [22].

10.6.3.3 Tenonplasty

In eyes with severe grade chemical burns with limbal and scleral ischemia, tenonplasty may help in reestablishing conjunctivalization of the ischemic area, thus preventing scleral necrosis and perforation of the adjacent cornea [23, 24]. After debridement of necrotic tissue from the sclera, advancement of viable, vascular Tenon's layer tissue up to the limbus can be performed. This can be combined with an AMT over the adjacent cornea with or without lamellar corneal patch grafting [25].

10.6.3.4 Autologous Serum Drops

Autologous and umbilical cord serum have epithelial growth factors and may promote epithelialization of PEDs [26, 27]. However, the procurement and storage of these drops are the significant challenges faced in clinical practice.

10.6.3.5 IOP Management

The rise of IOP may be immediate or delayed following chemical injury due to the inflammatory mediators penetrating the anterior chamber and causing tissue shrinkage and disruption of the trabecular meshwork and outflow channels [28, 29]. Additionally, topical steroids may precipitate a steroid response throughout treatment. Hence, regular IOP monitoring and timely initiation of anti-glaucoma medications is necessary.

10.6.3.6 Limbal Stem Cell Transplant

Allogeneic simple limbal epithelial transplantation (SLET) has recently gained popularity for enhancing epithelization in grades 4–6 of Dua's classification [30]. The goal is to achieve rapid epithelization of the cornea in the acute stage before stromal necrosis and other sequelae occur. In the chronic phase, autologous or allogeneic limbal stem cell transplantation (LSCT) in unilateral or bilateral cases, respectively, can be performed to restore the normal corneal epithelial layer.

10.7 Chronic Phase

Treatment in the chronic phase requires an integrated approach to address the cicatricial changes and LSCD that may occur. The treatment modalities are primarily surgical to restore ocular surface anatomy and visual function (Fig. 10.3).

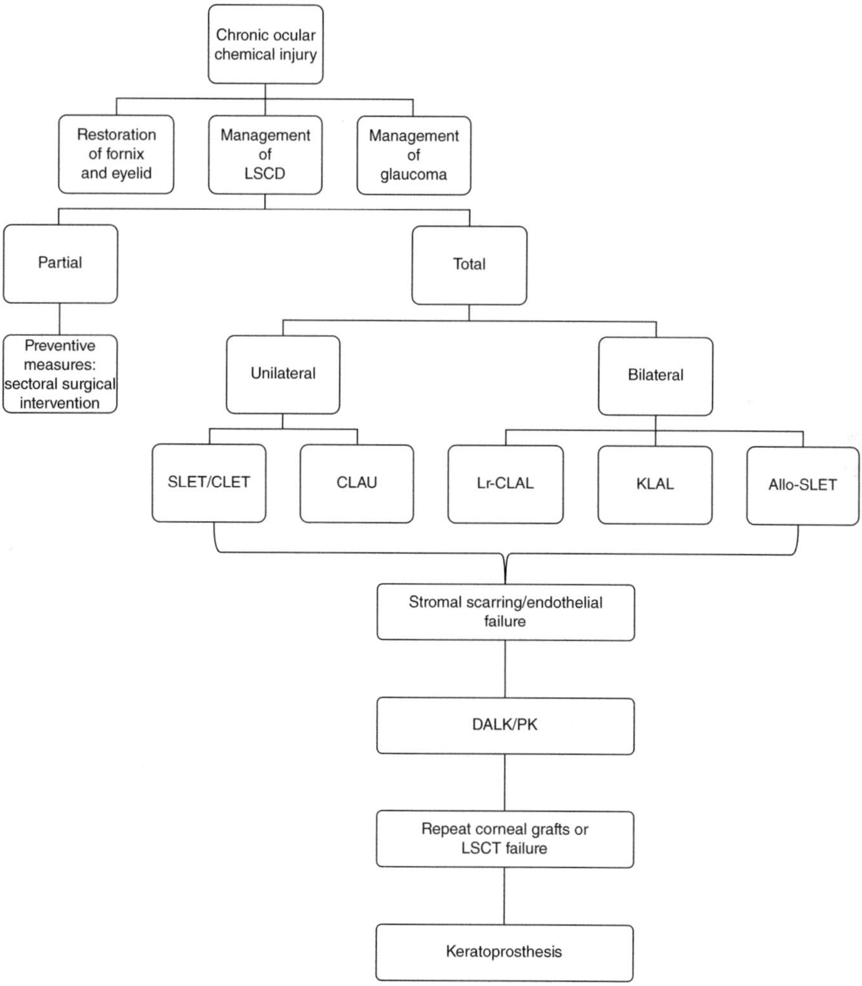

Fig. 10.3 Algorithm for management of ocular chemical burns in the chronic phase. *Lr-CLAL* live-related conjunctival limbal allograft, *KLAL* keratolimbal allograft, *SLET* simple limbal epithelial transplantation, *CLAU* conjunctival limbal autograft

10.7.1 Limbal Stem Cell Transplant

Clinical findings of LSCD include a loss of the palisades of Vogt, an opaque epithelium, whorl-like epithelial staining, recurrent and/or persistent epithelial defects, and superficial corneal neovascularization [31]. Conjunctivalization of the corneal surface is a hallmark of LSCD.

The treatment of LSCD depends on the laterality and extent of corneal involvement. For unilateral LSCD, surgical modalities such as SLET, conjunctival limbal autograft (CLAU), and cultivated limbal epithelial transplantation (CLET), which harvests healthy limbus from the contralateral eye, can be performed. CLAU and SLET have anatomical success rates of 78% and 81%, respectively, in eyes with unilateral LSCD secondary to OCBs [32]. Ideally, all adnexal abnormalities such as symblepharon, entropion, and trichiasis should be first addressed before planning for LSCT [33]. Bilateral LSCD can be addressed with LSCT performed with limbus harvested from cadaveric donor corneas or a living related donor. The long-term success of LSCT largely depends on tear film status, prior correction of adnexal abnormalities, and adequate immunosuppression [34, 35].

10.7.2 Keratoplasty and Keratoprosthesis

In eyes without significant limbal disease but with resultant corneal scarring from an OCB, deep anterior lamellar keratoplasty (DALK) or PKP can be performed depending on the extent of the disease. Eyes with deep corneal scarring which extends beyond Descemet's membrane or deep neovascularization cannot undergo DALK. Corneal transplantation, and specifically full-thickness penetrating keratoplasty (PK), has very poor outcomes in eyes with severe OCBs due to concomitant LSCD [36, 37]. In eyes with significant corneal scars, LSCD should ideally first be addressed with LSCT, and then PK should be attempted [38]. Simultaneous LSCT with PK can be attempted in eyes with a very thin cornea or corneal perforation [39]. In eyes with superficial scars, DALK can be performed after LSCT [40].

A keratoprosthesis (KPro) is indicated as a primary option in monocular patients with total LSCD and a wet surface or in patients who have undergone multiple keratoplasties post OCB [41, 42]. Adnexal issues must be addressed prior to the KPro. The advantage of a KPro is that no systemic immunosuppression is required, and good visual acuity is attained in the immediate postoperative period. However, close lifelong care is needed after KPro as complications can be severe and can develop anytime. There are several variations of the KPro available. In cases of extremely dry eyes, severe ocular surface keratinization, or non-functional eyelids, a Boston type 2 KPro, LVP KPro, or modified osteo-odonto-keratoprosthesis (MOOKP) may be needed [34].

10.7.3 Management of Glaucoma

In eyes with severe OCB, evaluation of the optic nerve may not be possible until corneal surgery clears any opacities. Glaucoma in the chronic phase may result from synechiae and angle closure and long-term use of topical corticosteroids. Corneal surgery itself, particularly KPro, can cause or worsen glaucoma. Glaucoma may occur after corneal surgeries required for visual rehabilitation, with reported rates of 10–53%, including after newer procedures such as Boston keratoprosthesis placement. A combination of IOP measurements and optic nerve head evaluation when media is clear must guide aggressive treatment of glaucoma with medications and procedures.

Summary
Chemical burns can cause devastating ocular surface damage. Prompt treatment is essential for preserving vision. The goal of treatment is to restore the ocular surface anatomy and visual function with medical and surgical interventions.

10.8 Stevens-Johnson Syndrome/Toxic Epidermal Necrolysis

Stevens-Johnson syndrome (SJS) and toxic epidermal necrolysis (TEN) are severe cutaneous adverse drug reactions that predominantly involves the skin and mucous membranes. Both are rare, affecting approximately 1–2 per million population annually [43]. These are considered medical emergencies in the acute phase as they can be life-threatening [44]. The most widely accepted definition of these conditions is based on the amount of skin detachment [45]. The disease is associated with mortality rates that range from 1% to 5% in SJS and 25% to 35% in TEN [43]. Therefore, much attention is directed toward life-saving measures during the acute stage of the illness.

Drugs are the primary cause of SJS/TEN. High-risk drug classes include antibiotics, particularly sulfonamide antibiotics, anti-epileptics, and allopurinol [46]. There appears to be genetic susceptibility to SJS/TEN, with certain HLA genotypes conferring increased risk of drug-specific SJS/TEN [47].

Multiple organ systems, including the eye, are affected in both the acute and chronic phases of SJS/TEN [48]. Ocular involvement occurs in up to 100% of patients, with varying degrees of severity [49–52].

10.9 Etiopathogenesis

1. **Cellular and molecular immunological mechanism**

   SJS/TEN is strongly associated with the dysregulation of innate immune system, with neoantigen formation leading to a T-cell-mediated hypersensitivity reaction [53]. Other mediators of cell death include granulysin, cytotoxic T lymphocytes, and natural killer cells [54]. The exact mechanism of disease in SJS/TEN is unknown.

2. **Genetic mechanism**
   2.1 Specific alleles at the HLA-A and HLA-B loci increase the risk of drug-induced SJS/TEN in different subsets of the Asian and European populations [55]. The strongest association between HLA type and a drug causing SJS/TEN has been found between HLA-B*15:02 and carbamazepine in the Han-Chinese [56]. Similar associations have been found in Thai and Malaysian populations [57, 58]. Strong associations have also been made between HLA-B*58:01 and allopurinol in several different ethnic/racial populations [59].
   2.2 Human ocular surface epithelial cells explicitly express Toll-like receptor (TLR-3), and several single nucleotide polymorphisms (SNPs) of the *TLR-3* gene are associated with the ocular surface complications from SJS/TEN [60].
   2.3 Genome-wide association studies have shown SNPs in prostaglandin E receptor (*EP3*) genes leading to the loss of its function. This may also play a role in the pathogenesis of SJS/TEN. Ocular complications may result from dysregulated epistatic interactions between TLR3 and EP3 [61].

10.10 Clinical Features

Acute Phase The most common ocular manifestations include conjunctival hyperemia (100%), lid margin epithelial denudation (85%), conjunctival pseudomembranes (40%), conjunctival epithelial defects (80%), and corneal epithelial defects (56%) [62]. A careful ocular examination with fluorescein staining is mandatory to evaluate the entire ocular surface [63].

Chronic Phase The chronic stage of the disease may be characterized by persistent and prolonged ocular surface inflammation. In the chronic phase, the lid margin changes that are seen are meibomian gland atrophy, distortion of the lid margin architecture, posterior mucocutaneous junction (MCJ) migration, and lid margin keratinization [64] (Fig. 10.4). Cicatricial entropion, distichiasis, and trichiasis are also common [65]. Severe dry eye is multifactorial and occurs due to cicatrization of the conjunctiva affecting lacrimal gland outflow, ocular surface inflammation, and meibomian gland dropout [66]. The combination of a dry ocular surface with lid margin keratinization can lead to the development of keratopathy, corneal vascularization and scarring, and eventually corneal perforation. The loss of LESCs due to lid-wiper keratopathy caused by the keratinized lid margin leads to LSCD. If these sequelae are not addressed expediently, end-stage disease and bilateral corneal blindness in the form of a dry and keratinized ocular surface may result, precluding corneal transplantation, type 1 KPro, and LSCT [67, 68].

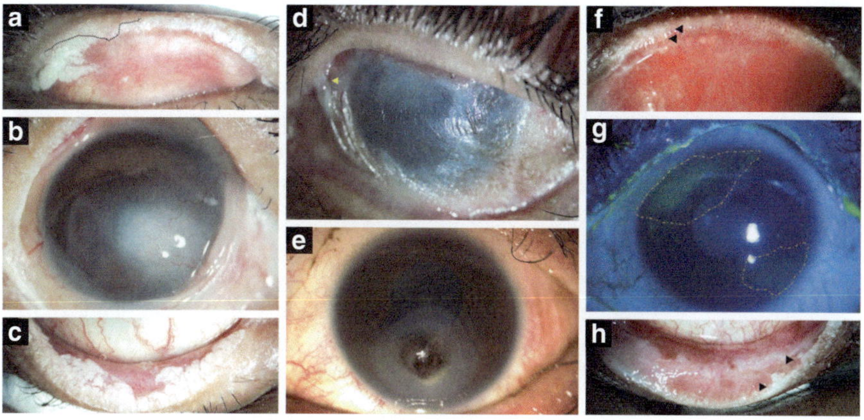

Fig. 10.4 Images illustrating the different ocular clinical features of Stevens-Johnson syndrome. (**a**–**c**) Everted upper and lower eyelids showing keratinization of the lid margin (**a**, **b**), with posterior migration of the mucocutaneous junction (dotted line). The cornea shows a leukomatous paracentral scar with superficial and deep vascularization (**c**). (**d**) Dry and keratinized ocular surface with an ankyloblepharon (yellow arrow head). (**e**) Paracentral sterile corneal perforation. (**f**–**h**) Lids show keratinization of the lid margin (black arrow heads, **f**, **h**) with punctate keratopathy in corresponding areas of the cornea (dotted yellow lines, **g**)

Sotozono et al. described a simple scoring system based on slit-lamp biomicroscopy of ocular findings for grading the extent and severity of ocular involvement in SJS/TEN [69]. The surface complications were graded on a scale of 0–3 based on the severity of involvement. The corneal complications included superficial punctate keratopathy, epithelial defect, loss of the palisades of Vogt, conjunctivalization, neovascularization, opacification, and keratinization. The conjunctival complications included hyperemia and symblepharon formation. Eyelid complications included trichiasis, MCJ involvement, meibomian gland involvement, and punctal damage. Such a grading system is useful in prognosticating the disease and assessing various medical and surgical treatment options.

10.11 Diagnosis

The diagnosis in the acute stage is based on the combination of skin and mucosal findings, history, and skin biopsy [70]. However, if a patient presents in the chronic stage of the disease, without appropriate documentation of the acute phase, or did not have access to healthcare in the acute phase, it is important to be able to identify the cause of the cicatricial eye disease as SJS/TEN. Shanbhag et al. have provided a scoring system that entails eliciting a detailed medical history with a careful systemic and ocular examination of patients presenting with chronic cicatricial conjunctivitis to identify patients with chronic stage SJS/TEN [71]. The correct diagnosis aids cornea specialists in providing appropriate care to the patients.

10.12 Management

Apart from the skin and the eyes, SJS/TEN affects many organ systems of the body, including the oral, otorhinolaryngologic, pulmonary, gastrointestinal, genitourinary, and gynecologic systems. Hence, SJS/TEN requires a multidisciplinary approach to not only improve survival of the patient but also improve morbidity, mortality, and mental health in survivors of the acute phase [48].

A. **Systemic management**

   Detailed systemic management in the acute phase is beyond the scope of this chapter. Briefly, identification and immediate discontinuation of the culprit drug, admission to an intensive care unit for supportive care and immunosuppressive management, and multidisciplinary care with a team of burn surgeons, dermatologists, ophthalmologists, gynecologists, and urologists are critical [43].

B. **Ocular management**

   In the acute phase of SJS/TEN, an ophthalmic consult is mandatory to prevent irreversible vision-threatening ocular complications. Chronic ocular complications are among the most severe and feared after SJS/TEN [72].

1. **Acute phase:** The goal of treatment in the acute phase is to minimize ocular surface inflammation, protect the ocular surface, and, to some extent, prevent symblepharon formation. Shanbhag et al. have published favorable long-term outcomes of a protocol for the management of ocular surface complications in the acute phase, which include the usage of topical steroids, topical antibiotics, topical lubricants, and AMT when indicated [72].
   1.1 **Topical medications**: Topical steroids, antibiotics, and preservative-free lubricants are used in the acute phase. Topical steroids help in reducing ocular surface inflammation [73]. Sotozono et al. reported better visual outcomes in patients with SJS/TEN using topical steroids compared to those not using them [74]. Topical antibiotics are given prophylactically and in the setting of ocular surface epithelial defects to prevent secondary infections. Preservative-free lubricants aid in the re-epithelization and provide symptomatic relief to the patient.
   1.2 **Amniotic membrane transplantation:** AM (amniotic membrane) has anti-inflammatory, anti-fibrotic, and anti-angiogenic properties and is widely used to treat various ocular surface disorders. AMT can be performed as a bedside procedure (sutureless with cyanoacrylate glue) and has been recommended in all cases of SJS/TEN with Sotozono grade 2 or above, that is, eyes with conjunctival pseudomembranes or conjunctival and corneal epithelial defects [62, 72, 75, 76]. It has proven to provide better long-term visual acuity and reduce the incidence of vision-threatening complications such as LSCD, corneal scars, corneal vascularization, and keratinization of the ocular surface [62].
2. **Chronic stage:** Treatment at this stage addresses chronic disease of the cornea, conjunctiva, and eyelids, which reduces vision and visual functioning.

Treatment strategies revolve around preventing continuous insult to the ocular surface and visual rehabilitation with surgical procedures.

2.1 **Topical medications:** Preservative-free lubricants play an imperative role in providing symptomatic relief in the chronic stage as most patients suffer from dry eye. Steroids are occasionally used depending on the presence of ocular inflammation. While topical steroids use should be limited in duration, long-term use is sometimes necessary in cases of chronic inflammation. Titration to lower potency steroids can be attempted.

2.2 **Scleral contact lens:** Scleral contact lenses play an essential role in managing ocular sequelae of SJS/TEN [77]. The prosthetic replacement of the ocular surface ecosystem (PROSE) device is a gas-permeable, large-diameter scleral lens that vaults the cornea and submerges the entire corneal surface in a pool of oxygenated artificial tears. Because of its high oxygen permeability, fluid-filled reservoir, lack of corneal contact, positional stability on the eye, and protection from lid-related shear forces, a PROSE device creates an environment that supports healing and maintenance of the corneal epithelium. Each prosthetic device is custom designed and manufactured per eye using a computer-aided design (available in diameter ranging from 15.5 to 23 mm). These lenses increase patient comfort by reducing photophobia, reducing the effect of the lid margin on the cornea, and providing relief from the underlying dry eye [67, 68]. Additionally, they improve vision by masking irregular astigmatism and improving corneal epithelial irregularities.

2.3 **Mucous membrane grafting (MMG)**: In eyes with posterior migration of the MCJ and subsequent lid margin keratinization, persistent microtrauma to the corneal epithelium occurs with every blink. If left untreated, this can lead to persistent corneal epithelial defects, microbial keratitis, corneal neovascularization and scarring, LSCD, and corneal perforation. Hence, replacing the keratinized lid margin with healthy labial/buccal mucosa in the form of MMG eliminates the lid-wiper keratopathy and restores a normally functioning lid margin [78]. An ideal case for lid-margin MMG is when the eye has posterior migration of MCJ with lid margin keratinization with early lid-related keratopathy with some wetness of the ocular surface (ideally a Schirmer‘s score > 5 mm at 5 min, without anesthesia) [79].

2.4 **Salivary gland transplantation for dry eye:** The severity of dry eye is the major prognostic factor of the final visual outcome in the chronic stage. The transplantation of minor salivary glands (harvested from the labial mucosa of the upper or lower lip) to the sclera has been shown to improve symptoms of severe dry eye, corneal transparency, and corneal neovascularization [80].

2.5 **Limbal stem cell transplantation and cultivated oral mucosal epithelial transplantation (COMET):** Patients with a relatively wet ocular surface are candidates for LSCT and COMET. Usually, both of these procedures have a relatively poor outcome in SJS/TEN due to persistent ocular inflammation, dry eye, and a higher risk of rejection (due to aberrant immune response) despite immunosuppression [81]. COMET, and some forms of LSCT, require cultivation of tissue in a lab, which significantly limits its use.

3. **End-stage disease**

   Patients with end-stage SJS/TEN have corneal blindness due to progressive keratinization and dermalization of a xerotic ocular surface. Corneal transplantation cannot be performed in these eyes, and KPro remains the only viable option for visual rehabilitation. Because of the xerotic surface, only a Boston KPro type II, MOOKP, LVP KPro, Moscow Eye Microsurgery Complex in Russia (MICOF) KPro, or the osteo-odonto KPro can be implanted [82–84]. Though these interventions are often the only hope for visual rehabilitation for patient with end-stage ocular SJS/TEN, they are fraught with complications and require close and lifelong follow-up. Only a few centers in the world specialize in these procedures.

10.13 Conclusion

SJS/TEN is a severe multisystem, immune-mediated mucocutaneous disease commonly involving the ocular surface that has the potential to result in corneal blindness. Early ophthalmology consultation and aggressive acute management is necessary to mitigate chronic disease. Even with aggressive acute management, chronic disease does still occur. Management strategies to improve vision and visual rehabilitation progressively become more invasive and complex with increased duration and severity of disease, but therapies to improve vision and visual quality of life do exist.

10.14 Future Directions

In both OCBs and SJS/TEN, the future lies in the prevention of disease. In the case of OCBs, large public health campaigns, particularly in areas with high incidence of OCBs, must be undertaken to alert the general public to the dangers of specific chemical substances and the necessity of protective eyewear. In certain parts of the developing world, where children are exposed to common household goods that can cause severe chemical injury, public health campaigns must occur at the community level. SJS/TEN is far less common than OCBs and has a genetic basis. Personalized medicine based on the detection of drug-specific genetic susceptibility will decrease exposure to culprit drugs in at-risk individuals and populations.

References

1. Wagoner MD. Chemical injuries of the eye: current concepts in pathophysiology and therapy. Surv Ophthalmol. 1997;41(4):275–313.
2. Eslani M, Baradaran-Rafii A, Movahedan A, Djalilian AR. The ocular surface chemical burns. J Ophthalmol. 2014;2014:196827.

3. White ML, Chodosh J, Jang J, Dohlman C. Incidence of Stevens-Johnson syndrome and chemical burns to the eye. Cornea. 2015;34(12):1527–33.
4. Kuckelkorn R, Makropoulos W, Kottek A, Reim M. Retrospective study of severe alkali burns of the eyes. Klin Monatsbl Augenheilkd. 1993;203(6):397–402.
5. Hong J, Qiu T, Wei A, Sun X, Xu J. Clinical characteristics and visual outcome of severe ocular chemical injuries in Shanghai. Ophthalmology. 2010;117(12):2268–72.
6. Ahmmed AA, Ting DSJ, Figueiredo FC. Epidemiology, economic and humanistic burdens of ocular surface chemical injury: a narrative review. Ocul Surf. 2021;20:199–211.
7. Hughes WF Jr. Alkali burns of the eye; clinical and pathologic course. Arch Ophthalmol. 1946;36:189–214.
8. Friedenwald JS, Hughes WF Jr, Herrmann H. Acid burns of the eye. Arch Ophthalmol. 1946;35:98–108.
9. Vazirani J, Nair D, Shanbhag S, Wurity S, Ranjan A, Sangwan V. Limbal stem cell deficiency-demography and underlying causes. Am J Ophthalmol. 2018;188:99–103.
10. Roper-Hall MJ. Thermal and chemical burns. Trans Ophthalmol Soc U K. 1965;85:631–53.
11. Dua HS, King AJ, Joseph A. A new classification of ocular surface burns. Br J Ophthalmol. 2001;85(11):1379–83.
12. Kam KW, Patel CN, Nikpoor N, Yu M, Basu S. Limbal ischemia: reliability of clinical assessment and implications in the management of ocular burns. Indian J Ophthalmol. 2019;67(1):32–6.
13. McCulley JP. Chemical injuries. In: Smolin GTR, editor. The cornea: scientific foundation and clinical practice. Boston: Little, Brown; 1987.
14. Rodrigues Z. Irrigation of the eye after alkaline and acidic burns. Emerg Nurse. 2009;17(8):26–9.
15. Baradaran-Rafii A, Eslani M, Haq Z, Shirzadeh E, Huvard MJ, Djalilian AR. Current and upcoming therapies for ocular surface chemical injuries. Ocul Surf. 2017;15(1):48–64.
16. Davis AR, Ali QK, Aclimandos WA, Hunter PA. Topical steroid use in the treatment of ocular alkali burns. Br J Ophthalmol. 1997;81(9):732–4.
17. Reim M, Bahrke C, Kuckelkorn R, Kuwert T. Investigation of enzyme activities in severe burns of the anterior eye segment. Graefes Arch Clin Exp Ophthalmol. 1993;231(5):308–12.
18. Gabler WL, Creamer HR. Suppression of human neutrophil functions by tetracyclines. J Periodontal Res. 1991;26(1):52–8.
19. Pfister RR, Haddox JL, Lank KM. Citrate or ascorbate/citrate treatment of established corneal ulcers in the alkali-injured rabbit eye. Invest Ophthalmol Vis Sci. 1988;29(7):1110–5.
20. Lim L, Lim EWL. Therapeutic contact lenses in the treatment of corneal and ocular surface diseases-a review. Asia-Pac J Ophthalmol (Phila). 2020;9(6):524–32.
21. Bouchard CS, John T. Amniotic membrane transplantation in the management of severe ocular surface disease: indications and outcomes. Ocul Surf. 2004;2(3):201–11.
22. Liu T, Zhai H, Xu Y, Dong Y, Sun Y, Zang X, et al. Amniotic membrane traps and induces apoptosis of inflammatory cells in ocular surface chemical burn. Mol Vis. 2012;18:2137–46.
23. Kuckelkorn R, Schrage N, Reim M. Treatment of severe eye burns by tenonplasty. Lancet. 1995;345(8950):657–8.
24. Sharma S, Kate A, Donthineni PR, Basu S, Shanbhag SS. The role of tenonplasty in the management of limbal and scleral ischemia due to acute ocular chemical burns. Indian J Ophthalmol. 2022;70(9):3203–12.
25. Kuckelkorn R, Redbrake C, Reim M. Tenonplasty: a new surgical approach for the treatment of severe eye burns. Ophthalmic Surg Lasers. 1997;28(2):105–10.
26. Poon AC, Geerling G, Dart JK, Fraenkel GE, Daniels JT. Autologous serum eyedrops for dry eyes and epithelial defects: clinical and in vitro toxicity studies. Br J Ophthalmol. 2001;85(10):1188–97.
27. Vajpayee RB, Mukerji N, Tandon R, Sharma N, Pandey RM, Biswas NR, et al. Evaluation of umbilical cord serum therapy for persistent corneal epithelial defects. Br J Ophthalmol. 2003;87(11):1312–6.
28. Lin MP, Ekşioğlu Ü, Mudumbai RC, Slabaugh MA, Chen PP. Glaucoma in patients with ocular chemical burns. Am J Ophthalmol. 2012;154(3):481–5.e1.

29. Chen X, Lei F, Zhou C, Chodosh J, Wang L, Huang Y, et al. Glaucoma after ocular surgery or trauma: the role of infiltrating monocytes and their response to cytokine inhibitors. Am J Pathol. 2020;190(10):2056–66.
30. Iyer G, Srinivasan B, Agarwal S, Tarigopula A. Outcome of Allo simple limbal epithelial transplantation (alloSLET) in the early stage of ocular chemical injury. Br J Ophthalmol. 2017;101(6):828–33.
31. Utheim TP. Limbal epithelial cell therapy: past, present, and future. Methods Mol Biol. 2013;1014:3–43.
32. Shanbhag SS, Nikpoor N, Rao Donthineni P, Singh V, Chodosh J, Basu S. Autologous limbal stem cell transplantation: a systematic review of clinical outcomes with different surgical techniques. Br J Ophthalmol. 2020;104(2):247–53.
33. Shanbhag SS, Patel CN, Goyal R, Donthineni PR, Singh V, Basu S. Simple limbal epithelial transplantation (SLET): review of indications, surgical technique, mechanism, outcomes, limitations, and impact. Indian J Ophthalmol. 2019;67(8):1265–77.
34. Vazirani J, Mariappan I, Ramamurthy S, Fatima S, Basu S, Sangwan VS. Surgical management of bilateral limbal stem cell deficiency. Ocul Surf. 2016;14(3):350–64.
35. Miri A, Al-Deiri B, Dua HS. Long-term outcomes of autolimbal and allolimbal transplants. Ophthalmology. 2010;117(6):1207–13.
36. Brown SI, Tragakis MP, Pearce DB. Corneal transplantation for severe alkali burns. Ophthalmology. 1972;76(5):1266–74.
37. Brown SI, Bloomfield SE, Pearce DB. A follow-up report on transplantation of the alkali-burned cornea. Am J Ophthalmol. 1974;77(4):538–42.
38. Sangwan VS, Matalia HP, Vemuganti GK, Ifthekar G, Fatima A, Singh S, et al. Early results of penetrating keratoplasty after cultivated limbal epithelium transplantation. Arch Ophthalmol. 2005;123(3):334–40.
39. Kunapuli A, Fernandes M. Successful outcome of simultaneous allogeneic simple limbal epithelial transplantation with therapeutic penetrating keratoplasty (PKP) for limbal stem cell deficiency and sterile keratolysis after chemical injury. Cornea. 2021;40(6):780–2.
40. Singh D, Vanathi M, Gupta C, Gupta N, Tandon R. Outcomes of deep anterior lamellar keratoplasty following autologous simple limbal epithelial transplant in pediatric unilateral severe chemical injury. Indian J Ophthalmol. 2017;65(3):217–22.
41. Shanbhag SS, Saeed HN, Paschalis EI, Chodosh J. Boston keratoprosthesis type 1 for limbal stem cell deficiency after severe chemical corneal injury: a systematic review. Ocul Surf. 2018;16(3):272–81.
42. Saeed HN, Shanbhag S, Chodosh J. The Boston keratoprosthesis. Curr Opin Ophthalmol. 2017;28(4):390–6.
43. Kohanim S, Palioura S, Saeed HN, Akpek EK, Amescua G, Basu S, et al. Stevens-Johnson syndrome/toxic epidermal necrolysis – a comprehensive review and guide to therapy. I. Systemic disease. Ocul Surf. 2016;14(1):2–19.
44. Harr T, French LE. Toxic epidermal necrolysis and Stevens-Johnson syndrome. Orphanet J Rare Dis. 2010;5:39.
45. Bastuji-Garin S, Rzany B, Stern RS, Shear NH, Naldi L, Roujeau JC. Clinical classification of cases of toxic epidermal necrolysis, Stevens-Johnson syndrome, and erythema multiforme. Arch Dermatol. 1993;129(1):92–6.
46. Roujeau JC, Kelly JP, Naldi L, Rzany B, Stern RS, Anderson T, et al. Medication use and the risk of Stevens-Johnson syndrome or toxic epidermal necrolysis. N Engl J Med. 1995;333(24):1600–7.
47. Chen P, Lin JJ, Lu CS, Ong CT, Hsieh PF, Yang CC, et al. Carbamazepine-induced toxic effects and HLA-B*1502 screening in Taiwan. N Engl J Med. 2011;364(12):1126–33.
48. Shanbhag SS, Chodosh J, Fathy C, Goverman J, Mitchell C, Saeed HN. Multidisciplinary care in Stevens-Johnson syndrome. Ther Adv Chronic Dis. 2020;11:2040622319894469.
49. Gueudry J, Roujeau JC, Binaghi M, Soubrane G, Muraine M. Risk factors for the development of ocular complications of Stevens-Johnson syndrome and toxic epidermal necrolysis. Arch Dermatol. 2009;145(2):157–62.

50. Jongkhajornpong P, Lekhanont K, Siriyotha S, Kanokrungsee S, Chuckpaiwong V. Factors contributing to long-term severe visual impairment in stevens-Johnson syndrome and toxic epidermal necrolysis. J Ophthalmol. 2017;2017:2087578.
51. Yip LW, Thong BY, Lim J, Tan AW, Wong HB, Handa S, et al. Ocular manifestations and complications of Stevens-Johnson syndrome and toxic epidermal necrolysis: an Asian series. Allergy. 2007;62(5):527–31.
52. Yang MS, Lee JY, Kim J, Kim GW, Kim BK, Kim JY, et al. Incidence of Stevens-Johnson syndrome and toxic epidermal necrolysis: a nationwide population-based study using national health insurance database in Korea. PLoS One. 2016;11(11):e0165933.
53. Ueta M, Kinoshita S. Ocular surface inflammation is regulated by innate immunity. Prog Retin Eye Res. 2012;31(6):551–75.
54. Chung WH, Hung SI, Yang JY, Su SC, Huang SP, Wei CY, et al. Granulysin is a key mediator for disseminated keratinocyte death in Stevens-Johnson syndrome and toxic epidermal necrolysis. Nat Med. 2008;14(12):1343–50.
55. Pavlos R, Mallal S, Phillips E. HLA and pharmacogenetics of drug hypersensitivity. Pharmacogenomics. 2012;13(11):1285–306.
56. Chung WH, Hung SI, Hong HS, Hsih MS, Yang LC, Ho HC, et al. Medical genetics: a marker for Stevens-Johnson syndrome. Nature. 2004;428(6982):486.
57. Tassaneeyakul W, Tiamkao S, Jantararoungtong T, Chen P, Lin SY, Chen WH, et al. Association between HLA-B*1502 and carbamazepine-induced severe cutaneous adverse drug reactions in a Thai population. Epilepsia. 2010;51(5):926–30.
58. Chang CC, Too CL, Murad S, Hussein SH. Association of HLA-B*1502 allele with carbamazepine-induced toxic epidermal necrolysis and Stevens-Johnson syndrome in the multi-ethnic Malaysian population. Int J Dermatol. 2011;50(2):221–4.
59. Hung SI, Chung WH, Liou LB, Chu CC, Lin M, Huang HP, et al. HLA-B*5801 allele as a genetic marker for severe cutaneous adverse reactions caused by allopurinol. Proc Natl Acad Sci USA. 2005;102(11):4134–9.
60. Ueta M, Sotozono C, Inatomi T, Kojima K, Tashiro K, Hamuro J, et al. Toll-like receptor 3 gene polymorphisms in Japanese patients with Stevens-Johnson syndrome. Br J Ophthalmol. 2007;91(7):962–5.
61. Ueta M, Sotozono C, Yokoi N, Inatomi T, Kinoshita S. Prostaglandin E receptor subtype EP3 expression in human conjunctival epithelium and its changes in various ocular surface disorders. PLoS One. 2011;6(9):e25209.
62. Shanbhag SS, Hall L, Chodosh J, Saeed HN. Long-term outcomes of amniotic membrane treatment in acute Stevens-Johnson syndrome/toxic epidermal necrolysis. Ocul Surf. 2020;18(3):517–22.
63. Jain R, Sharma N, Basu S, Iyer G, Ueta M, Sotozono C, et al. Stevens-Johnson syndrome: the role of an ophthalmologist. Surv Ophthalmol. 2016;61(4):369–99.
64. Singh S, Jakati S, Shanbhag SS, Elhusseiny AM, Djalilian AR, Basu S. Lid margin keratinization in Stevens-Johnson syndrome: review of pathophysiology and histopathology. Ocul Surf. 2021;
65. Singh S, Narang P, Mittal V. Labial mucosa grafting for lid margin, anterior lamellar, and posterior lamellar correction in recurrent cicatricial entropion. Orbit. 2021;40(4):301–5.
66. Singh S, Mishra DK, Shanbhag S, Vemuganti G, Singh V, Ali MJ, et al. Lacrimal gland involvement in severe dry eyes after Stevens-Johnson syndrome. Ophthalmology. 2021;128(4):621–4.
67. Basu S, Shanbhag SS, Gokani A, Kedar R, Bahuguna C, Sangwan VS. Chronic ocular sequelae of Stevens-Johnson syndrome in children: long-term impact of appropriate therapy on natural history of disease. Am J Ophthalmol. 2018;189:17–28.
68. Shanbhag SS, Shah S, Singh M, Bahuguna C, Donthineni PR, Basu S. Lid-related keratopathy in Stevens-Johnson syndrome: natural course and impact of therapeutic interventions in children and adults. Am J Ophthalmol. 2020;219:357–65.
69. Sotozono C, Ang LP, Koizumi N, Higashihara H, Ueta M, Inatomi T, et al. New grading system for the evaluation of chronic ocular manifestations in patients with Stevens-Johnson syndrome. Ophthalmology. 2007;114(7):1294–302.

70. Seminario-Vidal L, Kroshinsky D, Malachowski SJ, Sun J, Markova A, Beachkofsky TM, et al. Society of dermatology hospitalists supportive care guidelines for the management of Stevens-Johnson syndrome/toxic epidermal necrolysis in adults. J Am Acad Dermatol. 2020;82(6):1553–67.
71. Shanbhag SS, Chanda S, Donthineni PR, Sane SS, Priyadarshini SR, Basu S. Clinical clues predictive of Stevens-Johnson syndrome as the cause of chronic cicatrising conjunctivitis. Br J Ophthalmol. 2020;104(7):1005–9.
72. Shanbhag SS, Rashad R, Chodosh J, Saeed HN. Long-term effect of a treatment protocol for acute ocular involvement in Stevens-Johnson syndrome/toxic epidermal necrolysis. Am J Ophthalmol. 2019;208:331–41.
73. Shammas MC, Lai EC, Sarkar JS, Yang J, Starr CE, Sippel KC. Management of acute Stevens-Johnson syndrome and toxic epidermal necrolysis utilizing amniotic membrane and topical corticosteroids. Am J Ophthalmol. 2010;149(2):203–13.e2
74. Sotozono C, Ueta M, Koizumi N, Inatomi T, Shirakata Y, Ikezawa Z, et al. Diagnosis and treatment of Stevens-Johnson syndrome and toxic epidermal necrolysis with ocular complications. Ophthalmology. 2009;116(4):685–90.
75. Shanbhag SS, Chodosh J, Saeed HN. Sutureless amniotic membrane transplantation with cyanoacrylate glue for acute Stevens-Johnson syndrome/toxic epidermal necrolysis. Ocul Surf. 2019;17(3):560–4.
76. Sotozono C, Ueta M, Nakatani E, Kitami A, Watanabe H, Sueki H, et al. Predictive factors associated with acute ocular involvement in Stevens-Johnson syndrome and toxic epidermal necrolysis. Am J Ophthalmol. 2015;160(2):228–37.e2.
77. Papakostas TD, Le HG, Chodosh J, Jacobs DS. Prosthetic replacement of the ocular surface ecosystem as treatment for ocular surface disease in patients with a history of Stevens-Johnson syndrome/toxic epidermal necrolysis. Ophthalmology. 2015;122(2):248–53.
78. Iyer G, Pillai VS, Srinivasan B, Guruswami S, Padmanabhan P. Mucous membrane grafting for lid margin keratinization in Stevens–Johnson syndrome: results. Cornea. 2010;29(2):146–51.
79. Shanbhag SS, Singh S, Koshy PG, Donthineni PR, Basu S. A beginner's guide to mucous membrane grafting for lid margin keratinization: review of indications, surgical technique and clinical outcomes. Indian J Ophthalmol. 2021;69(4):794–805.
80. Vazirani J, Bhalekar S, Amescua G, Singh S, Basu S. Minor salivary gland transplantation for severe dry eye disease due to cicatrising conjunctivitis: multicentre long-term outcomes of a modified technique. Br J Ophthalmol. 2020;
81. Shimazaki J, Satake Y, Higa K, Yamaguchi T, Noma H, Tsubota K. Long-term outcomes of cultivated cell sheet transplantation for treating total limbal stem cell deficiency. Ocul Surf. 2020;18(4):663–71.
82. Basu S, Nagpal R, Serna-Ojeda JC, Bhalekar S, Bagga B, Sangwan V. LVP keratoprosthesis: anatomical and functional outcomes in bilateral end-stage corneal blindness. Br J Ophthalmol. 2018;
83. Iyer G, Pillai VS, Srinivasan B, Falcinelli G, Padmanabhan P, Guruswami S, et al. Modified osteo-odonto keratoprosthesis–the Indian experience–results of the first 50 cases. Cornea. 2010;29(7):771–6.
84. Sharma S, Donthineni PR, Iyer G, Chodosh J, de la Paz MF, Maskati Q, et al. Keratoprosthesis in dry eye disease. Indian J Ophthalmol. 2023;71(4):1154–66.

Keratoconus

11

Mohammadali Ashraf, Yamiko J. Chanza, Kanika Agarwal, Abdelrahman M. Elhusseiny, and Hajirah N. Saeed

Key Points

- Keratoconus is a progressive disease of the cornea that can lead to irregular astigmatism and decreased visual acuity.
- Until recently, management options included strategies for visual rehabilitation including glasses, contact lenses, intracorneal ring segments, and corneal transplantation, none of which prevent further progression of disease.
- The advent of corneal collagen cross-linking (CXL) has allowed for a treatment modality that prevents disease progression. The epithelium-off Dresden protocol for CXL is considered the current gold standard.
- Investigations into other or supplementary treatments for KCN include developing effective epithelium-on CXL techniques, Bowman's layer transplantation, noninvasive modalities such as eye drops to strengthen the cornea, and gene therapy.

The authors Mohammadali Ashraf and Yamiko J. Chanza have contributed equally to this chapter.

M. Ashraf
Department of Ophthalmology and Visual Sciences, Illinois Eye and Ear Infirmary, University of Illinois Chicago, Chicago, IL, USA
e-mail: mashra7@uic.edu

Y. J. Chanza
Department of Ophthalmology, Massachusetts Eye and Ear Infirmary, Harvard Medical School, Boston, MA, USA

Loma Linda University School of Medicine, Loma Linda, CA, USA
e-mail: ychanza@students.llu.edu

K. Agarwal
Department of Ophthalmology, Massachusetts Eye and Ear Infirmary, Harvard Medical School, Boston, MA, USA
e-mail: Kanika_agarwal@meei.harvard.edu

H. N. Saeed, R. B. Singh (eds.), *Corneal Disorders*, Current Practices in Ophthalmology, https://doi.org/10.1007/978-981-96-5294-5_11

11.1 Introduction

Keratoconus (KCN) is a corneal disorder characterized by progressive corneal stromal thinning and steepening and can lead to irregular astigmatism and decreased visual acuity [1]. KCN usually manifests in the second to fourth decade of life and has an incidence as high as 4% in some Middle Eastern cohorts [2, 3]. It may begin unilaterally but is bilateral in 96% of cases and often asymmetric in severity and progression between the two eyes [1]. While the exact pathogenesis of KCN is unknown, genetics is thought to play a role in 20% of patients based on positive family history [3, 4]. Down syndrome, eye rubbing, and atopic disease are also associated with the development of KCN [1, 4].

The management of KCN has drastically changed since the advent of corneal collagen cross-linking (CXL), providing patients with a treatment strategy that can prevent disease progression. Still, additional interventions are often needed for visual rehabilitation, including contact lenses, intrastromal corneal ring segments, and corneal transplantation. This chapter briefly reviews the clinical signs of KCN, details management options, and then discusses current and future investigations into novel treatments for KCN.

11.2 Diagnosis

Early diagnosis is difficult in mild cases of KCN as the slit-lamp examination and visual acuity are often normal. Early symptoms may include fluctuating vision, seeing lights or halos around objects, photophobia, eye strain, and decreased uncorrected visual acuity [1]. Once signs of KCN are seen on slit-lamp examination, the patient is likely symptomatic. These signs include:

- Thinning of the corneal stroma
- Iron deposition in the basal epithelium, known as Fleischer's ring
- Vertical lines in the posterior stroma at the apex of the cone, known as Vogt's striae

A. M. Elhusseiny
Department of Ophthalmology, Boston Children's Hospital, Harvard Medical School, Boston, MA, USA

Department of Ophthalmology, Harvey and Bernice Jones Eye Institute, University of Arkansas for Medical Sciences, Little Rock, AR, USA
e-mail: Amelhusseiny@uams.edu

H. N. Saeed (✉)
Department of Ophthalmology and Visual Sciences, Illinois Eye and Ear Infirmary, University of Illinois Chicago, Chicago, IL, USA

Department of Ophthalmology, Massachusetts Eye and Ear Infirmary, Harvard Medical School, Boston, MA, USA

Department of Ophthalmology, Loyola University Medical Center, Maywood, IL, USA
e-mail: hnsaeed@uic.edu

- Protrusion of the ectatic cornea pushing the lower lid out in a V-shape in downgaze, known as Munson's sign
- Breaks in Descemet's membrane and Bowman's layer

The Global Consensus on Keratoconus and Ectatic Disease established the following criteria for diagnosing keratoconus: posterior corneal elevation abnormalities, abnormal distribution of corneal thickness, and noninflammatory corneal thinning. There are many devices available for topographic and tomographic analyses of these parameters [5].

Historically, imaging for KCN was done using Placido disk technology, keratometry, photokeratoscopy, and computer-assisted videokeratoscopy. Imaging systems have since evolved from Placido disk to slit scanning and Scheimpflug imaging devices [6].

Elevation-based topography (tomography) systems are currently the most widely used systems in the diagnosis of KCN. Some devices also include software such as the Belin-Ambrosio Enhanced Ectasia Display and the ABCD keratoconus grading system on the Pentacam (Oculus Optikgeräte GmbH, Wetzlar, Germany) to diagnose keratoconus based on various corneal indices.

More recently, swept-source/Fourier domain OCT devices have been used to diagnose KCN, though it is not in common practice, and further validation of results needs to be performed [5].

Topographic and tomographic images in manifest KCN will reveal increased corneal curvature in the form of asymmetric bow-tie astigmatism or a cone with inferior steepening and associated inferior corneal thinning. The overall corneal power and inferior-superior (I-S) index are increased due to inferior steepening. Posterior corneal surface elevation is also a very sensitive marker for KCN [1].

While most corneal thinning is seen in the central cornea and the inferotemporal quadrant, atypical cases of "superior keratoconus" can also occur, where topographic and tomographic signs of corneal steepening and thinning occur in the superior cornea [7, 8].

11.3 Management

Depending on the degree and nature of corneal pathology, various treatment strategies may be employed to halt or reduce the progression of KCN and/or improve visual acuity.

11.3.1 Corneal Collagen Cross-linking (CXL)

The only treatment known to halt the progression of KCN is CXL. CXL involves applying riboflavin and ultraviolet A (UVA, 370 nm) light onto the cornea to create oxygen-free radicals, activating the physiologic lysyl oxidase pathway [9]. After exposure to UVA, the excited riboflavin molecules can produce either free radicals or singlet oxygen molecules, inducing covalent bonds, and cross-linking and strengthening the collagen in the cornea [10]. Riboflavin also acts as a masking agent to protect other ocular structures such as the corneal endothelium, lens, and retina from UVA radiation. A dose response in relation to UVA irradiation intensity is thought to be linked to increased resistance of stromal tissue to enzymatic digestion by matrix metalloproteinases [9].

UVA is cytotoxic and mutagenic, causing keratocyte apoptosis and corneal endothelial cell damage at high doses. Cell culture studies with endothelial cells have shown a cytotoxicity at UVA irradiation levels greater than 0.35 mW/cm^2. However, the standard parameters that are used in the United States (UVA dosage of 3 mW/cm^2 for 30 min in the setting of corneal thickness greater than 400 μm) result in endothelium irradiation of less than 0.18 mW/cm^2, half of the cytotoxic level. This is clinically relevant as the anterior 400 μm of the cornea absorb more than 85% of the UVA before it reaches the endothelium. For this reason, CXL is only approved for use in corneas with a thickness of greater than 400 μm, making early diagnosis and treatment a critical window of opportunity [9, 11].

11.3.2 Epithelium-Off CXL

The most commonly performed CXL technique is that of the epithelium-off Dresden protocol [10]. In this technique, the central 7–9 mm of the corneal epithelium is removed to ensure adequate riboflavin penetration into the corneal stroma. Prior to epithelium removal, the corneal thickness should be greater than 450 μm (400 μm after de-epithelialization) [9]. Riboflavin dosage and diffusion time vary after epithelium removal, but, in general, riboflavin 0.1% 5-phosphate in 20% dextran is applied every 2–5 min for 30 min onto the cornea [10]. The cornea is then irradiated with UVA at 3 mW/cm^2 for 30 min, during which the riboflavin is applied to the stromal surface every 2–5 min [9]. If the corneal pachymetry is below 400 μm prior to UVA irradiation, hypotonic riboflavin drops can be applied to swell the cornea. Afterward, a bandage contact lens is applied onto the eye. The patient is treated with topical corticosteroids and antibiotics postoperatively. The epithelium-off CXL technique is now considered the gold standard in halting the progression of keratoconus. In the United States, the Glaukos epi-off iLink technique using the KXL system (Glaukos Corporation, Aliso Viejo, CA) is the only FDA-approved CXL technique. This technique follows the Dresden protocol but applies riboflavin to the cornea at 2-minute intervals [12]. While riboflavin suspension in 20% dextran is approved in the United States and used in many protocols internationally, new isotonic formulations containing hydroxypropyl methylcellulose (HPMC) have been studied to avoid stromal dehydration and corneal thinning [9, 13].

11.3.2.1 Modified CXL Techniques

Modified CXL techniques have been proposed to shorten procedure duration, reduce the amount of post-procedure pain, accelerate recovery, and optimize visual outcomes.

Epithelium-On CXL

The standard epithelium-off CXL procedure almost universally causes acute postoperative pain and also carries a risk for postoperative infection. Transepithelial or epithelium-on CXL avoids these complications and has been shown to increase corneal rigidity, but to a lesser extent—one third to one fifth the amount seen in epithelium-off CXL due to decreased riboflavin penetration [10]. Treatment depth is also reduced in epithelium-on CXL [10]. Adjunctive methods have been studied to increase riboflavin penetration through intact epithelium, such as using benzalkonium chloride (BAC), ethylenediaminetetraacetic acid (EDTA), and tris-hydroxymethyl aminomethane (trometamol) to weaken epithelial tight junctions and thus increase penetration. These results have been promising, but the efficacy of epithelium-on CXL largely does not appear to be equal to that of epithelium-off CXL, though the risk of infection is nearly eliminated [14].

Iontophoresis, phonophoresis (ultrasound-assisted drug penetration), and biocompatible riboflavin-based nano emulsion systems are currently being investigated to increase transepithelial penetration of riboflavin, along with the use of hypo-osmolar riboflavin with 0.44% sodium chloride [10].

11.3.3 Accelerated CXL

Accelerated CXL (A-CXL) is currently being investigated to shorten procedure duration by increasing the UVA light intensity. However, increasing the irradiation levels leads to an increased risk of endothelial cell toxicity. Several studies have shown promising results with no long-term endothelial cell damage using UVA irradiation levels ranging from 7 mW/cm^2 to 18 mW/cm^2 with treatment times ranging from 5 to 15 min [10]. Levels greater than 50 mW/cm^2 did not demonstrate greater rigidity of the cornea compared to lower irradiation levels [10]. There are conflicting results from different A-CXL studies; however, A-CXL with an irradiation dose of 10 mW/cm^2 for 9 min has shown better outcomes compared to other A-CXL protocols [15].

11.3.4 CXL for Thin Corneas

Conventional CXL is limited to eyes with a corneal thickness greater than 400 μm, but there are several techniques in use for thin corneas such as using hypo-osmolar riboflavin to swell the cornea [10], a riboflavin-soaked contact lens [14], and leaving epithelial cells in "islands" above the thinnest points [16]. The clinician should also take into account the severity of the KCN and balance potential damage to the endothelium during CXL with the likelihood of penetrating keratoplasty (PKP) as the latter will make preservation of the endothelium less relevant.

Another technique employed for thin corneas includes contact lens-assisted CXL using a non-UVA-filtering riboflavin-soaked bandage contact lens that is applied to the cornea during UVA irradiation. It has the advantage of bypassing the need to

induce corneal swelling during the procedure in contrast to the hypo-osmolar riboflavin technique [17].
Modified techniques may also be employed in vulnerable populations where CXL may need to be performed under general anesthesia and/or for both eyes of the same patient at the same time. These populations include children and patients with Down syndrome or other developmental disorders who may not be able to tolerate an in-clinic procedure [16].

11.3.5 CXL Combined with Other Modalities

Combining CXL with other modalities can allow for reduced pain, enhanced efficacy, and optimized visual outcomes. Excimer laser can be used as an alternative to mechanical debridement to remove epithelium with less severe postoperative discomfort [18]. Another technique, called pocket CXL, involves creating an intrastromal pocket with a femtosecond laser for riboflavin induction [19].
Photorefractive keratectomy (PRK) or topography-guided PRK (TG-PRK) and CXL can be performed together to achieve superior refractive and topographic outcomes in irregular astigmatism while halting disease progression (Athens protocol) [20]. CXL and PRK can be performed simultaneously or sequentially, each with their advantages and disadvantages [21]. Intracorneal ring segments (ICRS) can be inserted in conjunction with CXL to flatten the cornea and enhance visual acuity [22]. ICRS is explained further in this chapter as a distinct procedure for keratoconus. Another recent approach is mini asymmetric radial keratotomy (MARK) followed by CXL (Rome protocol) to improve visual acuity while halting the progression of keratoconus. This technique offers the advantage of avoiding corneal thinning compared (as compared to the Athens protocol) while still improving visual acuity [23].

11.3.5.1 Complications and Postoperative Course

Patients may experience 24–72 h of severe ocular pain and several weeks of blurred vision following epithelium-off CXL. The pain and visual recovery time is lower in epithelium-on CXL. During the first 3 months after CXL, keratocytes repopulate the anterior and mid-stroma and increased density of the extracellular matrix occurs at 300–350 μm depth, forming the demarcation line seen on slit lamp examination [9]. Anterior stromal haze is seen during the first year after surgery and is thought to represent a physiologic wound-healing response [9]. Most post-CXL haze resolves over time due to repopulation of keratocytes and resolution of corneal edema. Figure 11.1 shows a case of post-CXL haze.

CXL has been proven safe and effective in studies with up to 15 years of follow-up [24]. However, complications can occur. Some patients may develop deterioration of visual acuity several months postoperatively due to late-onset persistent haze. This nonself-limiting haze can be treated with intensive topical steroid, which has been reported to be effective to some degree [25, 26]. Corneal scarring is another

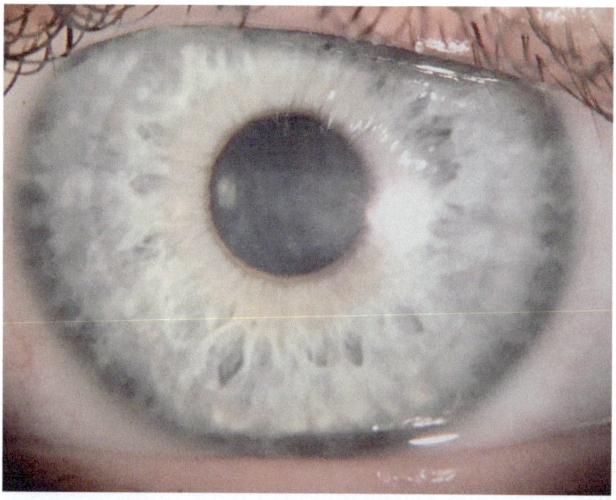

Fig. 11.1 Slit-lamp image demonstrating central corneal haze after corneal collagen cross-linking

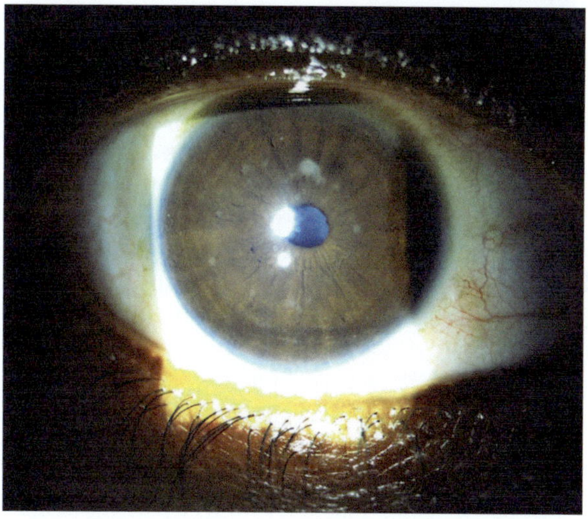

Fig. 11.2 Slit-lamp image demonstrating sterile corneal infiltrates of the central and mid-peripheral cornea

complication that can occur over the apex of the cone, particularly in extremely steep corneas (greater than 72 D) and thinner corneas [9]. However, scarring can occur even in mild KCN cases and in cases where photorefractive keratectomy (PRK) is followed by CXL [27, 28].

Sterile infiltrates can also occur in the first few weeks after CXL (Fig. 11.2) and tend to resolve within a month with topical steroids [29]. While sterile infiltrates are a common and minor complication, noninfectious keratitis and corneal melt are very rare, but serious complications can occur and may necessitate corneal transplantation [30, 31]. Infectious keratitis is rare and mostly occurs with the epithelium-off technique when the corneal stroma is at risk for bacterial infection [9]. While the incidence of infectious keratitis is low, it can be vision-threatening and is likely underreported. Patients should be counseled on the symptoms of infectious keratitis so they can seek expedient medical care.

Endothelial failure can occur, even in patients with pachymetry greater than 400 μm, and is thought to be due to stromal thinning associated with the use of hyper- and iso-osmolar riboflavin solutions or lack of uniform UVA delivery [9].

Lastly, failure to halt the progression of KCN occurs in a small percentage of patients after CXL, more often in cases of epithelium-on and accelerated epithelium-off techniques [32]. However, CXL can be repeated as long as the corneal thickness is sufficient [33].

11.3.5.2 Insurance Considerations

While CXL can halt the progression of KCN, it is not always covered by insurance in the United States. As such, patients who would have otherwise benefited from CXL often progress to needing corneal transplantation. The senior author (HNS) has found that conducting peer-to-peer discussions with the insurance company often results in approval for the procedure, even in cases of public aid insurance. However, it should be noted that only epithelium-off CXL, as approved by the FDA, is a covered procedure by insurance companies.

11.4 Intracorneal Ring Segments

Intracorneal ring segments (ICRS) can be used in patients with mild to moderate keratoconus to reduce astigmatism and delay or eliminate the need for keratoplasty. Patients should have a clear optical zone and be contact lens intolerant. Several different types of synthetic ICRS are available. The primary difference between them is the optical zone size. The primary ICRS used in the United States is INTACS (KeraVision Inc., Fremont, CA). INTACS consists of arc-like polymethyl methacrylate segments and has an optical zone of 7 mm. It is available in multiple thicknesses, which modulate the refractive effect of the segments [34].

When evaluating candidacy for INTACS, the steepest corneal reading should not exceed 58D and pachymetry should be greater than 450 μm at the 7 mm optical zone and/or the area of INTACS placement [35]. Poor candidates include patients with scarring in the visual axis, pachymetry less than 450 μm, and unstable progressive keratoconus [35].

The segments are placed in the relevant optical zone, at approximately two thirds depth. INTACS on average achieves 2–3 diopters of flattening by reshaping the central anterior cornea [35]. In centrally located cones, two symmetrical INTACS are used to achieve maximal flattening effect. In oval type cones with greater curvature inferiorly, two different thicknesses may be used, with the thicker segment placed inferiorly. In patients with a relatively small cone that does not cross the horizontal meridian, a single INTACS can be placed inferiorly (Fig. 11.3) [35, 36].

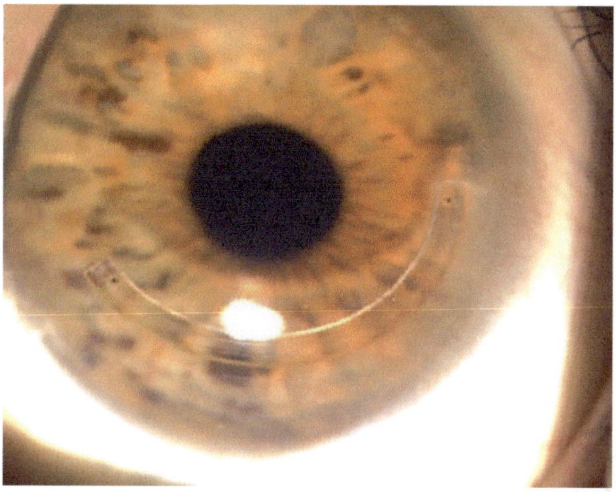

Fig. 11.3 Slit-lamp image demonstrating an inferiorly placed single INTACS intracorneal ring segment

Complications can occur from INTACS placement and include perforation of the segment into the anterior chamber, rotation or migration of the segment, infection, and erosion of the segment through the corneal stroma and extrusion through the epithelium with superficial placement [35]. Management usually consists of treatment with topical antibiotics in case of infection, explantation of the segment in case of erosion and extrusion or persistent infection, and suture fixation of the segment to the cornea in cases of segment migration [37].

Another ICRS that uses allogenic segments from donor cornea instead of synthetic material is called corneal allogenic intrastromal ring segments (CAIRS) [38]. In CAIRS, the allogenic segment is less rigid and more compatible for use in corneas with thickness less than 400 µm. The allogenic nature of CAIRS may offer better biocompatibility, reduced risk of extrusion and stromal necrosis, and lower rates of infection or inflammation compared to synthetic rings. Additionally, CAIRS can be tailored in terms of arc length, thickness, and placement, offering surgical flexibility for customized treatments. Early studies suggest favorable outcomes in visual acuity, corneal shape, and safety, although long-term comparative data are still emerging [39, 40].

11.5 Bowman's Layer Transplantation

Bowman's layer is an elastic acellular layer beneath the epithelial basement membrane of the cornea. It is hypothesized that Bowman's layer supports corneal structure and that disruption of this layer can cause weakening and steepening of the cornea, as seen in keratoconus. With these assumptions, Bowman's layer transplantation may be an option for reinforcement of the cornea.

The grafts in this technique can be harvested from donor corneal tissues as described by Groeneveld-van Beek, et al. [41] The advantage of preparing and using Bowman's layer is that it can be prepared from discarded donor tissue, tissue with poor endothelial quality, or from the remaining tissue after use in endothelial keratoplasty, increasing the efficiency of using donor cornea tissue grafts. There are two techniques for Bowman's layer transplantation: Bowman's layer inlay grafting and Bowman's layer onlay grafting. The difference between these techniques lies in where the Bowman layer tissue is transplanted. In the onlay method, the Bowman's layer graft is implanted subepithelially on the corneal surface instead of at the mid-stroma level as in the inlay technique. The onlay technique has the advantage of easier surgical technique, particularly in advanced keratoconus cases. Further studies are needed to evaluate the efficacy of either form of Bowman's layer transplantation [40].

11.6 Contact Lenses

Contact lenses are often needed for visual rehabilitation in patients with KCN. While soft contact lenses are typically used in forme-fruste or mild cases of KCN, specialty lenses for more advanced KCN have also been developed over the years with great success in fit, optical quality, tolerance, and patient satisfaction. Rigid lenses, which used to be the mainstay of treatment for KCN patients, can be classified into corneal, corneo-scleral, mini-scleral, and scleral lenses based on lens diameter and vault over the cornea [42]. A piggyback option, where a soft lens is worn under a rigid lens, also exists for highly irregular corneas. Hybrid lenses, which consist of a rigid center and a peripheral soft skirt, may be good options for patients with fitting difficulties or intolerance to rigid lenses [42].

It should be noted that contact lens wear is difficult in patients with developmental delay. As Down syndrome is strongly associated with KCN, clinicians should keep visual rehabilitation in mind when considering CXL, as early treatment with CXL may reduce the need for contact lenses and stabilize uncorrected visual acuity [43].

11.7 Corneal Transplantation

Patients who become contact lens intolerant, have severe corneal irregular astigmatism, and/or have stromal opacities or scars may require corneal transplantation for visual rehabilitation. PKP is most commonly done in these cases [44]. Graft rejection ranges from 7.8% to 31% [44]. A few studies have shown the recurrence of KCN 15–20 years after transplantation [44]. Deep anterior lamellar keratoplasty (DALK) may decrease some complications seen during and after PKP by preserving host endothelium. DALK has a reduced risk of rejection and fewer intraoperative complications such as wound dehiscence, expulsive hemorrhage, and endophthalmitis [44, 45]. However, the technique is more difficult to perform and may need to be converted to a PKP [44]. There is also the risk of poor visual outcome due to interface haze [45].

It should be noted that even after corneal transplantation, correction with contact lenses is often required for best corrected visual acuity. Hence, corneal transplantation is most useful in cases where contact lenses can be worn/tolerated postoperatively.

11.8 Future Directions

The near future of keratoconus management consists of changes in CXL technique, particularly with accelerated epithelium-on CXL. Other newer methods of improving visual acuity in KCN while halting progression include a three-step treatment consisting of ICRS, CXL, and a third step of either topography-guided transepithelial PRK or implantation of a toric posterior chamber phakic IOL [46, 47]. Studies on long-term outcomes with these treatments are necessary. Investigations into new forms of topical medications to strengthen the corneal stroma and address KCN through a less invasive approach are also underway [48]. Lastly, genetic screening and improved machine learning modalities may be able to identify individuals at risk for developing KCN and therefore aid in instituting early treatment [49].

References

1. Najmi H, Mobarki Y, Mania K, et al. The correlation between keratoconus and eye rubbing: a review. Int J Ophthalmol. 2019;12(11):1775–81. https://doi.org/10.18240/ijo.2019.11.17.
2. Gomes JAP, Rodrigues PF, Lamazales LL. Keratoconus epidemiology: a review. Saudi J Ophthalmol. 2022;36(1):3–6. https://doi.org/10.4103/sjopt.sjopt_204_21.
3. Godefrooij DA, de Wit GA, Uiterwaal CS, Imhof SM, Wisse RPL. Age-specific incidence and prevalence of keratoconus: a nationwide registration study. Am J Ophthalmol. 2017;175:169–72. https://doi.org/10.1016/j.ajo.2016.12.015.
4. Al-Amri AM. Prevalence of keratoconus in a refractive surgery population. J Ophthalmol. 2018;2018:1–5. https://doi.org/10.1155/2018/5983530.
5. Yip H, Chan E. Optical coherence tomography imaging in keratoconus. Clin Exp Optom. 2019;102(3):218–23. https://doi.org/10.1111/cxo.12874.
6. Matalia H, Swarup R. Imaging modalities in keratoconus. Indian J Ophthalmol. 2013;61(8):394–400. https://doi.org/10.4103/0301-4738.116058.
7. Romero-Jiménez M, Santodomingo-Rubido J, González-Méijome JM. The thinnest, steepest, and maximum elevation corneal locations in noncontact and contact lens wearers in keratoconus. Cornea. 2013 Mar;32(3):332–7. https://doi.org/10.1097/ICO.0b013e318259c98a.
8. Rogers GJ, Attenborough M. Bilateral superior keratoconus: two case reports. Eye (Lond). 2014;28(10):1254–7. https://doi.org/10.1038/eye.2014.146.
9. O'Brart DPS. Corneal collagen crosslinking for corneal ectasias: a review. Eur J Ophthalmol. 2017;27(3):253–69. https://doi.org/10.5301/ejo.5000916.
10. Sorkin N, Varssano D. Corneal collagen crosslinking: a systematic review. Ophthalmologica. 2014;232(1):10–27. https://doi.org/10.1159/000357979.
11. Spoerl E, Hoyer A, Pillunat LE, Raiskup F. Corneal cross-linking and safety issues. Open Ophthalmol J. 2011;11(5):14–6. https://doi.org/10.2174/1874364101105010014.
12. Belin MW, Lim L, Rajpal RK, Hafezi F, Gomes JAP, Cochener B. Corneal cross-linking: current USA status: report from the cornea society. Cornea. 2018;37(10):1218–25. https://doi.org/10.1097/ICO.0000000000001707.
13. Rapuano PB, Mathews PM, Florakis GJ, Trokel SL, Suh LH. Corneal collagen crosslinking in patients treated with dextran versus isotonic hydroxypropyl methylcellulose (HPMC) ribofla-

vin solution: a retrospective analysis. Eye Vis (Lond). 2018;10(5):23. https://doi.org/10.1186/s40662-018-0116-z.
14. Iqbal M, Gad A, Kotb A, Abdelhalim M. Analysis of the outcomes of three different cross-linking protocols for treatment of paediatric keratoconus: a multicentre randomized controlled trial. Acta Ophthalmol. 2024;102(1):e105–16. https://doi.org/10.1111/aos.15686. Epub 2023 May 4
15. Subasinghe SK, Ogbuehi KC, Dias GJ. Current perspectives on corneal collagen crosslinking (CXL). Graefes Arch Clin Exp Ophthalmol. 2018;256(8):1363–84. https://doi.org/10.1007/s00417-018-3966-0. Epub 2018 Apr 6
16. Fung SSM, Mason M, Gore DM, Mireskandari K, Ali A. Technique for pediatric corneal crosslinking under general anesthesia. J AAPOS. 2020;24(3):162–4. https://doi.org/10.1016/j.jaapos.2020.01.015.
17. Srivatsa S, Jacob S, Agarwal A. Contact lens assisted corneal cross linking in thin ectatic corneas – a review. Indian J Ophthalmol. 2020;68(12):2773–8. https://doi.org/10.4103/ijo.IJO_2138_20.
18. Alkayid H, Asena L, Yüce A, Yavuz Çolak M, Altınörs DD. Comparison of ocular discomfort after three different epithelial debridement techniques for corneal collagen cross-linking in keratoconus treatment. Ther Adv Ophthalmol. 2021;23(13):25158414211020147. https://doi.org/10.1177/25158414211020147.
19. Balidis M, Konidaris VE, Ioannidis G, Kanellopoulos AJ. Femtosecond-assisted intrastromal corneal cross-linking for early and moderate keratoconus. Eye (Lond). 2014;28(10):1258–60. https://doi.org/10.1038/eye.2014.155.
20. Kanellopoulos AJ. Ten-year outcomes of progressive keratoconus management with the Athens protocol (topography-guided partial-refraction PRK combined with CXL). J Refract Surg. 2019;35(8):478–83. https://doi.org/10.3928/1081597X-20190627-01.
21. Al-Mohaimeed MM. Combined corneal CXL and photorefractive keratectomy for treatment of keratoconus: a review. Int J Ophthalmol. 2019;12(12):1929–38. https://doi.org/10.18240/ijo.2019.12.16.
22. Park SE, Tseng M, Lee JK. Effectiveness of intracorneal ring segments for keratoconus. Curr Opin Ophthalmol. 2019;30(4):220–8. https://doi.org/10.1097/ICU.0000000000000582.
23. Abbondanza M, Abbondanza G, De Felice V, Wong ZSY. Long-term results of mini asymmetric radial keratotomy and corneal cross-linking for the treatment of keratoconus. Korean J Ophthalmol. 2019;33(2):189–95. https://doi.org/10.3341/kjo.2018.0028.
24. Raiskup F, Herber R, Lenk J, et al. Corneal crosslinking with riboflavin and UVA light in progressive keratoconus: fifteen-year results. Am J Ophthalmol. 2023;250:95–102. https://doi.org/10.1016/j.ajo.2023.01.022.
25. Peponis V, Kontomichos L, Chatziralli I, Kontadakis G, Parikakis E. Late onset corneal haze after corneal cross-linking for progressive keratoconus. Am J Ophthalmol Case Rep. 2019;14:64–6. https://doi.org/10.1016/j.ajoc.2019.02.008.
26. Omary R, Shehadeh-Mashor R. Late onset of persistent, deep stromal haze after corneal cross-linking in a patient with keratoconus. Can J Ophthalmol. 2017;52(2):e81–3. https://doi.org/10.1016/j.jcjo.2016.10.014.
27. Lim LS, Beuerman R, Lim L, Tan DT. Late-onset deep stromal scarring after riboflavin-UV-A corneal collagen cross-linking for mild keratoconus. Arch Ophthalmol. 2011;129(3):360–2. https://doi.org/10.1001/archophthalmol.2011.23.
28. Kymionis GD, Portaliou DM, Diakonis VF, et al. Posterior linear stromal haze formation after simultaneous photorefractive keratectomy followed by corneal collagen cross-linking. Invest Ophthalmol Vis Sci. 2010;51(10):5030–3. https://doi.org/10.1167/iovs.09-5105.
29. Çerman E, Özcan DÖ, Toker E. Sterile corneal infiltrates after corneal collagen cross-linking: evaluation of risk factors. Acta Ophthalmol. 2017;95(2):199–204. https://doi.org/10.1111/aos.13218.
30. Labiris G, Kaloghianni E, Koukoula S, Zissimopoulos A, Kozobolis VP. Corneal melting after collagen cross-linking for keratoconus: a case report. J Med Case Rep. 2011;5(1) https://doi.org/10.1186/1752-1947-5-152.

31. Chiu HH, Sade S, Chew HF. Corneal melt following collagen crosslinking and topography-guided customized ablation treatment for Keratoconus. Can J Ophthalmol. 2017;52(3):e88. https://doi.org/10.1016/j.jcjo.2016.11.007.
32. Lenk J, Herber R, Oswald C, Spoerl E, Pillunat LE, Raiskup F. Risk factors for progression of Keratoconus and failure rate after corneal cross-linking. J Refract Surg. 2021;37(12):816–23. https://doi.org/10.3928/1081597X-20210830-01.
33. Akkaya Turhan S, Aydın FO, Toker E. Clinical results of repeated corneal collagen cross-linking in progressive Keratoconus. Cornea. 2020;39(1):84–7. https://doi.org/10.1097/ICO.0000000000002128.
34. Alió JL, Shabayek MH, Artola A. Intracorneal ring segments for keratoconus correction: long-term follow-up. J Cataract Refract Surg. 2006;32(6):978–85. https://doi.org/10.1016/j.jcrs.2006.02.044.
35. Izquierdo L, Mannis MJ, Mejías Smith JA, Henriquez MA. Effectiveness of Intrastromal corneal ring implantation in the treatment of adult patients with keratoconus: a systematic review. J Refract Surg. 2019;35(3):191–200. https://doi.org/10.3928/1081597X-20190109-02.
36. Piñero DP, Alio JL. Intracorneal ring segments in ectatic corneal disease – a review. Clin Experiment Ophthalmol. 2010;38(2):154–67. https://doi.org/10.1111/j.1442-9071.2010.02197.x.
37. Barbara R, Barbara A. INTACS intracorneal ring segments complications in patients suffering from keratoconus. Int J Keratoconus Ectatic Corneal Dis. 2013;2(3):121–8. https://doi.org/10.5005/jp-journals-10025-1064.
38. Jacob S, Patel SR, Agarwal A, Ramalingam A, Saijimol AI, Raj JM. Corneal allogenic intrastromal ring segments (CAIRS) combined with corneal cross-linking for keratoconus. J Refract Surg. 2018;34(5):296–303. https://doi.org/10.3928/1081597X-20180223-01.
39. Ravishankar V, Jacob S. Corneal allogenic intrastromal ring segments C.A.I.R.S. In: Armia A, Mazzotta C, editors. Keratoconus. Cham: Springer; 2022. https://doi.org/10.1007/978-3-030-84506-3_10.
40. Dapena I, Parker JS, Melles GRJ. Potential benefits of modified corneal tissue grafts for keratoconus: Bowman layer 'inlay' and 'onlay' transplantation, and allogenic tissue ring segments. Curr Opin Ophthalmol. 2020;31(4):276–83. https://doi.org/10.1097/ICU.0000000000000665.
41. Groeneveld-van Beek EA, Parker J, Lie JT, et al. Donor tissue preparation for Bowman layer transplantation. Cornea. 2016;35(12):1499–502. https://doi.org/10.1097/ICO.0000000000000905.
42. Downie LE, Lindsay RG. Contact lens management of keratoconus. Clin Exp Optom. 2015;98(4):299–311. https://doi.org/10.1111/cxo.12300.
43. Netto MV, Cunha L. Corneal cross-linking in down syndrome patients. In: Almodin E, Nassaralla BA, Sandes J, editors. Keratoconus. Cham: Springer; 2022. https://doi.org/10.1007/978-3-030-85361-7_40.
44. Colin J, Velou S. Current surgical options for keratoconus. J Cataract Refract Surg. 2003;29(2):379–86. https://doi.org/10.1016/S0886-3350(02)01968-5.
45. Patil M, Mehta JS. Lamellar keratoplasty for advanced keratoconus. Asia-Pac J Ophthalmol. 2020;9(6):580–8. https://doi.org/10.1097/APO.0000000000000338.
46. He C, Joergensen JS, Knorz MC, McKay KN, Zhang F. Three-step treatment of keratoconus and post-LASIK ectasia: implantation of ICRS, corneal cross-linking, and implantation of Toric posterior chamber Phakic IOLs. J Refract Surg. 2020;36(2):104–9. https://doi.org/10.3928/1081597x-20191217-01.
47. Coskunseven E, Jankov MR, Grentzelos MA, Plaka AD, Limnopoulou AN, Kymionis GD. Topography-guided transepithelial PRK after intracorneal ring segments implantation and corneal collagen CXL in a three-step procedure for keratoconus. J Refract Surg. 2013;29(1):54–8. https://doi.org/10.3928/1081597x-20121217-01.
48. Molokhia S, Muddana SKK, Uehara H, Burr M, McCulloch J, Ambati BK. IVMED-80 eye drops for treatment of keratoconus. Invest Ophthalmol Vis Sci. 2018;59(9):4454.
49. Anogeianakis G. Genetics of keratoconus; how realistic is gene therapy? Acta Ophthalmol. 2022;100(S275) https://doi.org/10.1111/j.1755-3768.2022.15406.

Corneal Dystrophies 12

Patrick B. Rapuano, Zeba A. Syed, Beeran B. Meghpara, and Christopher J. Rapuano

- Corneal dystrophies are hereditary, bilateral conditions that affect the function of the cornea, typically causing pain and/or decreased vision.
- Corneal dystrophies are generally progressive disorders that can manifest themselves at birth or in adulthood.
- The diagnosis of corneal dystrophies can usually be made by a careful slit-lamp examination, although ancillary testing including corneal topography, pachymetry, anterior segment optical coherence tomography, and/or confocal microscopy may be helpful.
- Genetic testing, corneal histopathology, or electron microscopy may be necessary to make a definitive diagnosis.
- The prognosis for most corneal dystrophies is quite good. Depending on the dystrophy, treatments range from lubrication to excimer laser phototherapeutic keratectomy to corneal transplantation.

12.1 Introduction

A clear, smooth, and regular cornea is essential for optimal visual function. Corneal dystrophies include a wide variety of pathologies that affect the health of the cornea. As a rule, they are hereditary and bilateral, and for the most part, they have few systemic manifestations. Corneal dystrophies vary in prevalence and symptoms; some cause primarily ocular surface symptoms, while others present predominantly with vision loss. Corneal dystrophies may be categorized by the specific layer of the

P. B. Rapuano · Z. A. Syed · B. B. Meghpara · C. J. Rapuano (✉)
Wills Eye Hospital, Philadelphia, PA, USA
e-mail: zsyed@willseye.org; bmeghpara@willseye.org; cjrapuano@willseye.org

H. N. Saeed, R. B. Singh (eds.), *Corneal Disorders*, Current Practices in Ophthalmology, https://doi.org/10.1007/978-981-96-5294-5_12

cornea affected, and in this chapter, it will be discussed starting with the anterior corneal layers and proceeding posteriorly. We will focus on the most common corneal dystrophies except for Fuchs endothelial corneal dystrophy, which is covered elsewhere.

12.2 Epithelial Basement Membrane Dystrophy

Epithelial basement membrane dystrophy (EBMD), alternatively referred to as anterior basement membrane dystrophy, map-dot-fingerprint dystrophy, and Cogan microcystic epithelial dystrophy, is a common corneal dystrophy seen primarily in adults. While most cases have no documented inheritance and are likely degenerative, in two families, EBMD has been shown to be related to mutations in the transforming growth factor beta–induced (*TGFBI*) gene [1]. Patients are most commonly asymptomatic, although up to 10% present with recurrent corneal erosions, and a smaller percentage with painless visual distortion, shadowing of images, or monocular diplopia [2].

Slit-lamp biomicroscopy shows map-like lines, dots (microcysts), or fingerprint-like patterns in the corneal epithelium, all of which are best seen with either retroillumination or a broad slit beam. In many cases, "negative staining" from elevated areas of epithelium may be seen after the application of fluorescein dye (Figs. 12.1, 12.2 and 12.3) [3]. A much less common presentation is bleb-like changes (Fig. 12.4) [4]. Corneal topography, especially focusing on the Placido disc images, can reveal irregular astigmatism caused by subtle EBMD. In recent years, anterior segment optical coherence tomography (AS-OCT) has been used to diagnose subtle cases of symptomatic EBMD, which may not be very evident on slit-lamp biomicroscopy. AS-OCT can identify patients who may benefit from treatment who would otherwise go undiagnosed [5]. Light microscopy of pathology specimens shows excessive basement membrane material forming redundant sheets corresponding to map-like lines and intraepithelial pseudocysts containing cytoplasmic debris corresponding to dots [3]. Bowman layer is normal in this condition.

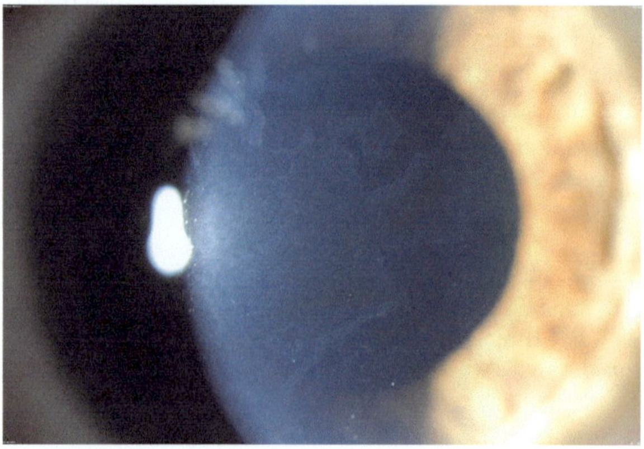

Fig. 12.1 Large patches of reduplicated epithelial basement membrane appear as gray areas ("maps") centrally in this eye with EBMD

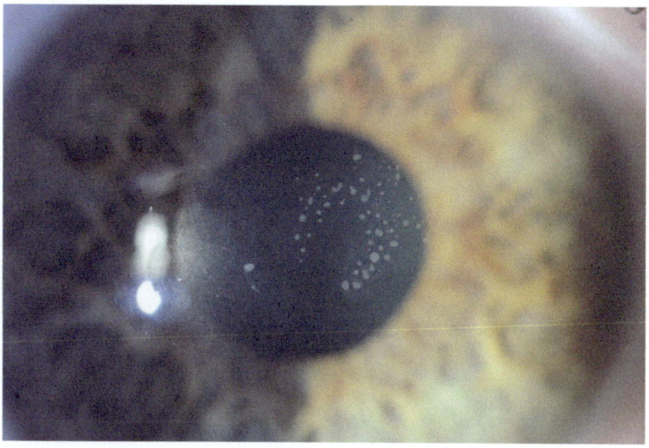

Fig. 12.2 Multiple epithelial inclusions ("dots") are present in the central cornea of this eye with visually significant EBMD

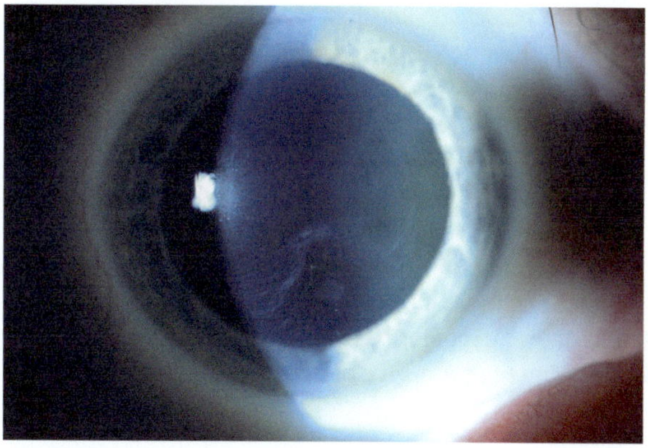

Fig. 12.3 A series of curvilinear parallel ("fingerprint") lines of EBMD are readily apparent inferiorly

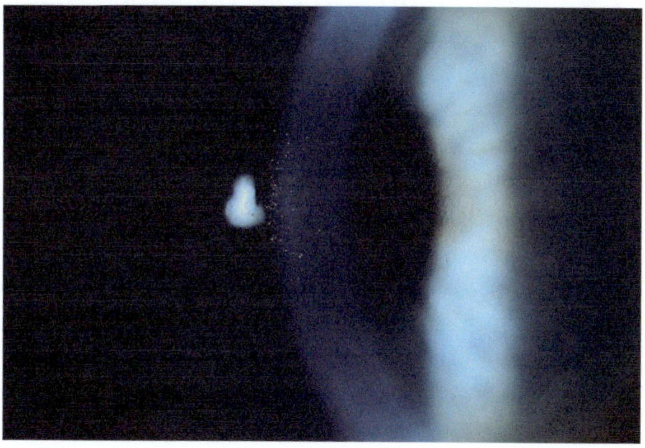

Fig. 12.4 Retroillumination off the iris demonstrates faint ovoid and globular irregularities in this eye with the rare bleb-like form of EBMD

Treatment options for EBMD include medical management or surgical removal of visually significant irregular epithelium. Painful erosions can be treated medically with lubrication, hypertonic drops and ointment, topical corticosteroids, doxycycline, or a bandage contact lens. Recurrent cases refractory to medical management can be treated with epithelial debridement with or without alcohol delamination, anterior stromal micropuncture, diamond burr polishing of Bowman membrane, or excimer laser phototherapeutic keratectomy (PTK) [6–9]. Patients with EBMD have a very good prognosis with appropriate treatment although some will have persistent recurrent erosions or visual symptoms despite treatment.

12.3 Epithelial Recurrent Erosion Dystrophies

Epithelial recurrent erosions dystrophies (EREDs), most notably variant Franceschetti corneal dystrophy (FRCD), are rare corneal epithelial dystrophies that typically present in the first decades of life. These dystrophies exhibit autosomal dominant inheritance, and recent studies have shown that some cases are associated with mutations in the *COL17A1* gene on 10q23-q24 [10–12]. EREDs present with painful episodes of recurrent corneal erosions (RCEs) in the first decades of life and progress to decreased vision due to scar formation. As visual decline progresses with age, episodes of recurrent erosions decrease in frequency.

Slit-lamp biomicroscopy in patients with FRCD, the most common of the EREDs, is unremarkable in youth, although progresses to diffuse central subepithelial opacification and fibrosis by middle age. Light microscopy of pathology specimens shows irregular basal epithelium and partial disruption of the Bowman layer.

Treatment options for patients with EREDs are identical to those discussed above for recurrent corneal erosions resulting from EBMD. Early treatment for patients with frequent RCEs may prevent scarring and subsequent visual symptoms.

12.4 Meesmann Corneal Dystrophy

Meesmann corneal dystrophy, alternatively referred to as juvenile hereditary corneal dystrophy, is a rare epithelial corneal dystrophy that typically presents in the first few years or decades of life. Meesmann corneal dystrophy demonstrates autosomal dominant inheritance and arises from mutations in keratin *K3* gene on chromosome 12q13; the Stocker-Holt variant arises from mutations in the keratin *K12* gene on chromosome 17q12 [13]. Patients are typically asymptomatic, although they may have mild glare and photophobia early in life and may develop pain related to recurrent corneal erosions in adulthood. Patients with the Stocker-Holt variant typically demonstrate more severe symptoms that present at an earlier age [14].

Slit-lamp biomicroscopy shows small gray epithelial lesions on direct illumination, and retroillumination reveals tiny, translucent, epithelial cysts that may be sectoral or may extend limbus-to-limbus (Fig. 12.5a, b) [15]. In the Stocker-Holt variant, patients have small gray epithelial opacities that stain weakly with

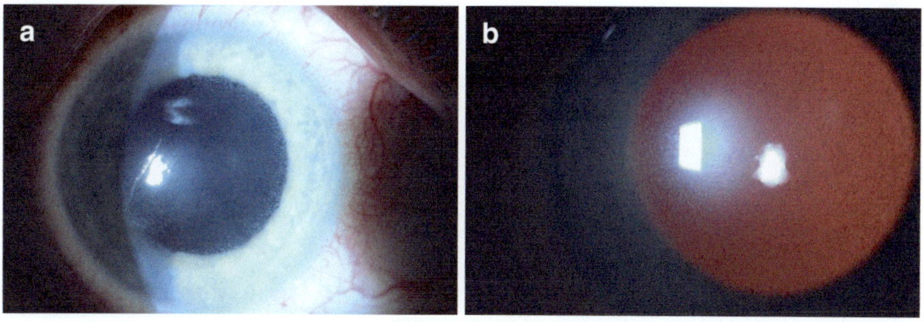

Fig. 12.5 (**a**) Myriad tiny translucent epithelial microcysts are seen throughout this eye with Meesmann corneal dystrophy, best seen in this photograph using broad illumination at the edge of the pupil. (**b**) Retroillumination off the retina highlights the microcysts in Meesmann corneal dystrophy in the eye seen in Fig. 12.5a

fluorescein throughout the entire cornea as well as fine linear opacities. Light microscopy of pathology specimens reveals many tiny vesicles containing periodic acid-Schiff (PAS)-positive "peculiar substance" in the epithelium [15].

Most patients require no treatment and have a good prognosis, although symptomatic patients may benefit from sunglasses for glare, and lubrication for irritation or RCEs. In severe cases, superficial keratectomy can be considered although the dystrophy typically recurs [16].

12.5 Lisch Epithelial Corneal Dystrophy

Lisch epithelial corneal dystrophy (LECD) is a rare epithelial dystrophy that may be found at any point in life. LECD is an X-linked dominant condition arising from mutations in chromosome 19p13.2 [17]. Patients are typically asymptomatic, although they may have mildly decreased vision if the central cornea is affected.

Slit-lamp biomicroscopy reveals gray-white epithelial opacities in a flame or feather-shaped pattern (Fig. 12.6a, b). The opacities can change shape over time, demonstrating progression or regression [18]. Confocal microscopy shows highly hyperreflective cytoplasm with hyporeflective nuclei [18]. AS-OCT shows normal thickness epithelial hyperreflectivity without stromal involvement [19]. Light microscopy of pathology specimens reveals PAS-positive vacuolated cells in the epithelium.

Patients with LECD have a good prognosis and most require no treatment, although for mild symptoms, sunglasses for glare and lubrication for mild irritation may be beneficial. There have been reports of cases of LECD regressing with soft contact lens use [20]. Rarely, patients with symptomatic cases can be treated with epithelial debridement, although the dystrophy typically recurs. Recently, superficial keratectomy combined with focal limbal cauterization has been successful in decreasing recurrence after keratectomy [21]. Excimer laser ablation with adjuvant mitomycin C has also been described [22].

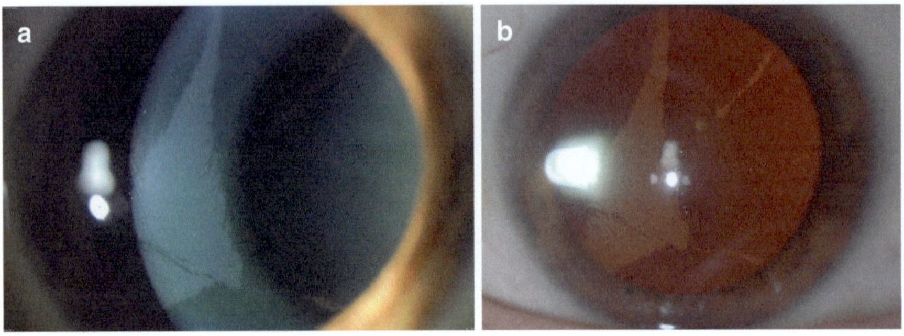

Fig. 12.6 (**a**) A large area of Lisch corneal dystrophy opacities can be seen with classic flame-shaped edges. (**b**) Retroillumination off the retina highlights the Lisch corneal dystrophy opacities seen in the patient in Fig. 12.6a

12.6 Gelatinous Drop-Like Dystrophy

Gelatinous drop-like dystrophy (GDLD) is a rare subepithelial corneal dystrophy that presents in the first or second decade of life and is somewhat more commonly seen in Japan [23]. GDLD demonstrates autosomal recessive inheritance and arises from mutation in the *TACSTD2* gene of chromosome 1p32 [24]. Patients present with significantly decreased vision, photophobia, tearing, redness, and irritation.

Slit-lamp biomicroscopy in GDLD can have a variety of presentations including relatively flat subepithelial opacities similar in appearance to band keratopathy, typical "mulberry" pattern grouped elevated nodules, or large "kumquat" nodular lesions (Figs. 12.7 and 12.8). Patients may have superficial and deep neovascularization and stromal opacification. Light microscopy of pathology specimens reveals subepithelial and stromal amyloid deposits [25].

Mild cases may be treated with lubrication alone, although more severe cases can be treated with bandage soft contact lenses, superficial keratectomy, excimer laser PTK, deep anterior lamellar keratoplasty (DALK), or penetrating keratoplasty (PK). In cases with multiple graft recurrences, a keratoprosthesis may be required. Patients with GDLD have a poor prognosis due to frequent and severe recurrence.

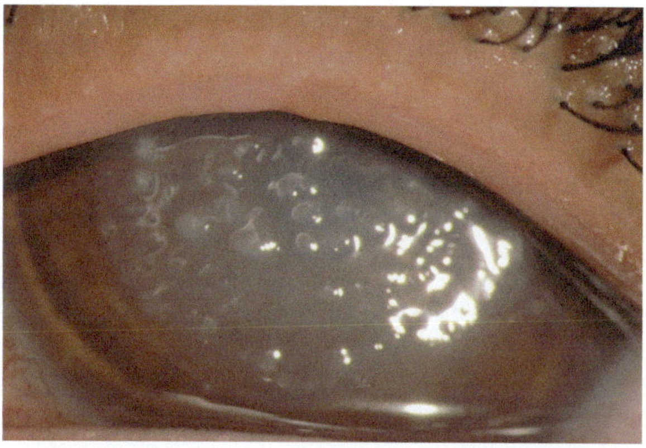

Fig. 12.7 Many elevated "mulberry-shaped" lesions of gelatinous drop-like dystrophy are evident in this very photosensitive patient

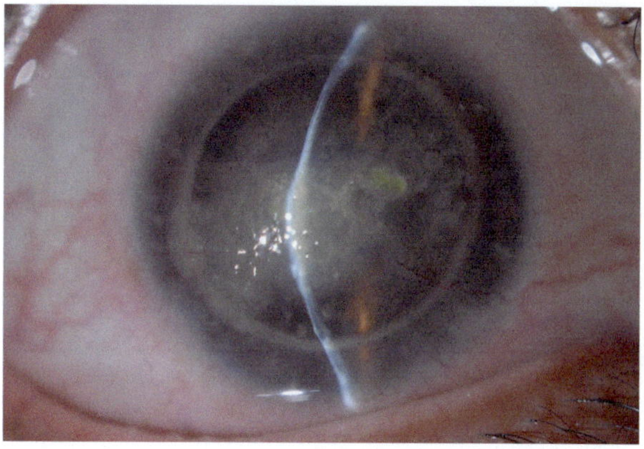

Fig. 12.8 Significant recurrence of gelatinous drop-like dystrophy can be seen after a penetrating keratoplasty

12.7 TGFBI-Associated Dystrophies

The transforming growth factor beta–induced (*TGFBI*) gene induces the expression of TGFBI protein (TGFBIp), which is ubiquitous in many human organs and tissues and is thought to play a role in cell adhesion, migration, proliferation, and differentiation [26]. TGFBIp expression was initially found to be upregulated in pathological corneal disease [27]. Subsequent genotypic analysis and the association of TGFBI with a group of similar corneal stromal dystrophies has played a large role in classifying corneal dystrophies. The TFGBI-associated corneal dystrophies discussed below all result from aberrant accumulation of TGFBIp or fragments of this protein depositing in the cornea.

Depending on the genotype and specific mutation in the *TGFBI* gene, these dystrophies manifest in different ways. Mutations in *TGFBI* have been associated with EBMD, lattice, granular types 1 and 2 (Avellino), Reis-Bücklers, and Thiel-Behnke corneal dystrophies [27, 28]. While these dystrophies present with different phenotypes and may respond somewhat differently to treatment, they have many clinical characteristics in common [29]. As genetic testing is becoming more common in the clinic, patients may begin to undergo testing for TGFBI more routinely as screening before refractive surgery [30].

12.7.1 Reis-Bücklers and Thiel-Behnke Corneal Dystrophies

Reis-Bücklers corneal dystrophy (RBCD), alternatively referred to as corneal dystrophy of Bowman layer type I (CDB 1), and Thiel-Behnke corneal dystrophy (TBCD), alternatively referred to as corneal dystrophy of Bowman layer type II (CDB 2), are uncommon dystrophies of Bowman membrane and the anterior stroma that present at a young age [28, 31]. Patients present early in life, including shortly after birth, with pain resulting from severe recurrent corneal erosions. Decreased vision typically occurs in the second to third decades of life. Symptoms are typically more severe in patients with Reis-Bücklers compared to those with Thiel-Behnke.

Slit-lamp biomicroscopy reveals a reticular subepithelial honeycomb appearance of the central cornea, often less dense or absent in the peripheral cornea, which may progress to involve the deeper stroma and peripheral cornea as the disease progresses. Although difficult to distinguish clinically, RBCD may display more irregular diffuse opacities with interceding clear cornea, whereas TBCD exhibits multiple flecks with reticular formation (Fig. 12.9). In recent years, in vivo confocal microscopy and AS-OCT have shown promise in their ability to help differentiate RBCD and TBCD during the patient's initial evaluation [32, 33]. Light microscopy of pathology specimens in RBCD shows Bowman layer replaced by subepithelial sheet of granular deposits that stain red with Masson trichrome, while TBCD shows furrowing of the anterior stroma with focal loss of Bowman layer, which gives a wavy sawtooth pattern appearance [34]. Transmission electron microscopy shows rod- or trapezoidal-shaped bodies in RBCD and curly fibers in TBCD [34].

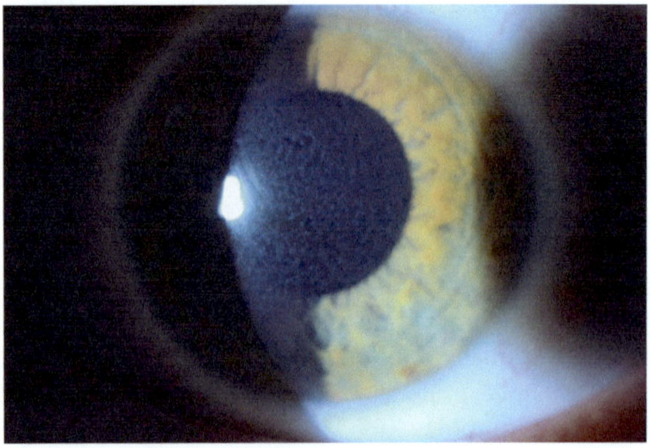

Fig. 12.9 Diffuse reticular opacities are present centrally in this relatively mild case of Reis-Bücklers corneal dystrophy

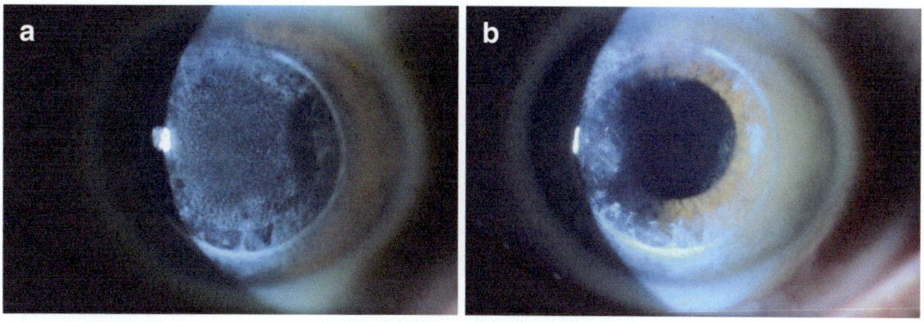

Fig. 12.10 (**a**) Moderate recurrence of Reis-Bücklers corneal dystrophy can be seen several years after penetrating keratoplasty. (**b**) One day after excimer laser PTK of the eye seen in Fig. 12.10a, the central cornea is much clearer with greatly improved vision

Mild cases may be treated with frequent lubrication, although more severe cases benefit from bandage soft contact lenses, superficial keratectomy, excimer laser PTK, DALK, or PK. Recurrence is common within several years after surgery, although excimer laser PTK can often be repeated and can be used to treat recurrence after keratoplasty (Fig. 12.10a, b) [35].

12.7.2 Lattice Corneal Dystrophies

There are several types of lattice corneal dystrophy. The most common is type 1 (LCD 1), alternatively referred to as Biber-Haab-Dimmer dystrophy, which is an uncommon epithelial-stromal dystrophy that typically presents in the first to second decades of life. LCD 1 demonstrates autosomal dominant inheritance [28, 36]. Patients may develop painful recurrent corneal erosions as early as the first or second decade of life, with vision beginning to decline in the third decade of life.

Lattice corneal dystrophy variants, previously designated type IIIA, I/IIIA, IV, and polymorphic amyloidosis, result from distinct heterozygous amyloidogenic mutations in *TGFBI* and tend to present somewhat later in life [37].

Slit-lamp biomicroscopy is similar for all types of LCD and shows superficial or deep, central, branching, refractile lines best seen with retroillumination as well as subepithelial white dots and diffuse anterior stromal haze early in the disease (Figs. 12.11 and 12.12a, b). Later in the disease, extensive subepithelial fibrosis and scarring may be seen. Light microscopy of pathology specimens shows amyloid deposits, which stain light red with Congo red dye, are metachromatic with crystal violet stain, and demonstrate apple-green birefringence under polarized light [38–40].

Mild cases are treated with lubrication alone to prevent recurrent corneal erosions. More severe cases can be managed with bandage contact lenses, superficial keratectomy, excimer laser PTK, or DALK, and PK in severe cases [41]. Recurrence is common in the donor graft within 5–10 years after corneal transplantation, as well as in residual stroma after excimer laser PTK. Recurrence occurs more slowly

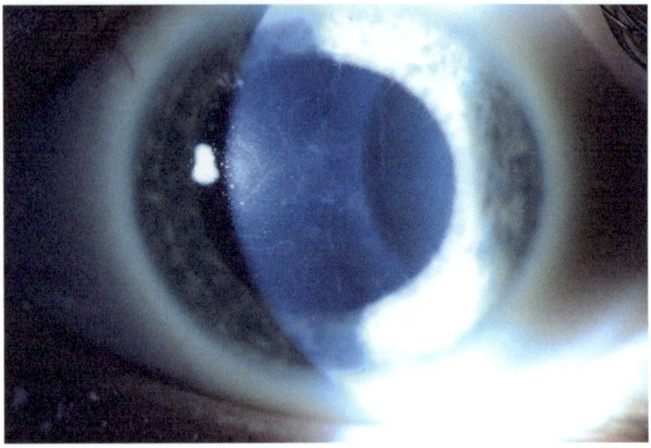

Fig. 12.11 Fairly mild refractile amyloid lines of lattice corneal dystrophy are present in this 17 year old woman

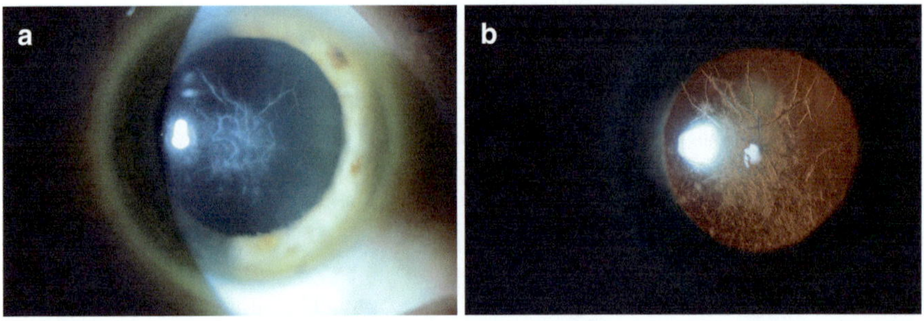

Fig. 12.12 (**a**) Moderate lattice lines along with central scarring from numerous recurrent erosions can be seen in this patient with lattice corneal dystrophy. (**b**) Retroillumination off the retina highlights the refractile amyloid lines and central scarring in the eye with lattice corneal dystrophy seen in Fig. 12.12a

than in RBCD or TBCD and consequently surgical treatment may provide years of improvement in symptoms and vision [16, 42]. Excimer laser PTK can be repeated in many cases and can be performed for recurrence after keratoplasty [35, 43].

12.7.3 Granular Corneal Dystrophies

There are two main forms of granular corneal dystrophy. Granular corneal dystrophy, type 1 (GCD 1), is an uncommon epithelial-stromal dystrophy that typically presents in the first and second decades of life. GCD 1 demonstrates autosomal dominant inheritance [28, 44]. Patients begin to develop decreased vision in the third to fifth decades of life as corneal opacities become confluent [45]. Painful recurrent corneal erosions are uncommon, although in some cases, they may begin prior to visual decline.

Slit-lamp biomicroscopy shows small discrete granules with a "crushed bread-crumb" appearance within the central anterior, and sometimes deep, stroma with

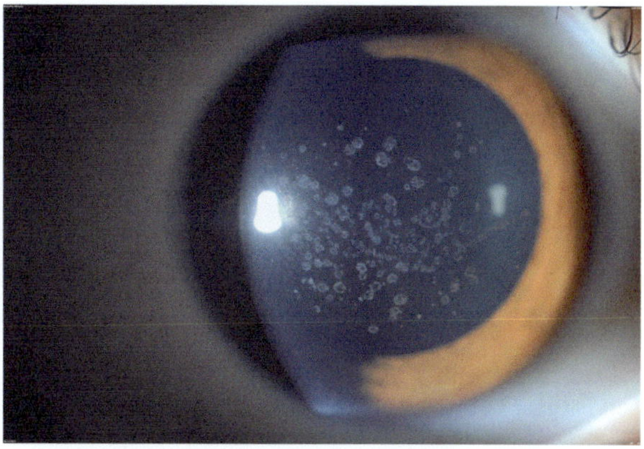

Fig. 12.13 Multiple small "crushed breadcrumb" creamy white opacities are present in the anterior stroma in this young woman with granular corneal dystrophy type 1. Note the clear intervening spaces

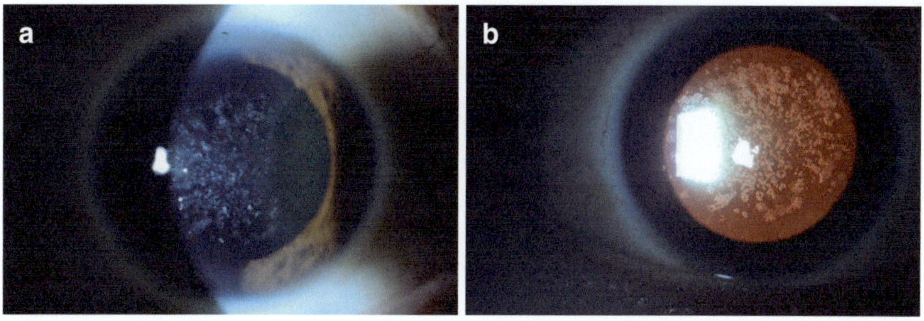

Fig. 12.14 (**a**) The central opacities in this older gentleman with granular corneal dystrophy type 1 have become more confluent and are now beginning to affect his visual function. (**b**) Retroillumination off the retina of the eye with granular corneal dystrophy type 1 seen in Fig. 12.14a highlights the fairly dense central opacities, but many clear spaces can still be seen

clear cornea between granules (Figs. 12.13 and 12.14a, b). With time, these granular deposits grow larger and more numerous and may become confluent, at which time, vision may be significantly affected [45, 46]. Light microscopy of pathology specimens shows stromal hyaline opacities that stain with Masson trichrome and extend from subepithelial stroma to Descemet membrane [46].

Mild cases may be treated with lubrication alone to prevent painful corneal erosions, although in more severe cases, bandage soft contact lens, superficial keratectomy, excimer laser PTK, DALK, or PK may be required. Patients with more superficial opacities can have significant improvement with excimer PTK, and while recurrence is common, it occurs more slowly than in RBCD or TBCD [16, 42]. PTK can often be repeated for superficial recurrences after PTK or corneal transplantation [35].

Granular corneal dystrophy, type 2 (GCD 2), also referred to as Avellino corneal dystrophy or combined granular lattice dystrophy, is a variant of GCD 1 with a similar presentation and clinical course and responds comparably to treatment [28, 47]. GCD 2 is a distinct entity from GCD 1 as slit-lamp biomicroscopy shows both

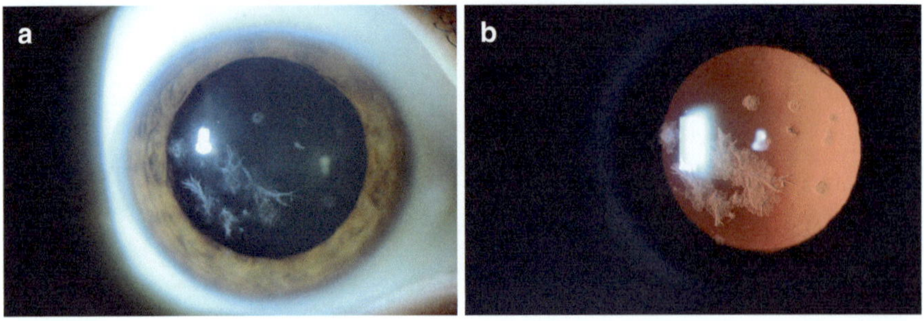

Fig. 12.15 (**a**) In this patient with granular dystrophy type 2, also known as Avellino dystrophy, both flat granular opacities and branching linear amyloid opacities are present. (**b**) Retroillumination off the retina of the eye with granular dystrophy type 2 seen in Fig. 12.15a highlights the more circular granular opacities and the refractile amyloid lines

anterior stromal "crushed breadcrumb" opacities typical of GCD 1 and deeper stromal refractile lines typical of LCD 1 (Fig. 12.15a, b) [45, 47]. Additionally, light microscopy of pathology specimens reveals both hyaline opacities typical of GCD 1 and amyloid deposits typical of LCD [47].

12.8 Macular Corneal Dystrophy

Macular corneal dystrophy (MCD) is a rare stromal dystrophy that presents in the first to third decades of life. MCD demonstrates autosomal recessive inheritance and arises from mutations in the *CHST6* gene of chromosome 16q22 [48]. MCD type 1 is more common and presents in childhood with glare and decreased vision, while MCD type 2 presents with similar symptoms in the second decade of life.

Slit-lamp biomicroscopy shows central, gray-white, poorly defined opacities with cloudiness of the intervening stroma, which over time progress to affect the entire cornea limbus-to-limbus (Fig. 12.16a) [49]. Central dense opacities are superficial, while more peripheral dense opacities are in the deep stroma (Fig. 12.16b). MCD is also associated with posterior corneal abnormalities such as Descemet membrane haze [50]. Corneal thinning is present in many cases and may be seen at the slit-lamp, on AS-OCT or with Scheimpflug imaging [50]. Light microscopy of pathology specimens shows acid mucopolysaccharide (glycosaminoglycan) deposits within the stroma that stain with Alcian blue and colloidal iron [51].

Vision is typically significantly affected by the third decade of life, and while excimer laser PTK may be useful to remove superficial central dense opacities, many patients require DALK or PK due to full-thickness corneal haze. PK is preferred in patients with significant posterior corneal abnormalities. Recurrence after either form of keratoplasty is uncommon, and when it does happen, it occurs much later than in the TGFBI gene–associated dystrophies [16, 42].

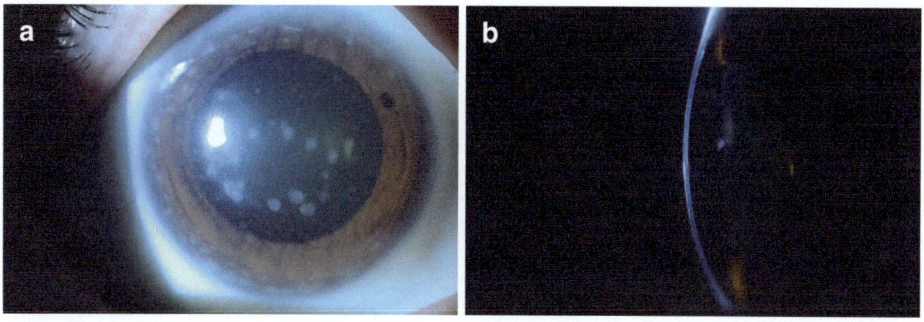

Fig. 12.16 (**a**) The entire cornea is diffusely hazy in this eye with macular corneal dystrophy, but more dense moderately large macules can be seen centrally and smaller macules peripherally. (**b**) The slit beam image of the eye with macular corneal dystrophy seen in Fig. 12.16a demonstrates that the central macules are located in the anterior cornea, while the peripheral macules are in the posterior cornea

12.9 Schnyder Corneal Dystrophy

Schnyder corneal dystrophy (SCD) is a rare stromal dystrophy that presents with clinical findings in the second and third decades of life, although it does not typically affect vision until years later. SCD demonstrates autosomal dominant inheritance and arises from mutations in the *UBIAD1* gene on chromosome 1p36 and is associated with hypercholesterolemia and hypertriglyceridemia and, in some patients, may be associated with xanthelasma and genu valgum [52, 53]. SCD typically does not manifest with symptoms until adulthood, when patients develop glare and, in advanced cases, decreased vision.

Slit-lamp biomicroscopy shows a fine ring of yellow-white, crystalline cholesterol deposits in the central anterior stroma, although this finding is only present in 50% of patients with SCD (Figs. 12.17 and 12.18) [54]. Typically, by the third and fourth decades, a prominent arcus lipoides is present on examination. In severe cases later in life, pan-stromal haze may develop [54]. Light microscopy of pathology specimens shows intracellular and extracellular phospholipid and cholesterol deposition that stains with Oil Red O and Sudan black.

SCD is a slowly progressive stromal dystrophy that may only present with glare early in life, and most patients maintain good vision despite corneal opacities seen on examination. Fasting cholesterol and triglyceride levels should be checked on all patients with suspected SCD [53]. Excimer laser PTK, DALK, or PK may be beneficial for patients with severe glare or decreased vision later in life, and visually significant recurrence of disease after treatment is rare.

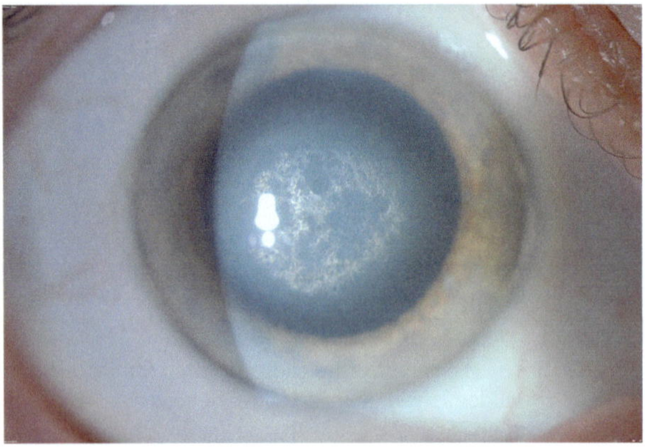

Fig. 12.17 Central crystalline opacities, central full thickness stromal haze, and peripheral arcus lipoides are all present in this eye with Schnyder corneal dystrophy

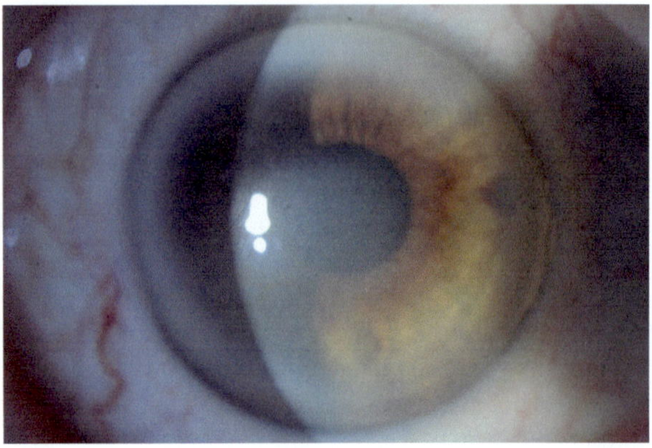

Fig. 12.18 This patient demonstrates the noncrystalline form of Schnyder corneal dystrophy, with central full thickness stromal haze and peripheral arcus lipoides. Other affected members of her family had the crystalline form

12.10 Congenital Stromal Corneal Dystrophy

Congenital stromal corneal dystrophy (CSCD) is an extremely rare stromal dystrophy that presents at birth. CSCD demonstrates autosomal dominant inheritance and arises from mutations in the decorin gene on chromosome 12q21.33 [55, 56]. Patients are born with diffuse bilateral corneal clouding and moderate to severe decrease in vision.

Slit-lamp biomicroscopy shows pan-stromal corneal opacities, equal in all areas of the corneal stroma (Fig. 12.19). Pachymetry may reveal mildly increased corneal thickness. Light microscopy of pathology specimens shows irregular stromal lamellae with intervening amorphous material.

Patients with severely decreased vision may benefit from DALK or PK. These patients have a fair visual prognosis and treatment is complicated by the many difficulties of performing corneal transplantation in children.

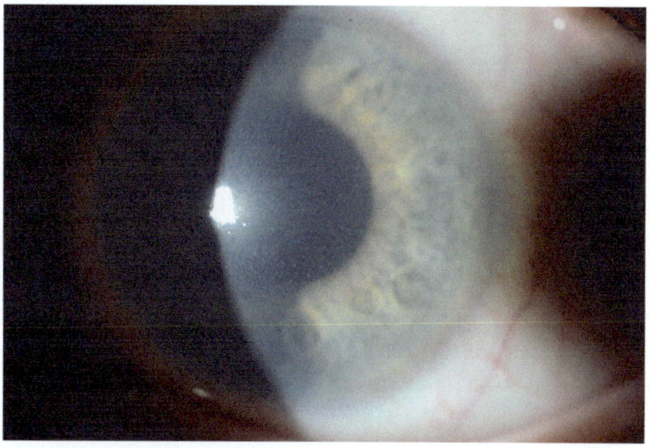

Fig. 12.19 This eye with congenital stromal corneal dystrophy reveals diffuse full-thickness stromal haze with some small scattered denser opacities

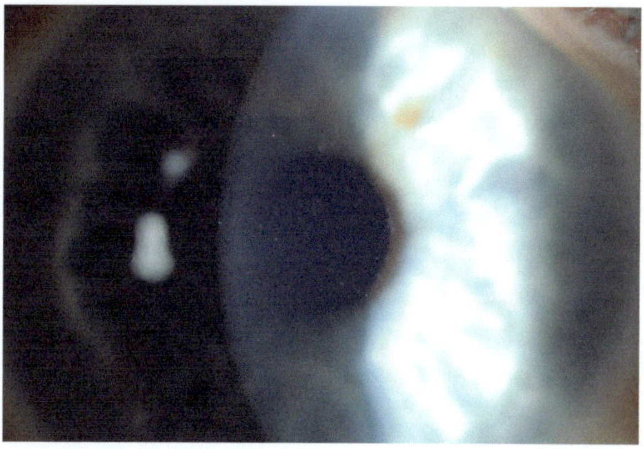

Fig. 12.20 Multiple small comma-shaped or ovoid gray-white opacities can be seen centrally in this eye with fleck corneal dystrophy

12.11 Fleck Corneal Dystrophy

Fleck corneal dystrophy (FCD) is a very rare stromal corneal dystrophy that may be seen in the first years of life. FCD demonstrates autosomal dominant inheritance and arises from mutations in the *PIKFYVE* gene on chromosome 2q35 [57]. Most patients remain asymptomatic, although some develop mild photophobia or decreased corneal sensitivity.

Slit-lamp biomicroscopy shows characteristic sharp-bordered, comma-shaped or oval flecks in all layers of the stroma extending limbus-to-limbus (Fig. 12.20). Light microscopy of pathology specimens shows vacuolated keratocytes containing glycosaminoglycans, which stain with Alcian blue, and complex lipids [58].

FCD is nonprogressive and typically does not require treatment.

12.12 Posterior Polymorphous Corneal Dystrophy

Posterior polymorphous corneal dystrophy (PPCD) is an uncommon endothelial dystrophy that can present with symptoms in early childhood but is often found incidentally in adulthood. PPCD has three subtypes which arise from mutations in different genes: PPCD 1 arises from mutations in 20p11.2-q11.2 affecting an unidentified gene, PPCD 2 arises from mutations in 1p34.3-p32.3 and mutations in *COL8A2*, and PPCD 3 arises from 10p11.22 and mutations in *ZEB1* [37]. PPCD can cause congenital corneal clouding and may also result in astigmatism in children. While many patients remain stable and asymptomatic, some patients develop corneal edema and subsequent blurred vision and, in rare cases, painful epithelial bullae if severe endothelial dysfunction develops. Approximately 15% of patients with PPCD will also have glaucoma, perhaps associated with iridocorneal adhesions and correctopia [59]. Rare cases may be associated with Alport syndrome in patients with nephritis and sensorineural hearing loss [60].

Slit-lamp biomicroscopy shows bilateral linear, bandlike, or vesicular endothelial irregularities with scalloping seen at the level of Descemet membrane and endothelium (Fig. 12.21a, b). Light microscopy of pathology specimens shows endothelial cells replaced by flat epithelium-like cells with microvilli that stain positive for keratin [61].

Patients with PPCD have a good visual prognosis and most are asymptomatic. If corneal edema develops and vision is significantly impaired, endothelial keratoplasty (EK) or PK should be considered and has a high success rate.

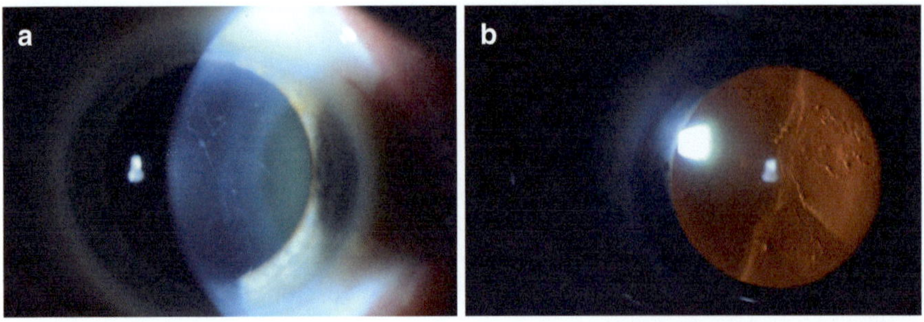

Fig. 12.21 (**a**) A large, serpiginous area of endothelial abnormality is evident in this eye with posterior polymorphous corneal dystrophy. (**b**) Retroillumination off the retina demonstrates the area of endothelial abnormality in the eye with posterior polymorphous corneal dystrophy seen in Fig. 12.21a

12.13 Congenital Hereditary Endothelial Dystrophy

Congenital hereditary endothelial dystrophy (CHED) is an extremely rare endothelial dystrophy that presents at birth. CHED demonstrates autosomal recessive inheritance and arises from mutations in 20p13 affecting the *SLC4A11* gene [62]. Patients present at birth with painless bilateral, often asymmetric, corneal clouding and nystagmus.

Slit-lamp biomicroscopy shows bilateral limbus-to-limbus severe corneal stromal edema with a blue-gray ground-glass appearance (Fig. 12.22). Corneal pachymetry may show a corneal thickness two to three times normal. Light microscopy of pathology specimens shows atrophic or absent endothelial cells with a thickened laminated Descemet membrane [63].

Patients with severe corneal edema from CHED may require EK or PK [62, 64]. These patients have a fair visual prognosis, and treatment is complicated by the many difficulties of performing corneal transplantation in children.

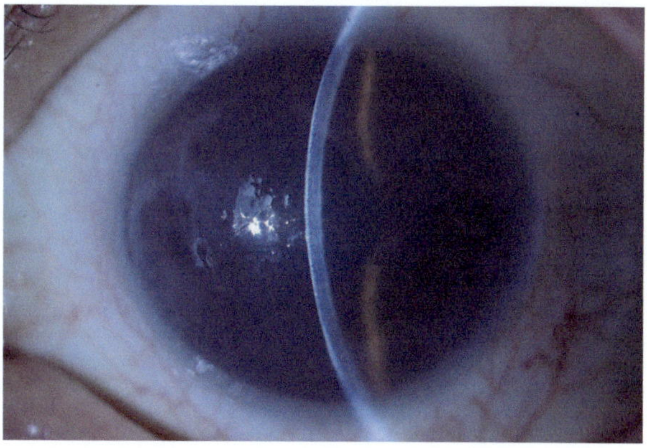

Fig. 12.22 Limbus-to-limbus severe corneal edema is apparent in the slit-beam image of this eye with congenital hereditary endothelial dystrophy

12.14 Future Directions

Our understanding of corneal dystrophies has been greatly enhanced in the last two decades by genetic sequencing, which has become common in research studies but not yet in clinical practice. As corneal dystrophy genetic panels develop in the coming years, genetics will continue to enhance our understanding of corneal dystrophies. A better appreciation of the genotype-phenotype connection in corneal dystrophies will help us to not only educate patients regarding what to expect with their specific dystrophy but also identify target genes in the cornea for therapeutic gene editing. CRISPR/Cas9-induced homology-directed repair, a commonly used research gene editing technology, has already shown the ability in vitro to repair the *TGFBI* gene known to cause multiple corneal dystrophies [65]. We hope that in the coming years, as gene editing technologies continue to mature, the last century of work identifying and characterizing corneal dystrophies will provide opportunities for patients with corneal dystrophies to be among the first to benefit from clinical gene therapy [66, 67].

References

1. Boutboul S, Black GCM, Moore JE, et al. A subset of patients with epithelial basement membrane corneal dystrophy have mutations in TGFBI/BIGH3. Hum Mutat. 2006;27(6):553–7.
2. Laibson PR. Recurrent corneal erosions and epithelial basement membrane dystrophy. Eye Contact Lens. 2010;36(5):315–7.
3. Laibson PR. Microcystic corneal dystrophy. Trans Am Ophthalmol Soc. 1976;74:488.
4. Bron AJ, Burgess SE. Inherited recurrent corneal erosion. Trans Ophthalmol Soc U K. 1981;101(Pt 2):239–43.
5. El Sanharawi M, Sandali O, Basli E, et al. Fourier-domain optical coherence tomography imaging in corneal epithelial basement membrane dystrophy: a structural analysis. Am J Ophthalmol. 2015;159(4):755–763.e1.
6. Miller DD, Hasan SA, Simmons NL, Stewart MW. Recurrent corneal erosion: a comprehensive review. Clin Ophthalmol (Auckland, N.Z.). 2019;13:325–35.
7. Dua HS, Lagnado R, Raj D, et al. Alcohol delamination of the corneal epithelium: an alternative in the management of recurrent corneal erosions. Ophthalmology (Rochester, Minn.). 2006;113(3):404–11.
8. Nagpal R, Maharana PK, Roop P, et al. Phototherapeutic keratectomy. Surv Ophthalmol. 2020;65(1):79–108.
9. Rapuano C. Excimer laser phototherapeutic keratectomy in eyes with anterior corneal dystrophies: short-term clinical outcomes with and without an antihyperopia treatment and poor effectiveness of ultrasound biomicroscopic evaluation. Cornea. 2005;24(1):20–31.
10. Jonsson F, Byström B, Davidson AE, et al. Mutations in collagen, type XVII, alpha 1 (COL17A1) cause epithelial recurrent erosion dystrophy (ERED). Hum Mutat. 2015;36(4):463–73.
11. Vahedi F, Chung DD, Gee KM, Chuephanich P, Aldave AJ. Epithelial recurrent erosion dystrophy secondary to COL17A1 c.3156C.T mutation in a non-white family. Cornea. 2018;37(7):909.
12. Lisch W, Weiss JS. Clinical and genetic update of corneal dystrophies. Exp Eye Res. 2019;186:107715.
13. Moore JE, McLean WHI, Swensson O, et al. Mutations in cornea-specific keratin K3 or K12 genes cause Meesmann corneal dystrophy. Nat Genet. 1997;16(2):184–7.

14. Stocker FW, Holt LB. Rare form of hereditary epithelial dystrophy: genetic, clinical, and pathologic study. AMA Arch Ophthalmol. 1955;53(4):536–41.
15. Javadi M, Rezaei-Kanavi M, Javadi A, Naghshgar N. Meesmann corneal dystrophy; a clinico-pathologic, ultrastructural and confocal scan report. J Ophthalmic Vis Res. 2010;5(2):122–6.
16. Dinh R, Rapuano CJ, Cohen EJ, Laibson PR. Recurrence of corneal dystrophy after excimer laser phototherapeutic keratectomy. Ophthalmology. 1999;106(8):1490.
17. Patterson K, Chong JX, Chung DD, et al. Lisch Epithelial Corneal Dystrophy Is Caused by Heterozygous Loss-of-Function Variants in MCOLN1. Am J Ophthalmol. 2024;258(2):183–95.
18. Kurbanyan K, Sejpal K, Aldave A, Deng S. In vivo confocal microscopic findings in Lisch corneal dystrophy. Cornea. 2012;31(4):437–41.
19. Pole C, Sise A, Joag M, et al. High-resolution optical coherence tomography findings of Lisch epithelial corneal dystrophy. Cornea. 2016;35(3):392–4.
20. Lisch W, Wasielica-Poslednik J, Lisch C, Saikia P, Pitz S. Contact lens-induced regression of Lisch epithelial corneal dystrophy. Cornea. 2010;29(3):342–5.
21. Salvador-Culla B, Alonso-Agesta M, Álvarez de Toledo J, Barraquer R. Combined keratectomy and localized limbal cauterization for treating Lisch epithelial corneal dystrophy. Cornea. 2019;38(2):243–5.
22. Wessel M, Sarkar J, Jakobiec F, et al. Treatment of Lisch corneal dystrophy with photorefractive keratectomy and mitomycin C. Cornea. 2011;30(4):481–5.
23. Tsujikawa M. Gelatinous drop-like corneal dystrophy. Cornea. 2012;31:37–40.
24. Paliwal P, Gupta J, Tandon R, et al. Identification and characterization of a novel TACSTD2 mutation in gelatinous drop-like corneal dystrophy. Mol Vis. 2010;16:729–39.
25. Weber FL, Babel J. Gelatinous drop-like dystrophy: a form of primary corneal amyloidosis. Arch Ophthalmol (1960). 1980;98(1):144–8.
26. Han KE, Choi S, Kim T, et al. Pathogenesis and treatments of TGFBI corneal dystrophies. Prog Retin Eye Res. 2016;50:67–88.
27. Lakshminarayanan R, Chaurasia SS, Anandalakshmi V, , et al. Clinical and genetic aspects of the TGFBI -associated corneal dystrophies. Ocul Surf 2014;12(4):234–251.
28. Munier FL, Korvatska E, Djemai A, et al. Kerato-epithelin mutations in four Sq31-linked corneal dystrophies. Nat Genet. 1997;15(3):247–51.
29. Gruenauer-Kloevekorn C, Braeutigam S, Froster U, Duncker G. Surgical outcome after phototherapeutic keratectomy in patients with TGFBI-linked corneal dystrophies in relation to molecular genetic findings. Graefes Arch Clin Exp Ophthalmol. 2009;247(1):93–9.
30. Chao-Shern C, Dedionisio LA, Jang J, et al. Evaluation of TGFBI corneal dystrophy and molecular diagnostic testing. Eye. 2019;33(6):874–81.
31. Small KW, Mullen L, Barletta J, et al. Mapping of Reis-Bücklers' corneal dystrophy to chromosome 5q. Am J Ophthalmol. 1996;121(4):384–90.
32. Kobayashi A, Sugiyama K. In vivo laser confocal microscopy findings for bowman's layer dystrophies (Thiel–Behnke and Reis–Bücklers corneal dystrophies). Ophthalmology (Rochester, Minn.). 2007;114(1):69–75.
33. Nishino T, Kobayashi A, Mori N, Yokogawa H, Sugiyama K. In vivo imaging of Reis–Bücklers and Thiel–Behnke corneal dystrophies using anterior segment optical coherence tomography. Clin Ophthalmol (Auckland, N.Z.). 2020;14:2601–7.
34. Küchle M, Green WR, Völcker HE, Barraquer J. Reevaluation of corneal dystrophies of Bowman's layer and the anterior stroma (reis-Bücklers and Thiel-Behnke types): a light and electron microscopic study of eight corneas and a review of the literature. Cornea. 1995;14(4):333–54.
35. Reddy JC, Rapuano CJ, Nagra PK, Hammersmith KM. Excimer laser phototherapeutic keratectomy in eyes with corneal stromal dystrophies with and without a corneal graft. Am J Ophthalmol. 2013;155(6):1111–1118.e2.
36. Holland EJ, Fishbaugh JA, Gorevic PD, et al. Three autosomal dominant corneal dystrophies map to chromosome 5q. Nat Genet. 1994;6(1):47–51.
37. Weiss J, Møller H, Aldave A, et al. IC3D classification of corneal dystrophies—edition 2. Cornea. 2015;34(2):117–59.

38. Dark A, Thomson D. Communications lattice dystrophy of the cornea: a clinical and microscopic study. Br J Ophthal. 1960;44:257.
39. Snead D, Mathews B. Differences in amyloid deposition in primary and recurrent corneal lattice dystrophy type 1. Cornea. 2002;21(3):308–11.
40. Smith M, Zimmerman L. Amyloid in corneal dystrophies: differentiation of lattice from granular and macular dystrophies. Arch Ophthalmol (1960). 1968;79(4):407–12.
41. Mohamed A, Chaurasia S, Ramappa M, Murthy S, Garg P. Outcomes of keratoplasty in lattice corneal dystrophy in a large cohort of Indian eyes. Indian J Ophthalmol. 2018;66(5):666–72.
42. Chen M, Xie L. Features of recurrence after excimer laser phototherapeutic keratectomy for anterior corneal pathologies in north China. Ophthalmology (Rochester, Minn.). 2013;120(6):1179–85.
43. Rapuano C. Phototherapeutic keratectomy: who are the best candidates and how do you treat them? Curr Opin Ophthalmol. 2010;21(4):280–2.
44. Klintworth G. Advances in the molecular genetics of corneal dystrophies. Am J Ophthalmol. 1999;128(6):747–54.
45. Han K, Chung W, Kim T, Kim K, Kim T, Kim E. Changes of clinical manifestation of granular corneal deposits because of recurrent corneal erosion in granular corneal dystrophy types 1 and 2. Cornea. 2013;32(5):e113–20.
46. Wittebol-Post D, van der Want JJ, Van Bijsterveld OP. Granular dystrophy of the cornea (Groenouw's type I). Ophthalmologica. 1987;195(4):169–77.
47. El-Ashry MFM, El-Aziz A, et al. A clinical, histopathological, and genetic study of Avellino corneal dystrophy in British families. Br J Ophthalmol. 2003;87(7):839.
48. Aldave AJ, Yellore VS, Thonar EJ, et al. Novel mutations in the carbohydrate sulfotransferase gene (CHST6) in American patients with macular corneal dystrophy. Am J Ophthalmol. 2004;137(3):465–73.
49. Aggarwal S, Peck T, Golen J, Karcioglu ZA. Macular corneal dystrophy: a review. Surv Ophthalmol. 2018;63(5):609–17.
50. Rubinstein Y, Weiner C, Einan-Lifshitz A, et al. Macular corneal dystrophy and posterior corneal abnormalities. Cornea. 2016;35(12):1605–10.
51. Micali A, Pisani A, Puzzolo D, et al. Macular corneal dystrophy. Ophthalmology (Rochester, Minn.). 2014;121(6):1164–73.
52. Orr A, Dubé M, Marcadier J, et al. Mutations in the UBIAD1 gene, encoding a potential prenyltransferase, are causal for Schnyder crystalline corneal dystrophy. PLoS One. 2007;2(8):e685.
53. Gaynor PM, Zhang W, Weiss JS, Skarlatos SI, Rodrigues MM, Kruth HS. Accumulation of HDL apolipoproteins accompanies abnormal cholesterol accumulation in Schnyder's corneal dystrophy. Arterioscler Thromb Vasc Biol. 1996;16(8):992.
54. Weiss JS. Schnyder crystalline dystrophy sine crystals: recommendation for a revision of nomenclature. Ophthalmology (Rochester, MN). 1996;103(3):465–73.
55. Bredrup C, Stang E, Bruland O, et al. Decorin accumulation contributes to the stromal opacities found in congenital stromal corneal dystrophy. Invest Ophthalmol Vis Sci. 2010;51(11):5578–82.
56. Bredrup C, Knappskog PM, Majewski J, Rodahl E, Boman H. Congenital stromal dystrophy of the cornea caused by a mutation in the decorin gene. Invest Ophthalmol Vis Sci. 2005;46(2):420–6.
57. Li S, Tiab L, Jiao X, et al. Mutations in PIP5K3 are associated with François-Neetens Mouchetée fleck corneal dystrophy. Am J Hum Genet. 2005;77(1):54–63.
58. Purcell JJ, Krachmer JH, Weingeist TA. Fleck corneal dystrophy. Arch Ophthalmol. 1977;95(3):440–4.
59. Rodrigues MM, Phelps CD, Krachmer JH, Cibis GW, Weingeist TA. Glaucoma due to endothelialization of the anterior chamber angle: a comparison of posterior polymorphous dystrophy of the cornea and Chandler's syndrome. Arch Ophthalmol (1960). 1980;98(4):688–96.
60. Nicklason E, Mack H, Beltz J, et al. Corneal endothelial cell abnormalities in X-linked Alport syndrome. Ophthalmic Genet. 2020;41(1):13–9.

61. Krachmer JH. Posterior polymorphous corneal dystrophy: a disease characterized by epithelial-like endothelial cells which influence management and prognosis. Trans Am Ophthalmol Soc. 1985;83:413–75.
62. Mittal V, Sehdev N, Mittal R. Descemet membrane endothelial keratoplasty in congenital hereditary endothelial dystrophy: initial experiences. Cornea. 2021;40(8):972–6.
63. Pearce WG, Tripathi RC, Morgan G. Congenital endothelial corneal dystrophy. Clinical, pathological, and genetic study. Br J Ophthalmol. 1969;53(9):577–91.
64. Ashar JN, Ramappa M, Vaddavalli PK. Paired-eye comparison of descemet's stripping endothelial keratoplasty and penetrating keratoplasty in children with congenital hereditary endothelial dystrophy. Br J Ophthalmol. 2013;97(10):1247–9.
65. Taketani Y, Kitamoto K, Sakisaka T, et al. Repair of the TGFBI gene in human corneal keratocytes derived from a granular corneal dystrophy patient via CRISPR/Cas9-induced homology-directed repair. Sci Rep. 2017;7(1):16713.
66. Williams KA, Irani YD. Gene therapy and gene editing for the corneal dystrophies. Asia-Pac J Ophthalmol (Philadelphia, Pa.). 2016;5(4):312–6.
67. Moore CBT, Christie KA, Marshall J, Nesbit MA. Personalised genome editing—the future for corneal dystrophies. Prog Retin Eye Res. 2018;65:147–65.

Ocular Surface Neoplasia 13

Jason A. Greenfield, Wathanee Sripawadkul, Anat Galor, and Carol L. Karp

Summary

- The three most common malignant ocular surface tumors are ocular surface squamous neoplasia (OSSN), conjunctival melanoma, and conjunctival lymphoma. Among the three, OSSN is the most prevalent, while melanoma is the most dangerous. Each of these tumors has distinctive clinical characteristics and treatment approaches.
- While histopathological analysis remains the gold standard for the diagnosis of OSSN, in-office anterior segment optical coherence tomography (AS-OCT) has become an important adjuvant tool that can aid in the diagnosis of ambiguous

The author Jason A. Greenfield and Wathanee Sripawadkul have contributed equally to this chapter.

J. A. Greenfield · C. L. Karp (✉)
Bascom Palmer Eye Institute, University of Miami Miller School of Medicine, Miami, FL, USA
e-mail: jason.greenfield@med.miami.edu; ckarp@med.miami.edu

W. Sripawadkul
Bascom Palmer Eye Institute, University of Miami Miller School of Medicine, Miami, FL, USA

Department of Ophthalmology, Faculty of Medicine, Srinakharinwirot University, Bangkok, Thailand
e-mail: wxs428@miami.edu

A. Galor
Bascom Palmer Eye Institute, University of Miami Miller School of Medicine, Miami, FL, USA

Surgical Services, Miami Veterans Affairs Hospital, Miami, FL, USA

Department of Ophthalmology, Miami Veterans Administration Medical Center, Miami, FL, USA
e-mail: AGalor@med.miami.edu

H. N. Saeed, R. B. Singh (eds.), *Corneal Disorders*, Current Practices in Ophthalmology, https://doi.org/10.1007/978-981-96-5294-5_13

lesions and detection of subclinical OSSN during the treatment course and follow-up. The term "optical biopsy" has become widely used to represent the benefits of AS-OCT.

- First-line treatment approaches for OSSN have shifted toward primary topical medical therapy with interferon α-2b (IFN), mitomycin (MMC), and 5-fluorouracil (5FU), as all provide high resolution rates with reasonable side effect profiles.
- Conjunctival melanoma and lymphoma can have systemic involvement. Therefore, a complete laboratory and imaging workup is recommended, as this affects the clinical staging of disease, the management approach, and the long-term prognosis.
- With the advent of new treatment modalities, personalized approaches are being applied to individuals with conjunctival melanoma and lymphoma based on the genetics of their disease. Examples of targeted therapies include BRAF/MEK (gene coding B-Raf/ mitogenactivated extracellular signal-regulated kinase) and immune checkpoint anti-PD1 (programmed death 1 protein), anti-PDL1 (programed death ligand 1), and anti-CLA4 (cytotoxic T-lymphocyte associated protein 4) inhibitors for melanoma, radioimmunotherapy, proteasome inhibitors, B cell receptor signaling inhibitors, and m-TOR (mammalian target of rapamycin) inhibitors for lymphoma.

13.1 Introduction

Malignant ocular surface neoplasia encompasses three main tumor types that are classified according to their cellular origins. These include epithelial tumors (ocular surface squamous neoplasia), melanocytic tumors (primary acquired melanosis with atypia and conjunctival melanoma), and conjunctival lymphoma. In this chapter, we focus on the clinical features, diagnosis, treatment options, and course of these three malignant lesions.

13.2 Ocular Surface Squamous Neoplasia

13.2.1 Etiology and Pathogenesis

Ocular surface squamous neoplasia (OSSN) is a term that represents an abnormal growth of squamous epithelial tissue on the cornea or conjunctiva. OSSN encompasses a wide spectrum of histopathologic abnormalities based on the depth of epithelial abnormalities, categorized as mild, moderate, or severe dysplasia; carcinoma in situ; and invasive squamous cell carcinoma [1–3]. Several risk factors have been associated with the development of OSSN, including ultraviolet (UV)-B light exposure (often by inducing a *p53* gene mutation), human papilloma virus (HPV) infection (mainly the 16 and 18 subtypes), HIV seropositivity status, xeroderma pigmentosa disease, and vitamin A deficiency [4–10]. These mechanisms can directly or indirectly cause DNA damage, reduce the function of DNA repair systems, or suppress the immune system, ultimately leading to tumor formation [5]. However, the pathogenesis of OSSN is likely due to a combination of these factors.

13.2.2 Clinical Characteristics

OSSN has various clinical characteristics. OSSN typically arises unilaterally and within the interpalpebral fissure, as this area accumulates the majority of UV light exposure [5]. Specifically, most cases are identified in the nasal quadrant of the limbus [11]. It typically presents as a slow-growing mass that can illicit no pain, mild discomfort, or severe pain [4]. OSSN can appear gelatinous, papilliform (abnormal vascularization, often with a "hairpin loop" appearance), opalescent (flat and opaque), leukoplakic (overlying white, keratinized plaque), or nodular (raised above the ocular surface) (Fig. 13.1) [12, 13]. However, OSSN can also present with a combination of these clinical descriptors. On gross examination, the lesions can be visualized as pink or white and either flat and diffuse appearing or elevated above the ocular surface [3, 14].

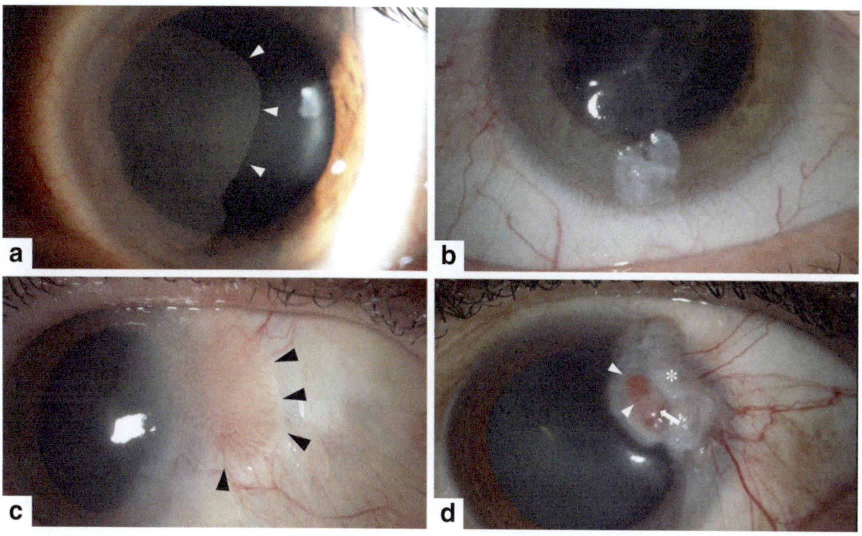

Fig. 13.1 Composite images of ocular surface squamous neoplasia (OSSN). (**a**) Slit-lamp image of a 56-year-old White Hispanic male. The left eye demonstrates an opalescent lesion on the cornea extending from the nasal limbus consistent with OSSN. White arrowheads show the lesion border. (**b**) Slit-lamp image of a 52-year-old White female. The right eye demonstrates a leukoplakic inferior corneal/limbal OSSN. (**c**) Slit-lamp image of the right eye of a 76-year-old White male demonstrates a papillomatous appearing OSSN with multiple hairpin vessels loops (black arrowheads). (**d**) Slit-lamp image of the left eye in a 68-year-old Hispanic male demonstrates an OSSN with gelatinous (asterisk), and papillomatous (arrowhead) components

13.2.3 Diagnostic Modalities

The gold standard for establishing a diagnosis of OSSN is through excisional or incisional biopsy and subsequent histopathological analysis. Upon examination of the lesion, the depth of epithelial dysplasia determines its classification. The criteria for mild, moderate, and severe dysplasia is less than 1/3, between 1/3 and 2/3, and greater than 2/3 of the epithelial thickness, respectively, while full-thickness epithelial dysplasia maintains preservation of the basement membrane and is termed carcinoma in situ [1]. Cytological studies of the specimen may show decreased differentiation with increasing dysplasia, and cellular features that include increased nuclei size, nuclear membrane atypia, hyperchromasia, and fine to coarse chromatin [1]. In addition, OSSN associated with HPV infection may show the presence of a koilocytosis [1].

OSSN may advance to invasive squamous cell carcinoma (SCC) if the epithelial basement membrane is breached. In this case, histopathological findings are significant for malignant cells penetrating the stromal tissue in an infiltrative or expansive architectural pattern [1]. These cells can display varying degrees of differentiation, with poorly differentiated tumors showing immature cells with high nucleus-to-cytoplasm ratios, pleomorphic nuclei, increased mitotic activity, and low levels of keratinization. In addition, rare variants of invasive SCC have been identified, and these include mucoepidermoid carcinoma, spindle cell carcinoma, papillary squamous cell carcinoma, and acantholytic/adenoid squamous cell carcinoma [1].

A diagnosis of OSSN can be suggested through information gathered from less-invasive in-office methods. First, vital dye staining can be performed to support a diagnosis of OSSN. Rose bengal, lissamine green, and toluidine blue stains may be applied topically, whereby positive staining identifies areas of abnormal epithelium and often stains leukoplakic lesions [15]. Although it is not specific to metabolically active or cancerous epithelial cells, it is useful for outlining areas of abnormality which are often larger than can be appreciated upon gross examination [15]. However, these vital dyes serve as auxiliary tools, as they are sensitive, but not specific, for OSSN and may stain other benign lesions such as pterygia, areas of dry eye, and actinic keratosis [15]. Next, impression or aspiration cytology techniques can be utilized to identify cellular atypia and have demonstrated promising results as screening tests for OSSN, with positive predictive results of 77–97% as compared to biopsy [16–18]. However, not all pathology laboratories possess the equipment needed to analyze these samples; furthermore, this diagnostic method reflects only the superficial cells and does not provide information on the depth of invasion or margin involvement.

Novel imaging modalities, such as anterior segment optical coherence tomography (AS-OCT) and in vivo confocal microscopy (IVCM), are also useful in supporting the diagnosis of OSSN. AS-OCT imaging is a noninvasive, in-office method that provides cross-sectional imaging of lesions on the ocular surface. The classic features of OSSN on AS-OCT include epithelial thickening and hyperreflectivity with abrupt transition of normal epithelium to OSSN (Fig. 13.2b) [19]. Overall, AS-OCT imaging aids in differentiating OSSN from other ocular surface lesions, with studies showing a sensitivity and specificity of 100% for a cutoff epithelial thickness of 120 μm using the commercially available Optovue AS-OCT device (RTVue, Optovue, Fremont, CA)

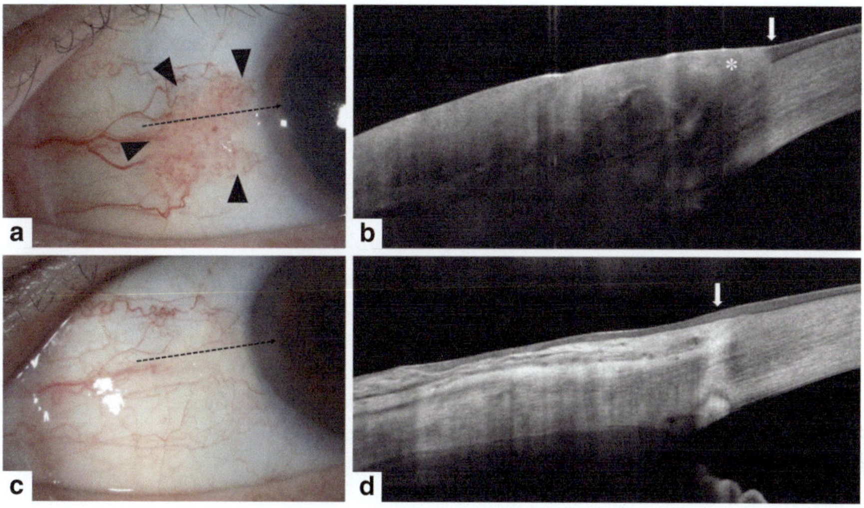

Fig. 13.2 A-D Composite images of an ocular surface squamous neoplasia (OSSN) pre- vs post-medical therapy in a 63-year-old White male. (**a**) Slit-lamp image of the left eye demonstrates a papillomatous OSSN on nasal bulbar conjunctiva (arrowheads). The black dotted arrow demonstrates the orientation of the anterior segment optical coherence tomography (AS-OCT) raster. (**b**) High-resolution AS-OCT image shows thickened hyperreflective epithelium (asterisk) with an abrupt transition from abnormal to normal (arrow). (**c**) Slit-lamp image of the same eye showing resolution after six 1-week cycles of 5-fluorouracil 1% topical eye drop treatment. The black dotted line demonstrates the orientation of the AS-OCT raster. (**d**) High-resolution AS-OCT image shows normal thickness epithelium (arrow) following treatment

[20]. It is also a technology easily learned, even by novices [21]. AS-OCT is also an important tool to monitor the effects of medical therapy and to screen for disease recurrence [22]. IVCM is a minimally invasive diagnostic method that has been applied to benign and malignant ocular surface lesions, with characteristics such as hyperreflective pleomorphic cells, enlarged and bright nuclei, prominent nucleoli, and basal cells containing ill-defined borders with a "starry night" appearance described in OSSN [15, 23]. However, studies have shown that these cellular features are nonspecific to OSSN, and therefore IVCM can serve as an adjunct to biopsy but cannot reliably distinguish OSSN from other ocular surface diseases [23].

13.2.4 Management

OSSN can be managed through surgical and medical interventions, or a combination of both. Surgical excision is commonly completed using a "no-touch" technique that reduces the likelihood of tumor cell seeding [3, 24]. This method consists of excising the tumor with wide margins (~4 mm) and applying cryotherapy to the conjunctival and limbal margins with a "double-freeze, slow-thaw" procedure that aims to rupture tumor cell membranes [3, 24]. An absolute alcohol epitheliectomy can be performed if there is corneal involvement, and a partial sclerectomy can be completed if the tumor is adherent to the sclera [25]. For closure, amniotic membrane transplantation following surgical excision of OSSN can promote healing of the ocular surface and allow for more extensive margins to be taken [26]. Disadvantages of surgical excision include the possibility of postoperative complications such as infection, symblepharon formation, corneal scarring, nonhealing epithelial defect, limbal stem cell deficiency, and hyphema [27]. Despite the surgeon's best efforts, residual margins may be positive, necessitating further treatment. For this reason, the use of topical chemotherapy has increased in favor over the past several years [28].

The three most established chemotherapeutic agents used for the treatment of OSSN are interferon α-2b (IFN), 5-fluorouracil (5FU), and mitomycin C (MMC). IFN can be applied topically as drops, through subconjunctival, perilesional injections, or both of these methods [29]. Topical applications and injections of IFN as primary treatment of OSSN are efficacious and have demonstrated total resolution of OSSN (with studies showing complete resolution rates ranging between 75 and 100%) with low rates of disease recurrence [29–33]. A major limitation of IFN is its high cost, where in the United States, the eyedrops may range from $500–800 per month for self-pay patients [14]. In other countries, such as India, interferon remains quite inexpensive. Another problem with IFN is that it is increasingly difficult to access. The usual dose for the eyedrops is 1 MIU/ml four times daily until resolved plus an additional month of treatment. In contrast, 5FU has a relatively low cost (approximately $50 per month) and has a similar efficacy profile to IFN, with studies showing complete tumor resolution rates between 82 and 100% (Fig. 13.2) [32]. 5FU is primarily administered topically as an eyedrop and causes minimal side effects, such as ocular pain or eyelid inflammation [32, 34–36]. It is cycled, usually at a frequency of 4–7 days per month, applied four times daily at a concentration of 1%, and then stopped for 3 weeks. Finally, MMC is utilized topically (0.02–0.04%) and has demonstrated rapid resolution rates as compared to IFN [37]. However, it has a greater level of toxicity to the ocular surface relative to both IFN and 5FU and may cause side effects such as pain, epitheliopathy, allergic conjunctivitis, conjunctival hyperemia, ectropion, punctal stenosis, and limbal stem cell deficiency [38]. In addition, MMC is more expensive than 5FU, at approximately $400 per bottle in the United States [14]. Each of these agents has been shown to be effective when utilized as a primary therapy and has demonstrated an ability to reduce the rate of recurrence when used as an adjunct to surgical excision [14, 39]. Other therapeutic interventions that should be noted include anti-vascular endothelial growth factor (anti-VEGF), retinoic acid, and aloe vera. However, the efficacy of these alternative treatments has yet to be established.

13.3 Primary Acquired Melanosis

13.3.1 Etiology and Pathogenesis

Primary acquired melanosis (PAM) is a hyperpigmented macule that can be found on the conjunctiva and cornea. In addition, it generally occurs unilaterally in light-skinned individuals. It has been found to be associated with patients who have

Southern European ancestry, dark brown hair, facial nevi, pingueculae or pterygia, and a history of smoking or hypertension [40]. PAM can exist in two forms that can be differentiated through histopathological analysis: PAM without atypia (a benign melanocytic hyperplasia) and PAM with atypia (an atypical melanocytic hyperplasia). PAM with atypia can be further subdivided into mild, moderate, and severe atypia based on the degree of melanocytic atypia and the extent of radial and vertical spread throughout the epithelium. In PAM with mild atypia, atypical melanocytes exist solely in the basal layer of the epithelium [41]. The criteria for PAM with severe atypia include hyperplasia of atypical melanocytes that have invaded the superficial epithelium or the presence of epithelioid cells [41]. Full-thickness PAM is also called "melanoma in situ." Damato et al. have referred to PAM of the conjunctiva as melanocytic intraepithelial neoplasia (c-MIN) [42]. The risk of progression to conjunctival melanoma increases with increasing atypia. Specifically, PAM without atypia does not progress to melanoma, while PAM with atypia has a 13–46% risk of transformation [41, 43].

13.3.2 Clinical Characteristics

PAM is clinically defined as a flat, pigmented, and non-cystic lesion that is at least 1 millimeter in diameter and can be found on the conjunctiva, cornea, and caruncle [44, 45]. PAM is usually brown and can be found in all racial and age groups but typically presents in white males at approximately 60 years of age [46]. It can appear in solitary, patchy, diffuse, and multifocal forms on the superficial conjunctiva (Fig. 13.3). These lesions must be differentiated from a conjunctival melanocytic nevus and complexion-associated melanosis (CAM, typically found bilaterally). When there is corneal involvement, PAM can show a speckled pigmentation on the affected corneal epithelium [44]. Finally, PAM can rarely present as a nonpigmented lesion, with a normal or thickened cornea, which makes establishing a clinical diagnosis significantly more challenging [47].

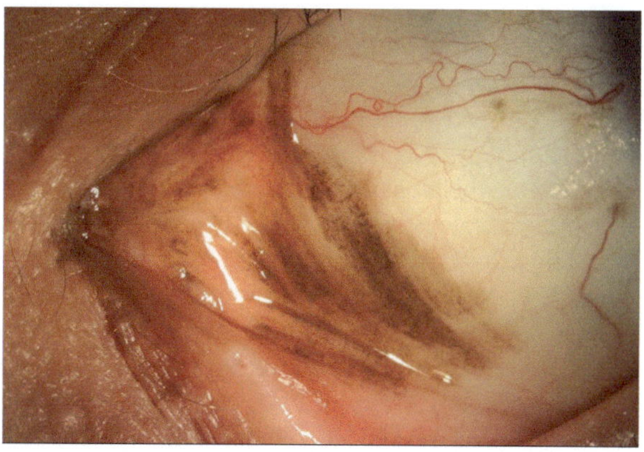

Fig. 13.3 Slit-lamp image of 44-year-old White female. The left eye demonstrates a patch of brown pigment with peppery appearance in the nasal bulbar area extending to the inferior fornix, plica semilunaris, caruncle, and eyelid margin. Histopathology was consistent with primary acquired melanosis (PAM) with moderate atypia

13.3.3 Diagnostic Modalities

No reliable method currently exists to differentiate PAM without atypia from PAM with atypia clinically, and thus histopathology is the gold standard for diagnosis. Through histopathological analysis, PAM without atypia demonstrates a diffuse melanocytic hyperplasia that is confined to the basal layer and show no signs of cytological abnormality [42]. In contrast, PAM with atypia appears as a melanocytic hyperplasia with a broad spectrum of cytological abnormality and pleomorphism [42]. Cytological studies can show melanocytes that vary in size, nucleolar prominence, amount of cytoplasm, and mitotic activity [42, 48]. In addition, they may exhibit different architectural features, such as clustering together into "nests" or demonstrating pagetoid spread [42]. Both increased cytological atypia and greater clock-hour involvement are significant predictive factors for the malignant transformation of PAM into invasive conjunctival melanoma [41].

Identifying features of PAM on AS-OCT include a hyperreflective band with normal overlying epithelium and no visualized cysts [48]. AS-OCT cannot differentiate between PAM with and without atypia, or differentiate PAM from CAM [48]. At this point, the resolution of the AS-OCT imaging limits its utility in PAM. It is mostly useful in that it rules out cysts, consistent with a nevus, or a subconjunctival mass.

13.3.4 Management

The optimal treatment approach for suspected PAM is dependent on the size and characteristics of the lesion. However, there is wide heterogeneity in management approaches across different groups [49]. In general, if the lesion involves less than 2 clock hours and mobile, it can be routinely monitored for changes in appearance [46]. "Waxing and waning" of the lesion can occur [49]. For lesions extending between 2 and 5 clock hours, wide excision should be performed using the "no-touch" technique described in the OSSN section. For larger and diffuse lesions (more than 5 clock hours of involvement), total surgical excision may not be the optimal approach due to the increased risk of inducing limbal stem cell deficiency (LSCD) and scarring. In these cases, conjunctival map biopsies can be performed, which consist of the procurement of several small biopsies in different areas of the lesion, after which decisive treatment is based on the pathological outcome.

Following the biopsy, the treatment modality for PAM is dependent on the results from histopathology. PAM without atypia can be managed with routine observation. In addition to surgical excision with intraoperative cryotherapy, postsurgical treatment of PAM with atypia can include cryotherapy and topical chemotherapy. Topical mitomycin-C (MMC) can be applied to the ocular surface prior or after surgical excision, for PAM that is not surgically excisable, or for recurrent disease [46]. It is typically prescribed in a cycle fashion with various regimens. The MMC (0.02% or 0.04%) is most commonly administered four times daily for 1–4 weeks followed by a 1–3-week period of treatment cessation [27, 50]. Punctal plugs are often inserted prior to MMC therapy to prevent punctal stenosis. Other chemotherapy agents, such as IFN-α2b, have not been robustly studied in individuals with PAM with atypia and are thus not routinely used. Inexcisable PAM may also be treated by cryotherapy, which can be done to focal areas of PAM recurrence or larger areas of inexcisable disease.

13.4 Conjunctival Melanoma

13.4.1 Etiology and Pathogenesis

Conjunctival melanoma is a serious and potentially lethal ocular tumor [27, 51, 52]. It accounts for 0.25% of overall melanoma, 5% of ocular melanoma [53], 2% of all ocular tumors, and 12% of all conjunctival tumors [54]. It has the highest incidence in non-Hispanic White individuals (incidence rate of 0.2–0.8 per million), followed by black individuals (0.18 per million) [55] and Asian individuals (0.15 per million) [56]. Previous studies have shown an age-adjusted, twofold increase in incidence of conjunctival melanoma over a 27-year period (between 1973 and 1999) [57, 58].

Conjunctival melanoma originates from melanocytes located in the basal conjunctival epithelium. Histopathological analysis has demonstrated that conjunctival melanoma can arise from PAM (32–77%) [51, 59–64], nevi (2–27%) [59, 61–64], and de novo (11–26%) [59, 61–64]. The tumor can be confined to the epithelium (melanoma in situ) or breach the epithelial basement membrane and invade the conjunctival stroma [27, 42]. These cellular features can be differentiated through histopathological analysis. Studies have shown that the incidence of conjunctival melanoma mirrors the incidence of cutaneous melanoma; thus, the linkage to a sunlight-related etiology has been proposed [58, 65]. To date, the risk factors of conjunctival melanoma have not been fully elucidated [27, 56]. However, the association between conjunctival melanoma and two other melanocytic lesions, conjunctival nevus and PAM, have been well established. Clinical studies have estimated that approximately 1 in 300 conjunctival nevi develops into melanoma [66]. In PAM, the presence of severe atypia and a greater area of involvement are significant risk factors for the transformation to conjunctival melanoma, and therefore routine follow-up care for individuals with PAM is recommended in order to detect early changes in appearance [67]. Recent studies in tumor genetics have shown that conjunctival melanoma can have similar genetic mutations (BRAF, NRAS, NF1, and TERT) to those identified in cutaneous melanoma; however, they are distinct from those found in uveal melanoma (GNAQ, GNA11, and BAP1) [68]. A *BRAF* mutation, particularly a V600E point mutation, is the most common mutation found in cutaneous melanoma (observed in approximately half of cutaneous melanoma cases), and the same gene mutation has been reported in about one third of conjunctival melanoma cases [61, 69]. Other gene mutations (*KIT* and *PTEN*) are less frequently identified [70, 71].

13.4.2 Clinical Characteristics

Conjunctival melanoma classically presents as a unilateral, painless, immobile, nodular, dark brown mass and commonly presents on the bulbar/limbal conjunctiva in patients aged 50–60 years old (Fig. 13.4) [72]. While less common in Asian and Black populations, when it occurs, it tends to affect younger patients [60]. In addition, it has been reported that the tumors demonstrate more aggressive features in Chinese individuals and are associated with a relatively poor prognosis [73]. Conjunctival melanoma most frequently affects the bulbar conjunctiva (53–97%), followed by the limbus (48–69%) [51, 62, 63, 74], palpebral conjunctiva (4–29%), fornix (3–29%), caruncle (1–13%), and plica semilunaris (1–13%) [51, 52, 60, 62–64, 74]. Tumors identified on extra-limbal locations carry worse prognoses for local recurrence, namely metastasis and death [52, 61, 75]. Although dark brown to black color is considered typical and found in 60–70% of conjunctival melanoma cases, they can also present with variable or mixed pigmentations, with previous reports of white, yellow, grey, pink, and red hues [60, 63]. Variation patterns in clinical presentations have been identified that are based on the tumor origin. Conjunctival melanoma that arises from PAM tends to occur in older patients and typically demonstrates greater clock hour involvement, whereas conjunctival melanoma that arises from a nevus is usually thicker and contains more feeder vessels [62]. Finally, it is possible that the conjunctival melanoma has invaded adjacent structures such as the eyelid and orbit upon the patient's initial presentation [27]. In such cases, the patient's prognosis is worse, and management often involves an oculoplastic specialist and extensive surgery. Conjunctival melanoma can spread via lymphatic or hematogenous routes, and common sites of metastasis include regional lymph nodes, the brain, lungs, and liver [27, 50–52].

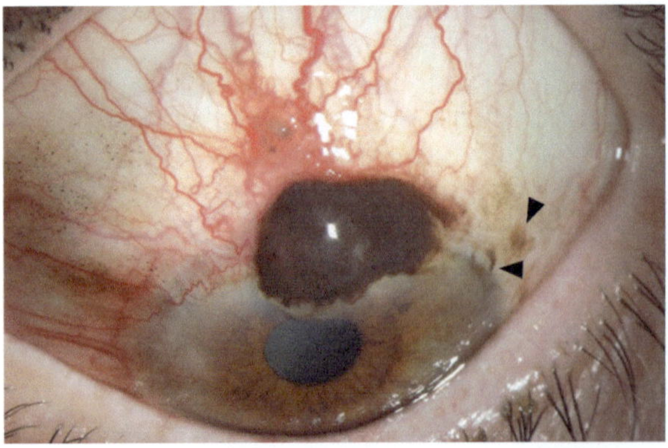

Fig. 13.4 Slit-lamp photo of a 60-year-old White Hispanic female. The left eye demonstrates an elevated, dark, brown mass along the superior limbus with feeder vessels from 11 to 2 o'clock. Dusting of pigment in the superior hemisphere and inferior bulbar conjunctival is seen. Histopathology was consistent with conjunctival melanoma and adjacent primary acquired melanosis (arrowheads)

13.4.3 Diagnostic Modalities

The diagnosis of conjunctival melanoma can be made after a complete ocular examination and histopathological analysis. Currently, clinical staging of the tumor (eighth edition of the American Joint Committee on Cancer, AJCC) is graded based on its location, quadrant involvement, and presence of local invasion (Table 13.1). Clinical studies on the outcomes of conjunctival melanoma found that tumors with higher clinical stages are associated with poorer outcomes [74, 77, 78]. Histopathology is the gold standard for confirming a diagnosis of conjunctival melanoma [27]. An excisional biopsy is recommended over an incisional biopsy due to the increased risk of recurrence and metastasis in the latter [46, 79]. Histopathological examination will show malignant melanocytic cells, which can be characterized by their nuclear atypia, lack of cellular organization, or prominent nucleoli. Four different malignant cell types have been identified, including spindle cells, balloon cells, small polyhedral cells, and round epithelioid cells [27]. In addition, the vertical tumor thickness and depth of invasion affect the pathologic staging [80].

The use of current imaging modalities, such as AS-OCT and ultrasound biomicroscopy (UBM), can support a diagnosis of conjunctival melanoma. One of the main advantages of AS-OCT is to differentiate epithelial and subepithelial lesions. Therefore, the diagnosis of amelanotic melanoma versus pigmented OSSN can be made by identifying which conjunctival layers the lesion involves [81]. AS-OCT findings in OSSN show thickened hyperreflective epithelium with an abrupt transition from normal to abnormal epithelium and can also have subepithelial involvement if the disease has advanced to invasive squamous cell carcinoma. In contrast, conjunctival melanoma shows a hyperreflective subepithelial lesion on AS-OCT with some overlying epithelial involvement of variable hyperreflectivity. One limitation of the use AS-OCT in the diagnosis of conjunctival melanoma is that the image quality can be reduced by the shadowing effect from thick and pigmented lesions that block light transmission. Therefore, details of the internal structural and posterior border of the tumor can be obscured. In this situation, UBM is a better tool to assess the tumor's dimensions and exclude scleral or intraocular invasion [81, 82].

13.4.4 Management

The goal of conjunctival melanoma treatment is to completely remove the tumor and prevent local recurrences and metastasis. The management of conjunctival melanoma is based on its disease stage, which consists of both local and systemic components. The gold standard treatment for conjunctival melanoma is excision of the lesion using the "no-touch" technique described in the OSSN section [24, 46, 83]. The first surgery is the most important, whereby the delicate and complete removal of the tumor will significantly minimize the risk for tumor seeding and is critical for preventing future recurrence, metastasis, and death [52, 63, 64, 83, 84]. In addition, tissue screening for melanoma biomarkers can be performed, if possible, as these markers are needed in planning any systemic treatments with targeted therapies [84].

Table 13.1 Conjunctival melanoma as defined by the eighth American Joint Committee on Cancer (AJCC) on cancer staging manual[a]

	Clinical tumor (cT)	Pathologic tumor (pT)
Tx	Primary tumor cannot be assessed	
T0	No evidence of primary tumor	
T1	Tumor of the bulbar conjunctiva	(Tis) Melanoma confined to conjunctival epithelium
T1a	$<$ 1 quadrant	Tumor of the bulbar conjunctiva with invasion of the substantia propria, not $>$2.0 mm in thickness
T1b	$\geq$ 1 to $<$2 quadrants	Tumor of the bulbar conjunctiva with invasion of the substantia propria, $>$ 2.0 mm in thickness
T1c	$\geq$ 2 to $<$3 quadrants	
T1d	$\geq$ Quadrants	
T2	Tumor of the nonbulbar (forniceal, palpebral, and tarsal) conjunctiva and tumor involving the caruncle	
T2a	Noncaruncular and $\leq$ 1 quadrant of the nonbulbar conjunctival involved	Tumor of the nonbulbar conjunctiva involved with invasion of the substantia propria, not $>$2.0 mm in thickness
T2b	Noncaruncular and $>$ 1 quadrant of the nonbulbar conjunctival involved	Tumor of the nonbulbar conjunctiva involved with invasion of the substantia propria, $>$ 2.0 mm in thickness
T2c	Caruncular and $\leq$ 1 quadrant of the nonbulbar conjunctival involved	
T2d	Caruncular and $>$ 1 quadrant of the nonbulbar conjunctival involved	
T3	Tumor of any size with local invasion	
T3a	Globe	
T3b	Eyelid	
T3c	Orbit	
T3d	Nasolacrimal duct, lacrimal sac, and/or paranal sinuses	
T4	Tumor of any size with invasion of the central nervous system	
Regional lymph node(N)		
Nx	Regional lymph nodes cannot be assessed	
N0	No regional lymph node metastasis	
N1	Regional lymph node metastasis	
Distant metastasis (M)		
M0	No distant metastasis	
M1	Distant metastasis	

[a]Reproduced with permission from Springer publishing [76]

Local adjuvant therapy can be used after excision to reduce the risk of local recurrence, particularly in cases where positive tumor margins are present after surgery [27, 56]. However, no consensus exists regarding a standardized treatment approach. Adjuvant therapies that are currently utilized include topical chemotherapy (MMC and 5FU), topical immunotherapy (IFN), and radiotherapy. Among the topical adjuvant options, MMC is the most studied agent and is preferred by most ophthalmologists for superficial disease [27, 56]. MMC can be used either intra- or postoperatively, but it is typically prescribed after surgery (after the surface has healed) in cases where positive superficial tumor margins are present. MMC is not a treatment for residual deep margins or a tumor identified in the scleral bed. MMC likely does not penetrate to tumor in the sclera, thus limiting its use to surface lesions [27]. Limited data currently exists on the efficacy of 5FU and IFN treatment for conjunctival melanoma, and therefore both agents are not the first choices for adjuvant therapy.

Brachytherapy, a type of radiotherapy, delivers a radioactive isotope via direct contact between the tumor and the radioactive source, either through a plaque, ring, or applicator. Common radioactive sources are strontium [85] and iodine-125 [56]. Brachytherapy has the advantage of treating both superficial and deep tissue compared with topical chemotherapy and is thus recommended in cases where positive deep margins are identified on histopathology. Overall, the frequency of complete resolution without recurrence or metastasis in brachytherapy is approximately 80%, and therefore it is considered an effective adjuvant therapy. The most common side effects of local radiation include pain, dry eye, symblepharon, ptosis, and cataract formation [86, 87]. Rarely, transient episcleritis, reduced peripheral corneal vascularization, corneal ulcers, and descemetocele can occur [86, 88].

In terms of systemic management, all patients with a conjunctival melanoma are seen by an oncologist. A complete physical examination should be performed including palpation of lymph nodes in the preauricular, parotid, submandibular, and cervical areas. Furthermore, additional investigations at baseline and annually are advised to search for early metastasis. Brain imaging (preferably MRI), chest CT, liver imaging, and, in some cases, whole body positron emission tomography-CT scanning may be performed as these are the sites for metastasis [46, 50, 56].

There is currently no consensus on the optimal approach for managing metastatic conjunctival melanoma [56], which occurs in 23–28% of T2 and T3 tumors at 5 years [74, 78]. If the tumor involves the orbit, orbital exenteration followed by adjuvant external radiation is one option, but may not provide any additional survival benefit [56].

Targeted therapy with a variety of novel therapeutics (BRAF, MEK inhibitors, and immune checkpoint inhibitors (anti-CTLA4 and anti-PD1)) have more recently been applied to individuals with metastatic conjunctival melanoma based on research identifying similar tumor genetics between cutaneous and conjunctival melanoma [50, 56, 68, 89]. The indication for immune checkpoint inhibitors is likely to expand to younger patients with advanced local disease and those who refuse orbital exenteration (even if metastasis has not been detected) [89]. Examples of medication in these classes are vemurafenib (BRAF inhibitor), dabrafenib, trametinib (MEK inhibitor), ipilimumab (anti-CTLA4), nivolumab, and pembrolizumab (anti-PD1) [68]. Due to its rarity compared with cutaneous melanoma, studies on the use of these new therapies are limited to case reports. However, outcomes in these patients might change the treatment paradigm for conjunctival melanoma in the near future [50, 56, 68].

13.5 Conjunctival Lymphoma

13.5.1 Etiology and Pathogenesis

Lymphoma is a malignant neoplasm derived from a monoclonal proliferation of lymphocytes. Ocular adnexal lymphoma (OAL) is defined as lymphoma that develops on the conjunctiva, eyelid, or orbital tissues. Conjunctival lymphoma (CL) accounts for 20–30% of OAL [85, 90, 91]. Overall, lymphomas can be divided into two major groups: Hodgkin lymphoma and non-Hodgkin lymphoma. The majority of OAL are non-Hodgkin B cell lymphomas (98%), while T cell, NK cell, and other cell type lymphomas are rarely encountered [90, 92, 93]. The four common histologic subtypes of OAL are extranodal marginal zone lymphoma (EMZL), follicular lymphoma (FL), diffuse large B cell lymphoma (DLBCL), and mantle cell lymphoma (MCL). The first two are low-grade subtypes, while the latter two are high-grade subtypes.

Several risk factors have been associated with CL. The most well-established risk factors are immunodeficiency (HIV seropositive patients or patients using immunosuppressive medications), autoimmune disease (Sjögren's syndrome, systemic lupus erythematosus, and rheumatoid arthritis), infections (*Chlamydia psittaci, Hepatitis C,* and *Helicobacter pylori*), genetic abnormalities (translocation, inactivating mutations, and trisomies), and prior radiation exposure [90, 93–97].

13.5.2 Clinical Characteristics

CL most commonly presents as a slightly elevated mass with a pink to yellow color. This pink coloration of the tumor is often described as a salmon patch (Fig. 13.5). Patients may present with a lump, irritation, redness, or they may be asymptomatic [93]. CL typically arises in the superior and inferior quadrant, rather than the horizontal limbus, where OSSN is usually seen [98]. A complete ophthalmic examination, including eyelid eversion, and thorough visualization of the bulbar and tarsal surface is warranted to search for tumors hidden in the midbulbar and forniceal areas [98]. Intrinsic tumor vessels are not usually seen [93]. Less commonly, CL may present as a chronic follicular conjunctivitis [99]. Most CL presents as an isolated disease, without evidence of prior or concurrent systemic involvement (67–90%) [93]. The exception is the MCL subtype, where systemic involvement is identified in approximately 50% of cases at the time of diagnosis [100, 101].

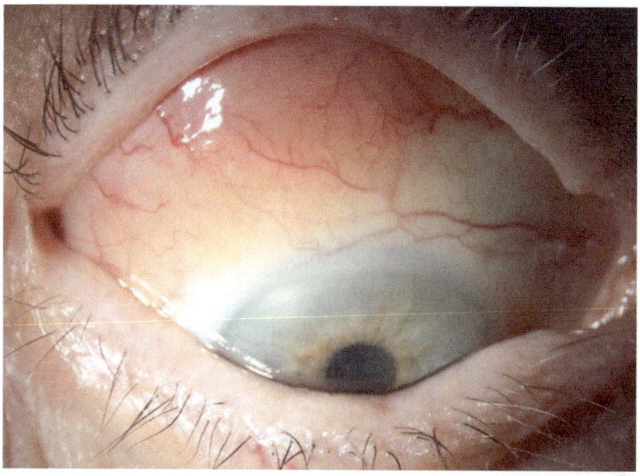

Fig. 13.5 Slit-lamp image a 92-year-old White female. The right eye demonstrates a large immobile, pink, fleshy ("salmon patch") mass in the supero-temporal quadrant. Histopathology was consistent with extranodal marginal zone lymphoma

EMZL, previously known as mucosa-associated lymphoid tissue (MALT) lymphoma, is the most common subtype and accounts for 68–80% of CL [90, 93, 100, 102, 103]. It typically affects females at a slightly higher frequency than males [93, 100]. The second most common subtype is FL, which is found in 8–16% of all CL and has no sex predilection. The shared clinical features of these low-grade subtypes are the patients' mean age (in 60 s), their unilateral presentations, the presence of the tumors for long periods prior to ophthalmic consultation (median 4–5 months duration), their occurrence as a primary disease (without systemic involvement), and their favorable prognosis. The high-grade subtypes, MCL and DLBCL, each accounts for 3–5% of all CL. In contrast, the patients' mean age is older (usually in their 70 s) and systemic involvement at diagnosis is present in about 25% of DLBCL cases and 50% of MCL cases. Due to the aggressive nature of these subtypes, the disease staging upon diagnosis is typically advanced.

13.5.3 Diagnosis

Clinical examination cannot differentiate conjunctival lymphoma from its benign counterpart, benign reactive lymphoid hyperplasia (BRLH); however, some clues can be gleaned from examining AS-OCT images. On AS-OCT, conjunctival lymphoma presents as a hyporeflective, homogenous, subepithelial mass with a smooth border and monomorphic dot-like infiltrate. The epithelial thickness is typically normal [104]. On the other hand, BRLH may have a more heterogenous quality, with variably reflective subepithelial tissue [104]. However, while AS-OCT may be suggestive, it is necessary to perform a tissue biopsy in every suspicious case of conjunctival lymphoma to differentiate between lymphoma and BRLH. The ocular pathologist will perform an array of special stains, including immunohistochemical staining. Fresh specimens are sent for analysis of flow cytometry and gene rearrangement [93]. Once the diagnosis of conjunctival lymphoma is confirmed, systemic laboratory and imaging workup to search for any systemic involvement is essential. This workup includes, but is not limited to, a complete blood count, serum chemistry, serum lactate dehydrogenase (LDH), CT/MRI of the orbit, full-body PET scan, bone marrow aspiration, and biopsy [93]. Clinical staging is determined by the Ann Arbor staging classification and the AJCC classification [76, 102] (Table 13.2).

13.5.4 Management

The main factors to consider in the management of conjunctival lymphoma treatment are clinical staging, histologic subtype, systemic involvement, and the general health of the patient [84, 93, 105]. A multidisciplinary approach involving an ophthalmologist, pathologist, and oncologist is necessary in order to perform a comprehensive workup on the patient. Overall, the treatment options for OAL include radiotherapy, chemotherapy, immunotherapy, combined therapy (immunochemotherapy and radioimmunotherapy), and other recent medical, oncological therapies.

The general approach in OAL treatment is radiotherapy for localized disease and systemic therapy in bilateral disease or OAL with systemic involvement. In isolated unilateral CL, external beam radiation therapy (EBRT) is the gold standard treatment [90, 93, 100, 103, 106, 107]. It is highly effective in treating low-grade OAL with overall local control rates ranging from 86 to 100% and local recurrence frequencies ranging between 0 and 15% [108–110]. To treat EMZL, a total radiation dose of 24–25 Gy divided into several fractions of 1.5–2.0 Gy is recommended [107]. The radiation dose for FL is slightly higher (24–36 Gy) [105, 111, 112].

Table 13.2 Conjunctival lymphoma as defined by the eighth American Joint Committee on Cancer on cancer staging manual[a]

Tumor (T)	
T0	No evidence of lymphoma
T1	Lymphoma involving the conjunctiva alone without orbital involvement
T2	Lymphoma with orbital involvement +/− any conjunctival involvement
T3	Lymphoma with preseptal eyelid involvement +/− orbital involvement +/− any conjunctival involvement
T4	Orbital adnexal lymphoma extending beyond orbit to adjacent structures, such as bone and brain
Regional lymph node (N)	
N0	No evidence of lymph node involvement
N1	Involvement of ipsilateral region lymph nodes
N2	Involvement of contralateral or bilateral regional lymph nodes
N3	Involvement of peripheral lymph nodes not draining ocular adnexal region
N4	Involvement of central lymph nodes
Distant metastasis (M)	
M0	No evidence of involvement of other extranodal sites
M1	Lymphomatous involvement in other organs recorded either at first diagnosis or subsequently

[a]Reproduced with permission from Springer publishing [76]

Recently, ultralow-dose radiotherapy in doses of 4 Gy (in 2 Gy fractions on consecutive days) have been applied in EMZL cases, which have demonstrated complete response rates of about 85% [113, 114]. Common side effects include eyelid irritation, mild conjunctivitis, dry eye syndrome, cataracts, glaucoma, orbital fat tissue atrophy, and radiation retinopathy [90, 93, 103, 107–109].

For *Chlamydia psittaci* positive OAL (EMZL subtype), oral doxycycline or clarithromycin treatment may be reasonable before considering more aggressive strategies [115–117]. Typical dosing of doxycycline is 100 mg twice daily for 3–6 weeks. Interestingly, even Chlamydia-negative OAL has been noted to respond to oral doxycycline [116].

Prior to the development of the anti-CD20 monoclonal antibody, rituximab, chemotherapy was the standard medication given to patients with lymphoma that has systemic involvement. Examples of these chemotherapy regimens include chlorambucil, cyclophosphamide (CHOP, hydroxydaunorubicin, oncovin, and prednisolone), and CVP (cyclophosphamide, vincristine, and prednisolone). The use of rituximab has improved the treatment outcomes in B cell originating lymphoma relative to chemotherapy agents, which are associated with several side effects. Therefore, it is currently used as a mainstay treatment and is indicated for high-grade subtypes, CL with bilateral or systemic involvement, and can either be administered alone or combined with conventional chemotherapy [90, 101, 105]. The usual route of rituximab administration is intravenous injection. However, successful cases of intralesional rituximab injections as monotherapy have also been reported [90, 118] but require multiple injections. IFN injections have also been showed to be effective in EMZL treatment [93, 118, 119].

Surgery is usually not effective due to the increased risk of microinfiltration of the surrounding tissue. One third of patients treated with surgery alone have been reported to have a relapse within 3 years of follow-up [90, 120, 121]. Finally, despite reports of spontaneous tumor regression, observation is not optimal as it carries a higher risk of progression [90, 105, 122].

High-grade OAL is still a disease with a poor prognosis and limited treatment strategies. The 5-year disease-specific survival for EMZL, FL, DLBCL, and MCL is 97%, 82%, 55%, and 9%, respectively [100]. Novel medications in the oncology field which target specific mechanisms of the disease are being investigated. Examples of these medications are 90-yttrium-ibritumomab tiuxetan (radioimmunotherapy), bortezomib (a proteasome inhibitor), ibrutinib (a B cell receptor signaling inhibitor), lenalidomide (an immunomodulating agent), and temsirolimus (an m-TOR inhibitor). The outcomes of these medications for OAL have yet to be determined.

13.6 Future Directions

The diagnosis and treatment of ocular surface tumors continue to evolve. The use of AS-OCT has aided the clinician in the differentiation of ocular surface lesions and in the monitoring of treatment [104, 123]. As this technology continues to develop, hopefully greater cellular resolution will occur. In addition, the advent of anterior segment optical coherence tomography angiography (AS-OCTA) may enhance the understanding of tumorigenesis. AS-OCTA can visualize the vascular networks in ocular surface lesions through capturing the motion of red blood cells and generating cross-sectional images. It has demonstrated an ability to characterize and quantify different vascular structures and patterns, such as increased vascular density, throughout OSSN lesions [12]. Next, the treatment options for ocular surface melanocytic tumors are rapidly changing with novel research in the field of oncology. Targeted therapies (that modify intracellular pathways based on specific tumor gene mutations) and immune checkpoint inhibition therapy (that augments the patient's immune system to attack tumor cells) are recent breakthroughs in the treatment of cutaneous melanoma and have shown promising outcomes in the treatment of conjunctival melanoma. Despite these advancements in individualized therapeutics, treatment-resistant cutaneous melanoma represents a current challenge where future investigation is needed. Additional research is necessary to determine the optimal combination of targeted therapies and checkpoint inhibitors where treatment resistance is minimized. Finally, it is hoped that advanced conjunctival lymphoma will also be treated with medications that target newly discovered, disease-specific mechanisms. Overall, the treatment trend in oncology is moving toward individualized therapy that will hopefully improve outcomes for patients.

Support NIH Center Core Grant P30EY014801 (Institution, CK, AG) RPB Unrestricted Award (CK), Dr. Ronald and Alicia Lepke Grant (CK), The Lee and Claire Hager Grant (CK), The Robert Farr Family Grant (CK), The Grant and Diana Stanton-Thornbrough (CK), The Robert Baer Family Grant (CK), The Emilyn Page and Mark Feldberg Grant (CK), The Calvin and Flavia Oak Support Fund (CK), The Robert Farr Family Grant (CK), The Jose Ferreira de Melo Grant (CK), The Richard and Kathy Lesser Grant (CK), The Michele and Ted Kaplan Grant (CK), The Roberto and Antonia Menendez Family Grant (CK), The Stephen Takach Grant (CK), The Christian Kathke Grant (CK), Dr. Tim and Cammy Ioannidis Grant (CK), The Ragheb Family Grant (CK), The Honorable A. Jay Cristol Grant (CK), The Carol Soffer Grant (CK), The Zvi Levin Grant (CK), and the Richard Azar Family Grant (institutional grants). Supported by the Department of Veterans Affairs, Veterans Health Administration, Office of Research and Development, Clinical Sciences R&D (CSRD) I01 CX002015 (AG), Biomedical Laboratory R&D (BLRD) Service I01 BX004893 (AG), Department of Defense Gulf War Illness Research Program (GWIRP) W81XWH-20-1-0579 (AG) and Vision Research Program (VRP) W81XWH-20-1-0820 (AG), National Eye Institute R01EY026174 (AG) and R61EY032468 (AG).

Conflict of Interest Authors Jason Greenfield, Wathanee Sripawadkul, Anat Galor, and Carol L. Karp declare that they have no conflict of interest.

References

1. Mittal R, Rath S, Vemuganti GK. Ocular surface squamous neoplasia – review of etio-pathogenesis and an update on clinico-pathological diagnosis. Saudi J Ophthalmol. 2013;27(3):177–86.
2. Margo CE, White AA. Ocular surface squamous neoplasia: terminology that is conceptually friendly but clinically perilous. Eye (Lond). 2014;28(5):507–9.
3. Cicinelli MV, et al. Clinical management of ocular surface squamous neoplasia: a review of the current evidence. Ophthalmol Therapy. 2018;7(2):247–62.
4. Kiire CA, Srinivasan S, Karp CL. Ocular surface squamous neoplasia. Int Ophthalmol Clin. 2010;50(3):35.
5. Gichuhi S, et al. Pathophysiology of ocular surface squamous neoplasia. Exp Eye Res. 2014;129:172–82.
6. Chauhan S, et al. Stratifin in ocular surface squamous neoplasia and its association with p53. Acta Ophthalmol. 2021;99:e1483.
7. Vempuluru VS, et al. Bilateral ocular surface squamous neoplasia: a study of 25 patients and review of literature. Eur J Ophthalmol. 2021;32:11206721211007109.
8. Scott IU, Karp CL, Nuovo GJ. Human papillomavirus 16 and 18 expression in conjunctival intraepithelial neoplasia. Ophthalmology. 2002;109(3):542–7.
9. Karp CL, et al. Conjunctival intraepithelial neoplasia. A possible marker for human immunodeficiency virus infection? Arch Ophthalmol. 1996;114(3):257–61.
10. Carrilho C, et al. p16 expression correlates with invasive ocular surface squamous neoplasms in HIV-infected mozambicans. Ocul Oncol Pathol. 2020;6(2):123–8.
11. Waddell KM, et al. Corneo-conjunctival carcinoma in Uganda. Eye (Lond). 2006;20(8):893–9.
12. Liu Z, et al. Role of optical coherence tomography angiography in the characterization of vascular network patterns of ocular surface squamous neoplasia. Ocul Surf. 2020;18(4):926–35.
13. Galor A, et al. Predictors of ocular surface squamous neoplasia recurrence after excisional surgery. Ophthalmology. 2012;119(10):1974–81.
14. Sayed-Ahmed IO, et al. Diagnosis and medical management of ocular surface squamous neoplasia. Exp Rev Ophthalmol. 2017;12(1):11–9.
15. Nanji AA, et al. Updates in ocular surface tumor diagnostics. Int Ophthalmol Clin. 2017;57(3):47–62.
16. Tananuvat N, et al. Role of impression cytology in diagnosis of ocular surface neoplasia. Cornea. 2008;27(3):269–74.
17. Grossniklaus HE, et al. Aspiration cytology of the conjunctival surface. Acta Cytol. 2003;47(2):239–46.
18. Nolan GR, Hirst LW, Bancroft BJ. The cytomorphology of ocular surface squamous neoplasia by using impression cytology. Cancer. 2001;93(1):60–7.
19. Thomas BJ, et al. Ultra high-resolution anterior segment optical coherence tomography in the diagnosis and management of ocular surface squamous neoplasia. Ocul Surf. 2014;12(1):46–58.
20. Nanji AA, et al. High-resolution optical coherence tomography as an adjunctive tool in the diagnosis of corneal and conjunctival pathology. Ocul Surf. 2015;13(3):226–35.
21. Yim M, et al. Ability of novice clinicians to interpret high-resolution optical coherence tomography for ocular surface lesions. Can J Ophthalmol. 2018;53(2):150–4.
22. Ong SS, Vora GK, Gupta PK. Anterior segment imaging in ocular surface squamous neoplasia. J Ophthalmol. 2016;2016:–5435092.
23. Nguena MB, et al. Diagnosing ocular surface squamous neoplasia in east africa: case-control study of clinical and in vivo confocal microscopy assessment. Ophthalmology. 2014;121(2):484–91.

24. Shields JA, Shields CL, De Potter P. Surgical management of conjunctival tumors. The 1994 Lynn B. McMahan Lecture. Arch Ophthalmol. 1997;115(6):808–15.
25. Mirzayev I, et al. Factors affecting recurrence after surgical treatment in cases with ocular surface squamous neoplasia. Int J Ophthalmol. 2019;12(9):1426–31.
26. Palamar M, et al. Amniotic membrane transplantation in surgical management of ocular surface squamous neoplasias: long-term results. Eye (Lond). 2014;28(9):1131–5.
27. Wong JR, et al. Management of conjunctival malignant melanoma: a review and update. Expert Rev Ophthalmol. 2014;9(3):185–204.
28. Adler E, Turner JR, Stone DU. Ocular surface squamous neoplasia: a survey of changes in the standard of care from 2003 to 2012. Cornea. 2013;32(12):1558–61.
29. Karp CL, et al. Subconjunctival/perilesional recombinant interferon α2b for ocular surface squamous neoplasia: a 10-year review. Ophthalmology. 2010;117(12):2241–6.
30. Karp CL, Moore JK, Rosa RH Jr. Treatment of conjunctival and corneal intraepithelial neoplasia with topical interferon alpha-2b. Ophthalmology. 2001;108(6):1093–8.
31. Kusumesh R, et al. Topical interferon α-2b as a single therapy for primary ocular surface squamous neoplasia. Asia Pac J Ophthalmol (Phila). 2015;4(5):279–82.
32. Venkateswaran N, et al. Comparison of topical 5-fluorouracil and interferon Alfa-2b as primary treatment modalities for ocular surface squamous neoplasia. Am J Ophthalmol. 2019;199:216–22.
33. Kim HJ, et al. Giant ocular surface squamous neoplasia managed with interferon alpha-2b as immunotherapy or immunoreduction. Ophthalmology. 2012;119(5):938–44.
34. Joag MG, et al. Topical 5-fluorouracil 1% as primary treatment for ocular surface squamous neoplasia. Ophthalmology. 2016;123(7):1442–8.
35. Sun Y, Hua R. Long-term efficacy and safety of subconjunctival/perilesional 5-fluorouracil injections for ocular surface squamous neoplasia. Drug Des Devel Ther. 2020;14:5659–65.
36. Chaugule SS, Park J, Finger PT. Topical chemotherapy for giant ocular surface squamous neoplasia of the conjunctiva and cornea: is surgery necessary? Indian J Ophthalmol. 2018;66(1):55–60.
37. Kusumesh R, et al. Retrospective comparative study of topical interferon α2b versus mitomycin C for primary ocular surface squamous neoplasia. Cornea. 2017;36(3):327–31.
38. Al Bayyat G, et al. Update on pharmacotherapy for ocular surface squamous neoplasia. Eye and Vision. 2019;6(1):24.
39. Viani GA, Fendi LI. Adjuvant treatment or primary topical monotherapy for ocular surface squamous neoplasia: a systematic review. Arq Bras Oftalmol. 2017;80(2):131–6.
40. Gloor P, Alexandrakis G. Clinical characterization of primary acquired melanosis. Invest Ophthalmol Vis Sci. 1995;36(8):1721–9.
41. Shields JA, et al. Primary acquired melanosis of the conjunctiva: experience with 311 eyes. Trans Am Ophthalmol Soc. 2007;105:61–72.
42. Damato B, Coupland SE. Conjunctival melanoma and melanosis: a reappraisal of terminology, classification and staging. Clin Experiment Ophthalmol. 2008;36(8):786–95.
43. Wong JR, et al. Management of conjunctival malignant melanoma: a review and update. Exp Rev Ophthalmol. 2014;9(3):185–204.
44. Shields JA, Shields CL. Eyelid, conjunctival, and orbital tumors: an atlas and textbook. Lippincott Williams & Wilkins; 2008.
45. DĘBicka-Kumela M, et al. The evaluation of the malignant characteristics of conjunctival lesions based on the dermatoscopic algorithm. Anticancer Res. 2021;41(2):895.
46. Oellers P, Karp CL. Management of pigmented conjunctival lesions. Ocul Surf. 2012;10(4):251–63.
47. Paridaens AD, McCartney AC, Hungerford JL. Multifocal amelanotic conjunctival melanoma and acquired melanosis sine pigmento. Br J Ophthalmol. 1992;76(3):163.
48. Alzahrani YA, et al. Primary acquired melanosis: clinical, histopathologic and optical coherence tomographic correlation. Ocular Oncol Pathol. 2016;2(3):123–7.
49. Cohen VML, O'Day RF. Management issues in conjunctival tumours: conjunctival melanoma and primary acquired melanosis. Ophthalmol Therapy. 2019;8(4):501–10.

50. Vora GK, et al. Advances in the management of conjunctival melanoma. Surv Ophthalmol. 2017;62(1):26–42.
51. Paridaens AD, et al. Prognostic factors in primary malignant melanoma of the conjunctiva: a clinicopathological study of 256 cases. Br J Ophthalmol. 1994;78(4):252–9.
52. Shields CL, et al. Conjunctival melanoma: risk factors for recurrence, exenteration, metastasis, and death in 150 consecutive patients. Arch Ophthalmol. 2000;118(11):1497–507.
53. Chang AE, Karnell LH, Menck HR. The national cancer data base report on cutaneous and noncutaneous melanoma: a summary of 84,836 cases from the past decade. The American College of Surgeons Commission on Cancer and the American Cancer Society. Cancer. 1998;83(8):1664–78.
54. Shields CL, et al. Conjunctival tumors in 5002 cases. comparative analysis of benign versus malignant counterparts. The 2016 James D. Allen Lecture. Am J Ophthalmol. 2017;173:106–33.
55. Hu DN, et al. Population-based incidence of conjunctival melanoma in various races and ethnic groups and comparison with other melanomas. Am J Ophthalmol. 2008;145(3):418–23.
56. Zeng Y, et al. Clinical treatment options for early-stage and advanced conjunctival melanoma. Surv Ophthalmol. 2021;66(3):461–70.
57. Tuomaala S, Kivelä T. Conjunctival melanoma: is it increasing in the United States? Am J Ophthalmol. 2003;136(6):1189–90. author reply 1190
58. Yu GP, et al. Conjunctival melanoma: is it increasing in the United States? Am J Ophthalmol. 2003;135(6):800–6.
59. Folberg R, McLean IW, Zimmerman LE. Malignant melanoma of the conjunctiva. Hum Pathol. 1985;16(2):136–43.
60. Jain P, et al. Conjunctival melanoma treatment outcomes in 288 patients: a multicentre international data-sharing study. Br J Ophthalmol. 2020;105:1358.
61. Larsen AC, et al. A retrospective review of conjunctival melanoma presentation, treatment, and outcome and an investigation of features associated with BRAF mutations. JAMA Ophthalmol. 2015;133(11):1295–303.
62. Pacheco RR, et al. Conjunctival melanoma: outcomes based on tumour origin in 629 patients at a single ocular oncology centre. Eye (Lond). 2021;36:603.
63. Shields CL, et al. Conjunctival melanoma: outcomes based on tumor origin in 382 consecutive cases. Ophthalmology. 2011;118(2):389–95.
64. Vaidya S, et al. Conjunctival melanoma: Risk factors for recurrent or new tumor in 540 patients at a single ocular oncology center. Eur J Ophthalmol. 2020;31:1120672120970393.
65. Kastelan S, et al. Conjunctival melanoma – epidemiological trends and features. Pathol Oncol Res. 2018;24(4):787–96.
66. Shields CL, et al. Conjunctival nevi: clinical features and natural course in 410 consecutive patients. Arch Ophthalmol. 2004;122(2):167–75.
67. Shields JA, et al. Primary acquired melanosis of the conjunctiva: experience with 311 eyes. Trans Am Ophthalmol Soc. 2007;105:61–71.
68. Brouwer NJ, et al. Conjunctival melanoma: new insights in tumour genetics and immunology, leading to new therapeutic options. Prog Retin Eye Res. 2021;86:100971.
69. Griewank KG, et al. Conjunctival melanomas harbor BRAF and NRAS mutations and copy number changes similar to cutaneous and mucosal melanomas. Clin Cancer Res. 2013;19(12):3143–52.
70. Sheng X, et al. Prognostic factors for conjunctival melanoma: a study in ethnic Chinese patients. Br J Ophthalmol. 2015;99(7):990–6.
71. Westekemper H, et al. Expression of HSP 90, PTEN and Bcl-2 in conjunctival melanoma. Br J Ophthalmol. 2011;95(6):853–8.
72. Shields CL, Shields JA. Ocular melanoma: relatively rare but requiring respect. Clin Dermatol. 2009;27(1):122–33.
73. Zhou C, et al. Conjunctival melanoma in chinese patients: local recurrence, metastasis, mortality, and comparisons with caucasian patients. Invest Ophthalmol Vis Sci. 2017;58(12):5452–9.

74. Shields CL, et al. Conjunctival melanoma: outcomes based on the american joint committee on cancer clinical classification (8th Edition) of 425 patients at a single ocular oncology center. Asia Pac J Ophthalmol (Phila). 2020;10(2):146–51.
75. Tuomaala S, et al. Population-based assessment of clinical characteristics predicting outcome of conjunctival melanoma in whites. Invest Ophthalmol Vis Sci. 2002;43(11):3399–408.
76. Amin MB, et al., editors. AJCC cancer staging manual. 8th ed. Springer International Publishing; 2017. p. 1032.
77. Esmaeli B, et al. Greater tumor thickness, ulceration, and positive sentinel lymph node are associated with worse prognosis in patients with conjunctival melanoma: implications for future AJCC classifications. Am J Surg Pathol. 2019;43(12):1701–10.
78. Jain P, et al. Multicenter, international assessment of the eighth edition of the american joint committee on cancer cancer staging manual for conjunctival melanoma. JAMA Ophthalmol. 2019;137(8):905–11.
79. Damato B, Coupland SE. An audit of conjunctival melanoma treatment in Liverpool. Eye (Lond). 2009;23(4):801–9.
80. Li Y, Fan X, Jia R. Conjunctival melanoma: update on management. Int Ophthalmol Clin. 2019;59(2):27–35.
81. Venkateswaran N, Sripawadkul W, Karp CL. The role of imaging technologies for ocular surface tumors. Curr Opin Ophthalmol. 2021;32(4):369–78.
82. Bianciotto C, et al. Assessment of anterior segment tumors with ultrasound biomicroscopy versus anterior segment optical coherence tomography in 200 cases. Ophthalmology. 2011;118(7):1297–302.
83. Shields JA, Shields CL, De Potter P. Surgical management of circumscribed conjunctival melanomas. Ophthalmic Plast Reconstr Surg. 1998;14(3):208–15.
84. Shields CL, et al. Conjunctival tumors: review of clinical features, risks, biomarkers, and outcomes – the 2017 J. Donald M. Gass lecture. Asia Pac J Ophthalmol (Phila). 2017;6(2):109–20.
85. Knowles DM, et al. Lymphoid hyperplasia and malignant lymphoma occurring in the ocular adnexa (orbit, conjunctiva, and eyelids): a prospective multiparametric analysis of 108 cases during 1977 to 1987. Hum Pathol. 1990;21(9):959–73.
86. Cohen VML, et al. The use of strontium-90 Beta radiotherapy as adjuvant treatment for conjunctival melanoma. J Oncol. 2013;2013:–349162.
87. Brouwer NJ, et al. Management of conjunctival melanoma with local excision and adjuvant brachytherapy. Eye. 2021;35(2):490–8.
88. Walsh-Conway N, Conway RM. Plaque brachytherapy for the management of ocular surface malignancies with corneoscleral invasion. Clin Experiment Ophthalmol. 2009;37(6):577–83.
89. Finger PT, Pavlick AC. Checkpoint inhibition immunotherapy for advanced local and systemic conjunctival melanoma: a clinical case series. J Immunother Cancer. 2019;7(1):83.
90. Kirkegaard MM, et al. Malignant lymphoma of the conjunctiva. Surv Ophthalmol. 2015;60(5):444–58.
91. Mannis MJ. Cornea fundamentals, diagnosis and management. 4th ed. Edinburgh: Elsevier; 2016.
92. Ferry JA, et al. Lymphoma of the ocular adnexa: a study of 353 cases. Am J Surg Pathol. 2007;31(2):170–84.
93. Tanenbaum RE, et al. Classification, diagnosis, and management of conjunctival lymphoma. Eye Vis (Lond). 2019;6:22.
94. Chan CC, et al. Helicobacter pylori (H. pylori) molecular signature in conjunctival mucosa-associated lymphoid tissue (MALT) lymphoma. Histol Histopathol. 2004;19(4):1219–26.
95. Ferreri AJ, et al. Evidence for an association between Chlamydia psittaci and ocular adnexal lymphomas. J Natl Cancer Inst. 2004;96(8):586–94.
96. Ferreri AJM, et al. Clinical implications of hepatitis C virus infection in MALT-type lymphoma of the ocular adnexa. Ann Oncol. 2006;17(5):769–72.
97. Lee S-B, Yang J-W, Kim C-S. The association between conjunctival MALT lymphoma and Helicobacter pylori. Br J Ophthalmol. 2008;92(4):534.
98. Shields CL, et al. Conjunctival lymphoid tumors: clinical analysis of 117 cases and relationship to systemic lymphoma. Ophthalmology. 2001;108(5):979–84.

99. Seker M, et al. Bilateral conjunctival MALT lymphoma mimicking chronic conjunctivitis. Onkologie. 2010;33(6):317–20.
100. Kirkegaard MM, et al. Conjunctival lymphoma – an international multicenter retrospective study. JAMA Ophthalmol. 2016;134(4):406–14.
101. Knudsen MKH, et al. Clinicopathological features of ocular adnexal mantle-cell lymphoma in an international multicenter cohort. JAMA Ophthalmol. 2017;135(12):1367–74.
102. Graue GF, et al. Ocular adnexal lymphoma staging and treatment: American Joint Committee on Cancer versus Ann Arbor. Eur J Ophthalmol. 2013;23(3):344–55.
103. Yen MT, et al. Treatments for ocular adnexal lymphoma: a report by the American academy of ophthalmology. Ophthalmology. 2018;125(1):127–36.
104. Venkateswaran N, et al. The use of high resolution anterior segment optical coherence tomography for the characterization of conjunctival lymphoma, conjunctival amyloidosis and benign reactive lymphoid hyperplasia. Eye Vis (Lond). 2019;6:17.
105. Mikkelsen LH, Würtz NS, Heegaard S. Recent advances in treating extra-ocular lymphomas. Exp Rev Ophthalmol. 2018;13(4):205–17.
106. Niwa M, et al. Radiotherapy alone for stage IE ocular adnexal mucosa-associated lymphoid tissue lymphomas: long-term results. Radiat Oncol. 2020;15(1):25.
107. Yahalom J, et al. Modern radiation therapy for extranodal lymphomas: field and dose guidelines from the International Lymphoma Radiation Oncology Group. Int J Radiat Oncol Biol Phys. 2015;92(1):11–31.
108. Decaudin D, et al. Ocular adnexal lymphoma: a review of clinicopathologic features and treatment options. Blood. 2006;108(5):1451–60.
109. Platt S, et al. Extranodal marginal zone lymphoma of ocular adnexa: outcomes following radiation therapy. Ocul Oncol Pathol. 2017;3(3):181–7.
110. Lee GI, et al. Low-dose radiation therapy for primary conjunctival marginal zone B-cell lymphoma. Cancer Res Treat. 2018;50(2):575–81.
111. Rasmussen PK, et al. Ocular adnexal follicular lymphoma: a multicenter international study. JAMA Ophthalmol. 2014;132(7):851–8.
112. Rasmussen PK, et al. Follicular lymphoma of the ocular adnexal region: a nation-based study. Acta Ophthalmol. 2015;93(2):184–91.
113. Pinnix CC, et al. Ultra-low-dose radiotherapy for definitive management of ocular adnexal B-cell lymphoma. Head Neck. 2017;39(6):1095–100.
114. Fasola CE, et al. Low-dose radiation therapy (2 Gy × 2) in the treatment of orbital lymphoma. Int J Radiat Oncol Biol Phys. 2013;86(5):930–5.
115. Sassone M, Ponzoni M, Ferreri AJ. Ocular adnexal marginal zone lymphoma: clinical presentation, pathogenesis, diagnosis, prognosis, and treatment. Best Pract Res Clin Haematol. 2017;30(1–2):118–30.
116. Ferreri AJ, et al. Bacteria-eradicating therapy with doxycycline in ocular adnexal MALT lymphoma: a multicenter prospective trial. J Natl Cancer Inst. 2006;98(19):1375–82.
117. Govi S, et al. Six-month oral clarithromycin regimen is safe and active in extranodal marginal zone B-cell lymphomas: final results of a single-centre phase II trial. Br J Haematol. 2010;150(2):226–9.
118. Blasi MA, et al. Intralesional interferon-α for conjunctival mucosa-associated lymphoid tissue lymphoma: long-term results. Ophthalmology. 2012;119(3):494–500.
119. Lachapelle KR, et al. Treatment of conjunctival mucosa-associated lymphoid tissue lymphoma with intralesional injection of interferon alfa-2b. Arch Ophthalmol. 2000;118(2):284–5.
120. Svendsen FH, Heegaard S. Lymphoma of the eyelid. Surv Ophthalmol. 2017;62(3):312–31.
121. Baldini L, et al. Treatment and prognosis in a series of primary extranodal lymphomas of the ocular adnexa. Ann Oncol. 1998;9(7):779–81.
122. Matsuo T, Yoshino T. Long-term follow-up results of observation or radiation for conjunctival malignant lymphoma. Ophthalmology. 2004;111(6):1233–7.
123. Atallah M, et al. Role of high resolution optical coherence tomography in diagnosing ocular surface squamous neoplasia with coexisting ocular surface diseases. Ocul Surf. 2017;15(4):688–95.

Artificial Intelligence for Corneal Disorders

14

Rohan Bir Singh, Uday Pratap Singh Parmar, Shawn Lin, and Hajirah N. Saeed

Summary

- Artificial intelligence platforms in various stages of development have shown high accuracy in the diagnosis and severity grading of corneal disorders.
- A standardized methodology and approach is required for swift progression and adoption of AI-based platforms in clinical settings.
- Machine learning algorithms should include heterogenous data for training to ensure high reliability and large-scale adoptability by the ophthal in eye clinics.

14.1 Introduction

Recent advances in artificial intelligence (AI) are rapidly transforming the diagnostics and management of disease across various specialties in medicine. As in other specialties, the application of AI in ophthalmology has significantly increased its

R. B. Singh · U. P. S. Parmar
Department of Ophthalmology, Massachusetts Eye and Ear, Harvard Medical School, Boston, MA, USA
e-mail: rohan_singh@meei.harvard.edu

S. Lin
Jules Stein Eye Institute, David Geffen School of Medicine at University of California at Los Angeles, Los Angeles, CA, USA
e-mail: slin@jsei.ucla.edu

H. N. Saeed (✉)
Department of Ophthalmology and Visual Sciences, Illinois Eye and Ear Infirmary, University of Illinois Chicago, Chicago, IL, USA

Department of Ophthalmology, Massachusetts Eye and Ear Infirmary, Harvard Medical School, Boston, MA, USA

Department of Ophthalmology, Loyola University Medical Center, Maywood, IL, USA
e-mail: hnsaeed@uic.edu

H. N. Saeed, R. B. Singh (eds.), *Corneal Disorders*, Current Practices in Ophthalmology, https://doi.org/10.1007/978-981-96-5294-5_14

footprint over the last several years. Newly developed AI-based platforms hold promise for wide adoption in ophthalmology due to the field's reliance on and utilization of imaging modalities for diagnosis and quantification of disease severity in day-to-day practice. Imaging-based diagnostic AI models focused on glaucoma, macular degeneration, and diabetic retinopathy have significantly evolved over the past decade, with clinical adoption imminent after the approval of the first AI-based autonomous diagnostic model for diabetic retinopathy by the US Food and Drug Administration [1–4]. Similar models for the diagnosis, quantification, and management of corneal disease are also rapidly developing.

Image preprocessing is a critical multistep process for AI applications in ophthalmology (Fig. 14.1). It involves various techniques to enhance the quality of images, making them suitable for further analysis and improving the accuracy of diagnostic models. Image preprocessing includes 1. image resizing to ensure that all images have a uniform size, which is important for training AI models; 2. image normalization to adjust the intensity values of images to a standard range, typically [0, 1] or [−1, 1], which helps reduce the impact of varying lighting conditions and contrast in the images; 3. image augmentation to apply transformations like rotation, flipping, zooming, and cropping to create variations of the original images; 4. noise reduction techniques to remove noise from images; 5. histogram equalization to adjust the contrast of the image by distributing intensity values more evenly to enhance the visibility of certain features in the image; 6. color space conversion to convert images from one color space to another (e.g., RGB to grayscale or HSV); 7. image segmentation to separate the image into different regions based on characteristics like intensity, color, or texture; 8. feature extraction to identify and extract key features from the image that are relevant for diagnosis; 9. registration to align images taken at different times or from different modalities to ensure that the images are comparable and that changes over time can be accurately detected; 10. image enhancement techniques like sharpening, contrast adjustment, and denoising to enhance the visual quality of images; and 11. removal of unwanted artifacts, such as reflections and shadows, that may have been introduced during image acquisition.

While a detailed discussion of algorithm platforms and model development is beyond the scope of this chapter, the clinician should know that various algorithms and machine learning models can be used to process raw data to predict outcomes [5]. The choice of algorithm will affect output and all have their benefits and drawbacks. Common algorithms in medicine and ophthalmology include neural networks (which include artificial neural networks, convoluted neural networks, and multilayer perceptron among others), support vector machines, tree-based classification and regression, and random forests [6, 7]. These are all mentioned below for specific models that have been trained. Each of these algorithms may have subsets of architectures that can further affect output, and no one platform universally performs the best in clinical ophthalmology.

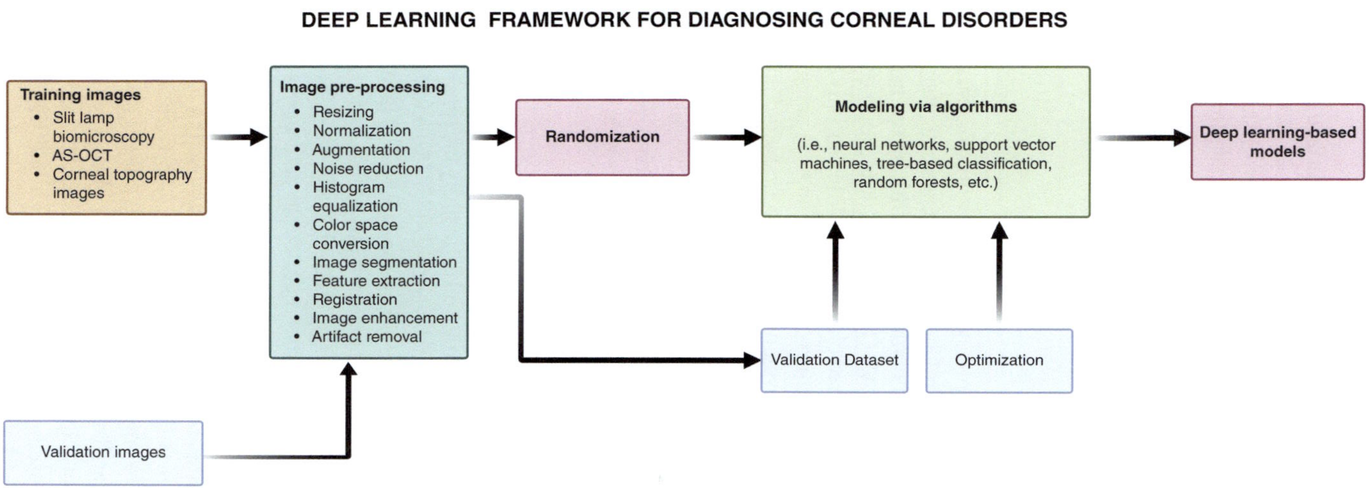

Fig. 14.1 Depiction of a deep learning framework for model development utilizing imaging modalities as the starting point. *AS-OCT* anterior segment optical coherence tomography

14.2 Dry Eye Disease

Dry eye disease (DED) is a disorder of the ocular surface that can present with an array of clinical signs and symptoms. Due to the multifactorial nature of DED, its diagnosis can be challenging for the ophthalmologist [8]. Moreover, there are no universally adopted and standardized diagnostic modalities for DED, and clinical presentation and symptomatology do not always correlate with disease quantification methods [9]. Therefore, AI-based modalities have the potential to aid in DED diagnosis and quantification of disease severity.

14.2.1 Diagnosis of DED

Recent studies have utilized complex neural networks (CNN) for the diagnosis of DED. An algorithm developed by Chase and colleagues to diagnose DED by detecting patterns in the corneal epithelium and tear film layers using anterior segment optical coherence tomography (AS-OCT) images was observed to be more accurate in DED diagnosis than established clinical modalities such as corneal and conjunctival fluorescein staining and Schirmer test, with an 85% accuracy, 86% sensitivity, and 82% specificity [10]. However, diagnostic accuracy did not correlate with ocular surface disease index score or tear breakup time. A set of CNN models developed by Maruoka and colleagues utilized confocal imaging for diagnosing meibomian gland dysfunction. The highly accurate models had an area under the curve of 0.981 when used in an ensemble configuration (i.e., combining multiple machine learning models) and 0.966 when used in a single configuration [11].

14.2.2 Assessing DED Severity

Recently, CNN models have been deployed to quantify the severity of DED. Recently, a slit-lamp photography–based model was utilized by Su and colleagues to quantify disease severity based on the grade of keratopathy [12]. The authors reported 97% accuracy in detecting keratopathy. However, this model had less than 80% sensitivity and specificity in determining the clinical grade of disease. A similar model assessing punctate epithelial erosions reported an area under the curve (AUC) of 0.940 and 77% grading accuracy [13]. Despite the relatively lower grading accuracy, the scores had strong clinical correlation with the slit-lamp images.

Other imaging-based parameters have also been used in the assessment of DED severity. Stegmann and colleagues used AS-OCT to train a CNN model for the quantification of low tear meniscus height through direct tear meniscus segmentation or evaluation of localized regions of interest [14]. They reported an accuracy, sensitivity, and specificity of >93% for both approaches. However, a custom-built AS-OCT system was used, making wide adoption and translation difficult. Deng and colleagues developed a CNN model based on corneal topography images for the quantification of tear meniscus height and reported sensitivity and F1 scores of

90% [15]. Wei and colleagues trained a CNN model to quantify subbasal corneal nerve fibers using confocal images and reported an AUC of 0.96 [16]. Several new models in various stages of development have also been used to quantify the extent of meibomian gland dysfunction by using meibography images [17–20].

14.3 Infectious Keratitis

Infectious keratitis is one of the leading causes of vision loss globally [21]. The diagnosis and management of infectious keratitis is often clinically challenging due to delayed patient presentation, suboptimal detection of underlying infectious etiology, no standardized staging or grading systems for disease, and a lack of tools to accurately assess the progression of corneal ulceration. Therefore, the development of AI-based platforms with high accuracy can aid the ophthalmologist in early and accurate disease detection and monitoring of disease progression.

14.3.1 Diagnosis Infectious Keratitis

Current AI models are primarily focused on the diagnosis of infectious keratitis as well as the identification of underlying etiologies. In 2003, Saini and colleagues evaluated the effectiveness of an artificial neural network (ANN) for classifying infectious keratitis. They trained a three-layer feed-forward neural network using input variables from 63 known bacterial or fungal ulcers. This trained neural network was then used to classify an additional set of 43 corneal ulcers. The ANN successfully classified all 63 ulcers in the training set and accurately identified 39 out of 43 ulcers in the test set. The specificity for bacterial and fungal categories was 76.47% and 100%, respectively. The neural network achieved an overall classification accuracy of 90.7%, significantly higher than the clinicians' predicted accuracy of 62.8% ($p < 0.01$) [22]. Using slit-lamp and smartphone photographs, Li and colleagues used a purpose-optimized, preexisting CNN to differentiate infectious keratitis from other corneal pathologies with an AUC of 0.998 [23]. Using heterogeneous data (slit-lamp photography) from the United States and India, Tiwari and colleagues deployed a trained CNN to differentiate infectious keratitis ulceration from healed scars. They trained and tested their algorithm using slit-lamp images from the Steroids for Corneal Ulcer Trial (SCUT), Mycotic Ulcer Treatment Trial (MUTT), and Byers Eye Institute at Stanford University. They reported an AUC of >0.94 [24]. Gu and colleagues developed a deep learning algorithm, which was trained using a dataset of 5325 ocular surface images. The algorithm's performance was then tested against 10 ophthalmologists using a prospective dataset consisting of 510 outpatients newly diagnosed with various corneal pathologies. The algorithm achieved an AUC of 0.930 for infectious keratitis, 0.934 for noninfectious keratitis, and 0.951 for a normal ocular surface [25]. Recently, a CNN model was used to diagnose 89 different corneal disorders by Xu and colleagues using slit-lamp photography [26]. The authors reported an accuracy of 80%, but the model fell short while differentiating the etiologic organisms based on presenting ophthalmological features. However, a CNN model trained on a larger dataset by Wang and colleagues was not only able to diagnose microbial keratitis but also able to detect the etiologic organisms and had an AUC of 0.959 and greater accuracy when compared to diagnosis by an ophthalmologist [27].

14.3.2 Detecting Etiology in Infectious Keratitis

Accurate detection of causative organisms based solely on clinical examination is often challenging for ophthalmologists due to a large degree of overlapping presentations. Additionally, polymicrobial infections and varying immune responses to infectious organisms further complicate diagnosis [28, 29]. This can lead to incorrect diagnoses and delays in the management of patients with infectious keratitis.

AI algorithms have been designed to help ophthalmologists to not only diagnose infectious keratitis but also detect the underlying organisms causing it. Using slit-lamp photographs, Koyama and colleagues trained a model to differentiate between bacterial, fungal, viral, and *Acanthamoeba* keratitis. The authors reported an 88% and 90% accuracy for multiclass and organism-type differentiation, respectively [30]. Conversely, Redd and colleagues reported significantly lower accuracy in a CNN model trained to differentiate between fungal and bacterial keratitis [31]. Their model had an 81% sensitivity when differentiating fungal from bacterial keratitis and 75% sensitivity vice versa, with an AUC of 0.81. In a similar approach using an ensemble CNN, Ghosh and colleagues reported a 77% sensitivity and 83% F1 score [32].

Several researchers have also explored the application of CNNs using confocal imaging for greater sensitivity and accuracy. Two studies that trained CNNs using confocal imaging for fungal keratitis reported high accuracies of 96% and 99.9% [33, 34]. Furthermore, Lv and colleagues used gradient-weighted class activation mapping to provide further insights by identifying fungal hyphae [34].

14.4 Keratoconus

Keratoconus (KCN) is an ectatic disorder characterized by the progressive thinning of the cornea [35]. The extent and area of the anatomical alterations in the cornea result in mild to severe loss of vision due to myopic shift, irregular astigmatism, and corneal opacity. The prevalence of the disease ranges from 1:500 to 1:2000 individuals [36]. Diagnosis is often delayed in KCN as the early form (i.e., forme fruste KCN) is asymptomatic, and visual symptoms often present in the later stages of the disease. Currently, the mainstay of diagnosis revolves around imaging techniques such as three-dimensional topographic imaging, Placido disk-based topographic imaging, and anterior segment optical coherence tomographic (AS-OCT) imaging systems. Various AI-based platforms in different stages of development have been trained using corneal topography images.

14.4.1 Early Diagnosis of KCN

Several trained CNN models have been deployed to differentiate between KCN, forme fruste KCN, and normal corneas based on corneal topography (Fig. 14.2). A hybrid CNN deep learning model was trained to identify features of KCN and then used in training a support vector machine to diagnose the disorder [37]. The authors reported an accuracy of 92% in detecting KCN compared to normal eyes. However, this model could only achieve 69% accuracy in differentiating between normal corneas, suspected KCN, and KCN patients. Abdelmotaal and colleagues reported an accuracy of 99% in differentiating between normal, KCN, and forme fruste corneas using corneal topographic images [38]. Meanwhile, a deep learning–based model using Pentacam (Oculus, Wetzlar, Germany) images demonstrated an accuracy of 95% [39]. Another CNN-based model trained by Zeboulon and colleagues to detect KCN from normal and post-refractive surgery eyes had 99% accuracy [40]. Shi and colleagues used multimodal imaging (corneal tomography and OCT) to differentiate between normal and forme fruste KCN and reported an AUC of 0.93 [41].

The rationale behind detecting forme fruste KCN over KCN is early diagnosis and management of the disorder before the clinical symptoms become apparent. Kuo and colleagues reported high AUC (>0.95) in three CNN-based models trained to detect normal, forme fruste KCN, and KCN corneas using corneal topography images [42]. The diagnosis of forme fruste KCN by the algorithm was performed by detecting established features of the disorder including the presence of a central cone, steepening of the cornea in the inferior quadrant, and asymmetric bowtie. Castro-Luna and colleagues used a random forest model, a machine learning technique for classification based on the construction of thousands of decision trees, to classify and predict subclinical KCN, and had an accuracy of 89% [43]. In a similar study, Cao and colleagues tested the diagnostic performance of models built from eight different machine learning methods after adding various clinical measures, such as axial length, graphic parameters, and spherical equivalent, to topographic data. The greatest AUC (0.97) was obtained by the random forest model and the

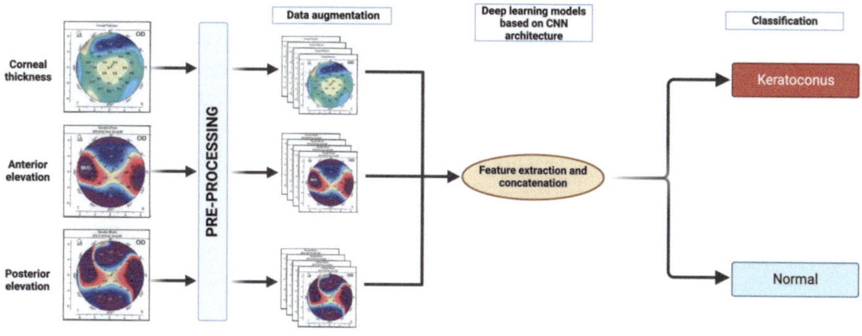

Fig. 14.2 Step-by-step processing of topography images depicting corneal thickness and anterior and posterior elevation in a model utilizing CNNs in the diagnosis of keratoconus. *CNN* convolutional neural network

highest sensitivity (0.94) and specificity (0.90) by the support vector machine and the k-nearest neighbor model, respectively [44]. In addition, Aatila and colleagues also found a random forest model to have the highest accuracy compared to other models for mild (98%) vs severe (95%) KCN, respectively [45].

14.4.2 KCN Grading

Malyugin and colleagues used a machine learning model based on the Amsler–Krumeich classification system, employing AS-OCT and visual acuity data to classify the severity of KCN [46]. The authors reported variable accuracy for different stages of KCN. The highest accuracy was reported for stage 4 of the disease (97%), whereas the lowest accuracy was reported for forme fruste KCN, with an AUC ranging between 0.95 to 1.00 for all stages. Ghaderi and colleagues trained an ensemble CNN using measurement data from AS-OCT and achieved 98% accuracy in differentiating between various stages of KCN [47]. Kamiya and colleagues reported 79% accuracy in the diagnosis and staging of KCN using topography images, whereas Chen and colleagues reported a comparatively higher (93%) accuracy using a similar dataset [48, 49].

14.4.3 KCN Progression

Several studies have been conducted to assess the progression of KCN using tomographic imaging; however, the classification of disease progression varies significantly among researchers. Kamiya and colleagues were the first to train a CNN model using AS-OCT images [50]. This model could differentiate progression from non-progression with 79% accuracy. The authors reported that posterior elevation map analysis was the most reliable parameter for detecting progression, whereas the pachymetry map had the lowest reliability. Kato and colleagues reported an AUC of 0.814 in a model trained to evaluate disease progression and the need for crosslinking using AS-OCT and demographic data [51]. Similarly, Yousefi and colleagues trained a machine learning model to predict the need for corneal transplantation in KCN patients using AS-OCT images. The algorithm was developed using multiple tomography, topography, and pachymetry parameters and was trained on 3156 eyes. During testing, their ML algorithm showed a specificity of 97.4% and a sensitivity of 96.3% [52].

14.4.4 KCN Prognosis

AI has been utilized to predict the outcomes of KCN management. A study by Valdés-Mas and colleagues introduced a novel machine learning approach to forecast vision improvement in KCN patients following intracorneal ring implantation. Vision enhancement was evaluated through the metrics of corneal curvature and astigmatism.

The best results were obtained using an artificial neural network based on a multilayer perceptron (i.e., consisting of multiple layers of neurons), but with a mean absolute error of 29% of the standard deviation for corneal curvature and 46% for astigmatism. Though the mean absolute error (MAE) is high, they correspond to 0.98D and 1D, respectively. Coupled with the range of dioptric power and astigmatism in KCN and high correlation coefficient of 0.93, the model may be a good predictor of outcome and likely needs further refinement and more robust data points [53].

14.5 Fuchs Endothelial Dystrophy

Fuchs endothelial dystrophy (FED) is a progressive hereditary corneal disorder characterized by the gradual, progressive deterioration of endothelial cells, resulting in the formation of guttae, which are excrescences of Descemet's membrane [54]. Several advanced AI algorithms have been developed to diagnose the disorder and detect its severity and progression using tools such as specular microscopy and AS-OCT to evaluate corneal endothelial cell count, thickness, and haze.

14.5.1 Detection of Fuchs Endothelial Dystrophy

The first model to diagnose FED without clinically apparent corneal edema was trained by Eleiwa and colleagues with AS-OCT images [53]. The authors reported an AUC of 0.97 in differentiating healthy corneas from early and late FED. In another CNN model, an AUC of 0.994 and 99% accuracy were reported using corneal edema as the feature of interest in AS-OCT images, for differentiating between FED and other corneal disorders with a similar presentation [55].

14.5.2 Assessing the Severity of FED

A few CNN models have been developed to assess the severity of FED by assessing corneal endothelial cell counts and their morphology based on specular microscopy imaging. Shilpashree and colleagues reported an AUC of 0.967 and 88% accuracy in detecting corneal endothelial cell density, cellular morphology variation, and guttae percentage [56].

14.6 Other Applications of AI in Cornea

14.6.1 Corneal Nerves

The cornea is one of the most densely innervated tissues in the human body [57]. The correlation between the morphometric parameters of corneal nerves (such as tortuosity and density) and various systemic diseases (like diabetic neuropathy) has been widely studied [58–60]. However, most current methods for quantifying corneal nerve parameters rely on manual or semiautomatic tracing of nerve fibers, a tedious and time-consuming process that lacks reproducibility. The development of AI-based algorithms for the rapid and reliable analysis of corneal nerves can be helpful in the screening and diagnosis of large cohorts of patients with these diseases.

Williams and colleagues developed a deep learning algorithm to aid in the diagnosis of diabetic neuropathy by quantifying nerve fiber properties. They trained and tested their algorithm using 1698 and 2137 corneal confocal microscopy images, respectively [61]. They reported an AUC of 0.83, specificity of 87%, and sensitivity of 68% for the classification of patients as with or without neuropathy. Scarpa and colleagues used a convolutional neural network system to classify images of the subbasal nerve plexus from healthy and diabetic subjects with neuropathy and reported a classification accuracy of 96% [62].

14.7 Conclusion

The past decade has seen rapid progression and application of AI in the field of ophthalmology. In this chapter, we highlighted recent developments in AI to aid in the diagnosis of major corneal disorders. Over the past few years, AI-based platforms have swiftly progressed from solely diagnosing corneal disorders to accurately grading and staging the severity of disease. However, most of these models are still in preclinical stages. Several hurdles remain before these models can be widely adopted in clinical practice. The primary limiting factor is the lack of reporting standardization and the resultant lack of trust in the modality by ophthalmologists.. Standardization will improve the transparency, validity, and comparability of algorithms and can help reduce this lack of trust [63]. Clinical trials are also needed to confirm the reliability and accuracy of models. Over time, AI researchers should develop techniques to prevent cross-contamination of data and ensure that variability in data reporting and biases are minimized. Lastly, diverse data sources and images across a diverse patient population must be used to train models to improve real-world performance and in any clinical setting. The swift progression of AI-based platforms in the field of cornea holds the potential to improve patient outcomes and physician workflow efficiency.

References

1. FDA permits marketing of artificial intelligence-based device to detect certain diabetes-related eye problems | FDA n.d.. https://www.fda.gov/news-events/press-announcements/fda-permits-marketing-artificial-intelligence-based-device-detect-certain-diabetes-related-eye. Accessed 31 May 2023.
2. Abràmoff MD, Lou Y, Erginay A, Clarida W, Amelon R, Folk JC, et al. Improved automated detection of diabetic retinopathy on a publicly available dataset through integration of deep learning. Invest Ophthalmol Vis Sci. 2016;57:5200. https://doi.org/10.1167/iovs.16-19964.

3. Ting DSW, Cheung CYL, Lim G, Tan GSW, Quang ND, Gan A, et al. Development and validation of a deep learning system for diabetic retinopathy and related eye diseases using retinal images from multiethnic populations with diabetes. JAMA J Am Med Assoc. 2017;318:2211. https://doi.org/10.1001/jama.2017.18152.
4. De Fauw J, Ledsam JR, Romera-Paredes B, Nikolov S, Tomasev N, Blackwell S, et al. Clinically applicable deep learning for diagnosis and referral in retinal disease. Nat Med. 2018;24:1342. https://doi.org/10.1038/s41591-018-0107-6.
5. Ting DSW, Pasquale LR, Peng L, Campbell JP, Lee AY, Raman R, et al. Artificial intelligence and deep learning in ophthalmology. Br J Ophthalmol. 2019;103:167–75. https://doi.org/10.1136/bjophthalmol-2018-313173.
6. Li JPO, Liu H, Ting DSJ, Jeon S, Chan RVP, Kim JE, et al. Digital technology, tele-medicine and artificial intelligence in ophthalmology: a global perspective. Prog Retin Eye Res. 2021;82:100900. https://doi.org/10.1016/j.preteyeres.2020.100900.
7. Ting DSW, Peng L, Varadarajan AV, Keane PA, Burlina PM, Chiang MF, et al. Deep learning in ophthalmology: the technical and clinical considerations. Prog Retin Eye Res. 2019;72:100759. https://doi.org/10.1016/j.preteyeres.2019.04.003.
8. Craig JP, Nichols KK, Akpek EK, Caffery B, Dua HS, Joo C-KK, et al. TFOS DEWS II definition and classification report. Ocul Surf. 2017;15(3):276–83. https://doi.org/10.1016/j.jtos.2017.05.008.
9. Amparo F, Schaumberg DA, Dana R. Comparison of two questionnaires for dry eye symptom assessment: The ocular surface disease index and the symptom assessment in dry eye. Ophthalmology. 2015;122:1498–503. https://doi.org/10.1016/J.OPHTHA.2015.02.037.
10. Chase C, Elsawy A, Eleiwa T, Ozcan E, Tolba M, Shousha MA. Comparison of autonomous as-oct deep learning algorithm and clinical dry eye tests in diagnosis of dry eye disease. Clin Ophthalmol. 2021;15:4281. https://doi.org/10.2147/OPTH.S321764.
11. Maruoka S, Tabuchi H, Nagasato D, Masumoto H, Chikama T, Kawai A, et al. Deep neural network-based method for detecting obstructive Meibomian gland dysfunction with in vivo laser confocal microscopy. Cornea. 2020;39:720. https://doi.org/10.1097/ICO.0000000000002279.
12. Su TY, Ting PJ, Chang SW, Chen DY. Superficial punctate keratitis grading for dry eye screening using deep convolutional neural networks. IEEE Sensors J. 2020;20:1672. https://doi.org/10.1109/JSEN.2019.2948576.
13. Qu J-H, Qin X-R, Li C-D, Peng R-M, Xiao G-G, Cheng J, et al. Fully automated grading system for the evaluation of punctate epithelial erosions using deep neural networks. Br J Ophthalmol. 2021;107:453. https://doi.org/10.1136/bjophthalmol-2021-319755.
14. Stegmann H, Werkmeister RM, Pfister M, Garhöfer G, Schmetterer L, dos Santos VA. Deep learning segmentation for optical coherence tomography measurements of the lower tear meniscus. Biomed Opt Express. 2020;11:11. https://doi.org/10.1364/boe.386228.
15. Deng X, Tian L, Liu Z, Zhou Y, Jie Y. A deep learning approach for the quantification of lower tear meniscus height. Biomed Signal Process Control. 2021;68:102655. https://doi.org/10.1016/j.bspc.2021.102655.
16. Wei S, Shi F, Wang Y, Chou Y, Li X. A deep learning model for automated sub-basal corneal nerve segmentation and evaluation using in vivo confocal microscopy. Transl Vis Sci Technol. 2020;9:32. https://doi.org/10.1167/tvst.9.2.32.
17. Khan ZK, Umar AI, Shirazi SH, Rasheed A, Qadir A, Gul S. Image based analysis of meibomian gland dysfunction using conditional generative adversarial neural network. BMJ Open Ophthalmol. 2021;6:6. https://doi.org/10.1136/bmjophth-2020-000436.
18. Prabhu SM, Chakiat ASS, Vunnava KP, Shetty R. Deep learning segmentation and quantification of Meibomian glands. Biomed Signal Process Control. 2020;57:101776. https://doi.org/10.1016/J.BSPC.2019.101776.
19. Setu MAK, Horstmann J, Schmidt S, Stern ME, Steven P. Deep learning-based automatic meibomian gland segmentation and morphology assessment in infrared meibography. Sci Rep. 2021;11:11. https://doi.org/10.1038/S41598-021-87314-8.

20. Wang J, Li S, Yeh TN, Chakraborty R, Graham AD, Yu SX, et al. Quantifying Meibomian gland morphology using artificial intelligence. Optom Vis Sci. 2021;98:1094. https://doi.org/10.1097/OPX.0000000000001767.
21. Singh RB, Das S, Chodosh J, Sharma N, Zegans ME, Kowalski RP, et al. Paradox of complex diversity: challenges in the diagnosis and management of bacterial keratitis. Prog Retin Eye Res. 2021;88:101028. https://doi.org/10.1016/J.PRETEYERES.2021.101028.
22. Saini JS, Jain AK, Kumar S, Vikal S, Pankaj S, Singh S. Neural network approach to classify infective keratitis. Curr Eye Res. 2003;27:111–6. https://doi.org/10.1076/ceyr.27.2.111.15949.
23. Li Z, Jiang J, Chen K, Chen Q, Zheng Q, Liu X, et al. Preventing corneal blindness caused by keratitis using artificial intelligence. Nat Commun. 2021;12:12. https://doi.org/10.1038/s41467-021-24116-6.
24. Tiwari M, Piech C, Baitemirova M, Prajna NV, Srinivasan M, Lalitha P, et al. Differentiation of active corneal infections from healed scars using deep learning. Ophthalmology. 2022;129:129. https://doi.org/10.1016/j.ophtha.2021.07.033.
25. Gu H, Guo Y, Gu L, Wei A, Xie S, Ye Z, et al. Deep learning for identifying corneal diseases from ocular surface slit-lamp photographs. Sci Rep. 2020;10:17851. https://doi.org/10.1038/s41598-020-75027-3.
26. Xu Y, Kong M, Xie W, Duan R, Fang Z, Lin Y, et al. Deep sequential feature learning in clinical image classification of infectious keratitis. Engineering. 2021;7:7. https://doi.org/10.1016/j.eng.2020.04.012.
27. Wang L, Chen K, Wen H, Zheng Q, Chen Y, Pu J, et al. Feasibility assessment of infectious keratitis depicted on slit-lamp and smartphone photographs using deep learning. Int J Med Inform. 2021;155:155. https://doi.org/10.1016/j.ijmedinf.2021.104583.
28. Bourcier T, Thomas F, Borderie V, Chaumeil C, Laroche L. Bacterial keratitis: predisposing factors, clinical and microbiological review of 300 cases. Br J Ophthalmol. 2003;87:834–8. https://doi.org/10.1136/bjo.87.7.834.
29. Singh RB, Zhu S, Yung A, Dohlman TH, Dana R, Yin J. Efficacy of cyanoacrylate tissue adhesive in the management of corneal thinning and perforation due to microbial keratitis. Ocular Surface. 2020;18:795–800. https://doi.org/10.1016/j.jtos.2020.08.001.
30. Koyama A, Miyazaki D, Nakagawa Y, Ayatsuka Y, Miyake H, Ehara F, et al. Determination of probability of causative pathogen in infectious keratitis using deep learning algorithm of slit-lamp images. Sci Rep. 2021;11:11. https://doi.org/10.1038/s41598-021-02138-w.
31. Redd TK, Prajna NV, Srinivasan M, Lalitha P, Krishnan T, Rajaraman R, et al. Image-based differentiation of bacterial and fungal keratitis using deep convolutional neural networks. Ophthalmol Science. 2022;2:2. https://doi.org/10.1016/j.xops.2022.100119.
32. Ghosh AK, Thammasudjarit R, Jongkhajornpong P, Attia J, Thakkinstian A. Deep learning for discrimination between fungal keratitis and bacterial keratitis: DeepKeratitis. Cornea. 2022;41:616. https://doi.org/10.1097/ICO.0000000000002830.
33. Liu Z, Cao Y, Li Y, Xiao X, Qiu Q, Yang M, et al. Automatic diagnosis of fungal keratitis using data augmentation and image fusion with deep convolutional neural network. Comput Methods Prog Biomed. 2020;187:187. https://doi.org/10.1016/j.cmpb.2019.105019.
34. Lv J, Zhang K, Chen Q, Chen Q, Huang W, Cui L, et al. Deep learning-based automated diagnosis of fungal keratitis with in vivo confocal microscopy images. Ann Transl Med. 2020;8:706. https://doi.org/10.21037/atm.2020.03.134.
35. Santodomingo-Rubido J, Carracedo G, Suzaki A, Villa-Collar C, Vincent SJ, Wolffsohn JS. Keratoconus: an updated review. Contact Lens Anterior Eye. 2022;45:101578. https://doi.org/10.1016/j.clae.2021.101559.
36. Godefrooij DA, de Wit GA, Uiterwaal CS, Imhof SM, Wisse RPL. Age-specific incidence and prevalence of Keratoconus: a Nationwide registration study. Am J Ophthalmol. 2017;175:169–72. https://doi.org/10.1016/j.ajo.2016.12.015.
37. Al-Timemy AH, Mosa ZM, Alyasseri Z, Lavric A, Lui MM, Hazarbassanov RM, et al. A hybrid deep learning construct for detecting Keratoconus from corneal maps. Transl Vis Sci Technol. 2021;10:16. https://doi.org/10.1167/tvst.10.14.16.

38. Abdelmotaal H, Mostafa MM, Mostafa ANR, Mohamed AA, Abdelazeem K. Classification of color-coded scheimpflug camera corneal tomography images using deep learning. Transl Vis Sci Technol. 2020;9:9. https://doi.org/10.1167/tvst.9.13.30.
39. Feng R, Xu Z, Zheng X, Hu H, Jin X, Chen DZ, et al. KerNet: a novel deep learning approach for Keratoconus and sub-clinical Keratoconus detection based on raw data of the Pentacam HR system. IEEE J Biomed Health Inform. 2021;25:25. https://doi.org/10.1109/JBHI.2021.3079430.
40. Zéboulon P, Debellemanière G, Bouvet M, Gatinel D. Corneal topography raw data classification using a convolutional neural network. Am J Ophthalmol. 2020;219:219. https://doi.org/10.1016/j.ajo.2020.06.005.
41. Shi C, Wang M, Zhu T, Zhang Y, Ye Y, Jiang J, et al. Machine learning helps improve diagnostic ability of subclinical keratoconus using Scheimpflug and OCT imaging modalities. Eye Vision. 2020;7:48. https://doi.org/10.1186/s40662-020-00213-3.
42. Kuo BI, Chang WY, Liao TS, Liu FY, Liu HY, Chu HS, et al. Keratoconus screening based on deep learning approach of corneal topography. Transl Vis Sci Technol. 2020;9:9. https://doi.org/10.1167/tvst.9.2.53.
43. Castro-luna G, Jiménez-rodríguez D, Castaño-fernández AB, Pérez-rueda A. Diagnosis of subclinical keratoconus based on machine learning techniques. J Clin Med. 2021;10:4281. https://doi.org/10.3390/jcm10184281.
44. Cao K, Verspoor K, Sahebjada S, Baird PN. Evaluating the performance of various machine learning algorithms to detect subclinical keratoconus. Transl Vis Sci Technol. 2020;9:24. https://doi.org/10.1167/TVST.9.2.24.
45. Aatila M, Lachgar M, Hamid H, Kartit A. Keratoconus severity classification using features selection and machine learning algorithms. Comput Math Methods Med. 2021;2021:1. https://doi.org/10.1155/2021/9979560.
46. Malyugin B, Sakhnov S, Izmailova S, Boiko E, Pozdeyeva N, Axenova L, et al. Keratoconus diagnostic and treatment algorithms based on machine-learning methods. Diagnostics. 2021;11:1933. https://doi.org/10.3390/diagnostics11101933.
47. Ghaderi M, Sharifi A, Jafarzadeh PE. Proposing an ensemble learning model based on neural network and fuzzy system for keratoconus diagnosis based on Pentacam measurements. Int Ophthalmol. 2021;41:41. https://doi.org/10.1007/s10792-021-01963-2.
48. Kamiya K, Ayatsuka Y, Kato Y, Shoji N, Mori Y, Miyata K. Diagnosability of Keratoconus using deep learning with Placido disk-based corneal topography. Front Med (Lausanne). 2021;8:8. https://doi.org/10.3389/fmed.2021.724902.
49. Chen X, Zhao J, Iselin KC, Borroni D, Romano D, Gokul A, et al. Keratoconus detection of changes using deep learning of colour-coded maps. BMJ Open Ophthalmol. 2021;6:6. https://doi.org/10.1136/bmjophth-2021-000824.
50. Kamiya K, Ayatsuka Y, Kato Y, Shoji N, Miyai T, Ishii H, et al. Prediction of keratoconus progression using deep learning of anterior segment optical coherence tomography maps. Ann Transl Med. 2021;9:10.21037/atm-21-1772.
51. Kato N, Masumoto H, Tanabe M, Sakai C, Negishi K, Torii H, et al. Predicting keratoconus progression and need for corneal crosslinking using deep learning. J Clin Med. 2021;10:10. https://doi.org/10.3390/jcm10040844.
52. Yousefi S, Takahashi H, Hayashi T, Tampo H, Inoda S, Arai Y, et al. Predicting the likelihood of need for future keratoplasty intervention using artificial intelligence. Ocular Surface. 2020;18:320. https://doi.org/10.1016/j.jtos.2020.02.008.
53. Eleiwa T, Elsawy A, Özcan E, Abou SM. Automated diagnosis and staging of Fuchs' endothelial cell corneal dystrophy using deep learning. Eye Vision. 2020;7:7. https://doi.org/10.1186/s40662-020-00209-z.
54. Ong Tone S, Kocaba V, Böhm M, Wylegala A, White TL, Jurkunas UV. Fuchs endothelial corneal dystrophy: the vicious cycle of Fuchs pathogenesis. Prog Retin Eye Res. 2021;80:80. https://doi.org/10.1016/j.preteyeres.2020.100863.

55. Zéboulon P, Ghazal W, Gatinel D. Corneal edema visualization with optical coherence tomography using deep learning: proof of concept. Cornea. 2021;40:40. https://doi.org/10.1097/ICO.0000000000002640.
56. Shilpashree PS, Suresh KV, Sudhir RR, Srinivas SP. Automated image segmentation of the corneal endothelium in patients with Fuchs dystrophy. Transl Vis Sci Technol. 2021;10:27. https://doi.org/10.1167/tvst.10.13.27.
57. Müller LJ, Marfurt CF, Kruse F, Tervo TMT. Corneal nerves: structure, contents and function. Exp Eye Res. 2003;76:521–42. https://doi.org/10.1016/S0014-4835(03)00050-2.
58. The EN, Fry GA, Lecture A. Ophthalmic markers of diabetic neuropathy. Optom Vis Sci. 2010;2011(88):661–83. https://doi.org/10.1097/OPX.0b013e3182171020.
59. Cruzat A, Pavan-Langston D, Hamrah P. In vivo confocal microscopy of corneal nerves: analysis and clinical correlation. Semin Ophthalmol. 2010;25:171–7. https://doi.org/10.3109/08820538.2010.518133.
60. Kallinikos P, Berhanu M, O'Donnell C, Boulton AJM, Efron N, Malik RA. Corneal nerve tortuosity in diabetic patients with neuropathy. Invest Opthalmol Vis Sci. 2004;45:418. https://doi.org/10.1167/iovs.03-0637.
61. Williams BM, Borroni D, Liu R, Zhao Y, Zhang J, Lim J, et al. An artificial intelligence-based deep learning algorithm for the diagnosis of diabetic neuropathy using corneal confocal microscopy: a development and validation study. Diabetologia. 2020;63:419–30. https://doi.org/10.1007/s00125-019-05023-4.
62. Scarpa F, Colonna A, Ruggeri A. Multiple-image deep learning analysis for neuropathy detection in corneal nerve images. Cornea. 2020;39:342–7. https://doi.org/10.1097/ICO.0000000000002181.
63. Kang L, Ballouz D, Woodward MA. Artificial intelligence and corneal diseases. Curr Opin Ophthalmol. 2022;33:33. https://doi.org/10.1097/ICU.0000000000000885.

MIX
Papier aus verantwortungsvollen Quellen
Paper from responsible sources
FSC® C105338

If you have any concerns about our products,
you can contact us on
ProductSafety@springernature.com

In case Publisher is established outside the EU,
the EU authorized representative is:
Springer Nature Customer Service Center GmbH
Europaplatz 3, 69115 Heidelberg, Germany

Printed by Libri Plureos GmbH
in Hamburg, Germany